BIOTECHNOLOGICAL ATTRIBUTES OF COAGULASE-NEGATIVE STAPHYLOCOCCI

By :

AMEER KHUSRO

ACKNOWLEDGEMENT

First and foremost, I thank Almighty for His showers of blessings throughout the completion of my research work.

Immeasurable appreciation and deepest gratitude for the help and support are extended to the following persons who in one way or another have contributed in making this research work possible.

I thank **Fr. G. Joseph Antony Samy, S.J., Fr. M. Arockiasamy Xavier, S.J., Fr. F. Andrew, S.J., (**Former Principals) and **Fr. A. Thomas, S.J.,** Principal, Loyola College, Chennai for providing me all the necessary amenities and invaluable support.

I wish to express my heartfelt gratitude to **Mr. L. Antoine Label** (Former Head of Department) and **Dr. R. Ravindhran**, Associate Professor and Head of Department of Plant Biology and Biotechnology, Loyola College, Chennai for their sincere and valuable encouragement.

I would like to thank **Dr. S. Vincent** (Former Dean of Research) and **Dr. J. Madhavan,** Dean of Research, Loyola College for their assistance and constant support during the research work.

I wish to express my sincere thank to my supervisor **Dr. Agastian Paul**, Associate Professor, Department of Plant Biology and Biotechnology, Loyola College, Chennai for providing me opportunity to do my doctoral research under his guidance.

I would like to acknowledge Maulana Azad National Fellowship (F1-17.1/ 2015-16/MANF-2015-17-BIH-60730), University Grants Commission (UGC), Delhi, India for providing me the fellowship for completion of this research work.

I extend my thanks to **Dr. S. Sheela** (Co-ordinator, PG Biotechnology) and **Mr. Preetam Raj J.P.** (Lab Instructor, PG Biotechnology) for their co-operation in various ways during the course of my research.

I thank Lab attenders of Department of Plant Biology and Biotechnology, Loyola College, Chennai for providing me with all the necessary facilities in the lab in order to complete my research work successfully.

I take the opportunity to record my sincere thanks to all the faculty members of Department of Plant Biology and Biotechnology and PG Biotechnology, Loyola College, Chennai for their support and encouragement.

Most importantly, heartfelt gratitude to my lab members (**Mr. T. Selvaraj, Mr. Stephen Nehru, Dr. K. Bharathi Kannan, Mr. Prince Clarance, Dr. J. Dhivahar, Mr. Venkatadri Babu, Mr. Jerin Sales, Ms. Chirom Aarti, Ms. Roja K, Ms. Benchilo Ezung, Mrs. L. Jebalsy Lalitha, Mrs. Saritha Valsalam,** and **Ms. R. Sagaya Jansi**) and friends from other departments of this college whose help has been a moral support in completion of my research work.

Last but not least I would like to thank my parents, my sisters, and other close family members for their constant support as a source of inspiration.

Ameer Khusro

CONTENT

Acronyms and Abbreviations

ANN:	Artificial neural network
ANOVA:	Analysis of variance
AT:	Adenine Thymine
ATP:	Adenosine triphosphate
AU:	Arbitrary unit
AuNPs:	Gold nanoparticles
BBD:	Box-Behnken Design
Bcl-2:	B-cell lymphoma type 2
Bcl-xL:	B-cell lymphoma-extra large
BLAST:	Basic local alignment search tool
BPNN:	Back propagation learning algorithm
BSA:	Bovine serum albumin
BSH:	Bile salt hydrolase
BSS:	Basal salt solution
C.V:	Coefficient of variation
CCD:	Central composite design
CDK2:	Cycline dependent kinase 2
CDK4:	Cycline dependent kinase 4
CFNS:	Cell free neutralized supernatant
cfu:	Colony forming unit
CNS:	Coagulase-negative staphylococci
CS:	Control strain
DLS:	Dynamic light scattering
DM:	Dry matter
DMD:	Degradable dry matter
DMEM:	Dulbecco's Modified Eagle Medium
DNA:	Deoxyribonucleic acid
dNTPs:	Deoxyribonucleotide triphosphates
DOE:	Design of experiments
EDX:	Energy-dispersive X-ray
EGFR:	Epidermal growth factor receptor

ELISA:	Enzyme-linked immunosorbent assay
EPS:	Exopolysaccharide
E-value:	Energy value
fcc:	face-centred cubic
FT-IR:	Fourier-transform infrared
GC:	Guanine Cytosine
GI:	Gastro-intestinal
GRAVY:	Grand average of hydropathocity
GSA:	γ-glutamate-semialdehyde
HIV:	Human immunodeficiency virus
LAB:	Lactic acid bacteria
LRP:	Luciferase reporter phase
MALDI-TOF:	Matrix-Assisted Laser Desorption/Ionization-Time of Flight
MDR:	Multi-drug resistant
MEGA:	Molecular Evolutionary Genetics Analysis
MFE:	Minimum free energy
MIC:	Minimum inhibitory concentration
MLP:	Multilayer perceptron
mRNA:	Messenger ribonucleic acid
MRS:	De Man, Rogosa and Sharpe
MS:	Mass spectrometry
MSE:	Mean squared error
MTCC:	Microbial type culture collection
MTT:	3-(4,5-dimethylthiazol-2-yl)-2,5-diphenyltetrazolium bromide
NCBI:	National Centre for Biotechnology Information
NJ:	Neighbor-joining
OA:	Orthogonal array
OD:	Optical density
OFAT:	One factor at a time
ORF:	Open reading frame
P5C:	Δ^1-pyrroline-5-carboxylate
P5CDH:	Δ^1-pyrroline-5-carboxylate dehydrogenase
P5CR:	Δ^1-pyrroline-5-carboxylate reductase
PBS:	Phosphate buffered saline

PCR:	Polymerase chain reaction
PDB:	Protein data bank
pI:	Isoelectric point
PMF:	Peptide mass fingerprinting
PRESS:	Prediction residual sum of squares
ProDH:	Proline dehydrogenase
RCSB:	Research Collaboratory for Structural Bioinformatics
RLU:	Relative light unit
RNA:	Ribonucleic acid
rpm:	Revolutions per minute
rRNA:	Ribosomal ribonucleic acid
RSM:	Response surface methodology
SAS:	Statistical analysis system
SD:	Standard variation
SDS-PAGE:	Sodium dodecyl sulfate–polyacrylamide gel electrophoresis
SEM:	Scanning electron microscopy
sp.:	Species
spp.:	Species pluralis
SPR:	Surface plasmon resonance
SS:	Stressed strain
TB:	Tuberculosis
UV:	Ultraviolet
UV-Vis:	Ultraviolet-visible
WHO:	World Health Organization
XDR:	Extensively drug resistant
XRD:	X-ray diffraction
YT:	Yeast extract-tryptone

Units and Symbols

% v/v: Percentage volume by volume

% w/v: Percentage weight by volume

%: Percentage

-: Negative/Hyphen/Subtraction

+: Positive/Plus/Addition

$<$: Less than

$>$: More than

$\leq$: Less than or equal to

°C: Degree Celsius

µg: Microgram

µL: Microlitre/Microlitres

µm: Micrometre

µmol: Micromole

°: Degrees

2D: Two dimensional

3D: Three dimensional

cm^{-1}: Per centimetre

d: Distance

D: Particle size

Da: Dalton

g/L: Gram per litre

g: Gram/Grams

g: Relative centrifugal force

h: Hour/Hours

k: Number of variables

k_B: Distribution Boltzmann constant

kcal/mol: Kilocalories per mole

kDa: Kilodalton

keV: Kiloelectron volts

kg: Kilogram/Kilograms

KJ/mol: Kilo Joule per mole

kV:	Kilovolt
L:	Electrode distance
L:	Litre/ Litres
m/z:	Mass by charge
M:	Molar/Molarity
m^3:	Cubic metre
mA:	Milliampere
mg/L:	Milligrams per litre
mg/mL:	Milligram/Milligrams per millilitre
mg:	Milligram/Milligrams
min:	Minute/Minutes
min^{-1}:	Per minute
mL:	Millilitre/Millilitres
mm:	Millimetre/Millimetres
mM:	Millimole/Millimolar
mV:	Millivolt
N:	Normal/Normality
n:	Number of experiments/Integers
ng:	Nanogram/Nanograms
nm:	Nanometre
pM:	Picomole
ppm:	Parts per million
r:	Radius
R^2:	Coefficient of determination
sec:	Second/Seconds
T:	Absolute temperature
U:	Electrophoretic mobility
v:	Particle speed
V:	Volt/Voltage
vs:	Versus
α:	Alpha
β:	Beta
γ:	Gamma
δ:	Delta

ε:	Epsilon/Dielectric constant
η:	Viscosity of solution
θ:	Theta/Angle of incidenace
λ:	Wavelength
ϕ:	Phi
Φ:	Ef
n:	Number of neurons

General Introduction

Fermentation of foods has been an immense area of interest since ancient periods. Fermentation is one of the oldest processes of biotechnology which represents the formation of certain products by the action of microorganisms. As a matter of fact, autochthonous microorganisms present in foods are not only involved in the fermentation process but also preserve the perishable foods and provide health-inducing benefits to consumers (Farhad *et al.*, 2010). Fermentation of foods is generally carried out by naturally or spontaneously, back-slopping or by the supplementation of active starter cultures. Fermentation provides several benefits to humankind by improving nutritional and sensorial qualities of foods. Research on fermented foods and its global productivity had escalated rapidly in the 21st century. Over the past few years, the demands of functional foods have increased tremendously again due to their medicinal values. Naturally fermented foods have nutritive as well as non-nutritive constituents, which have the potentiality to modulate specific target functions relevant to the human health (Thapa and Tamang, 2015).

Health beneficial aspects of Indian fermented foods have been investigated extensively in the past. In view of the techno-functional significance, traditional fermented foods occupy an important place in the diet of Indian people, particularly from southern regions of India. Ethnic people of Tamil Nadu (a southern state of India) prepare varieties of traditional fermented foods using locally available raw sources as ideal substrates. Vegetables, bamboo shoots, beans, milk, cereals, and millets are the most common substrates used for the preparation of fermented foods. Traditional fermented foods of Tamil Nadu are prepared with prominent knowledge of indigenous people which has auspicious market value due to enormous growing demand day by day (Thirumangaimannan and Gurumurthy, 2013). Despite the colossal health benefits of commonly consumed fermented food items, there are few other fermented foods which deserve research input and wide scientific attention as these foods have a huge impact on large population of Tamil Nadu.

Functional and non-functional microorganisms are the prime components of fermented foods (Tamang *et al.*, 2016). The chemical entities of foods associated raw substrates are being transformed by functional microorganisms during fermentation process, thereby causing enhancement of nutrients bioavailability, enrichment of sensory quality of foods, improvement of food safety, degradation of toxic components, production of therapeutic substances, stimulation of technological traits, and fortification of health-inducing bioactive constituents (Thapa and Tamang, 2015). Additionally, the functional attributes of microbes include probiotic traits, antagonistic characteristics, antioxidative properties, fibrinolytic activities, peptide productions etc. which can be selective criteria for the selection of ideal starter cultures towards the preparation of traditional fermented foods (Badis *et al.*, 2004).

Traditionally prepared fermented foods are generally considered to contain heterogeneous groups of probiotics. Probiotics are live fed microorganisms that when administered in adequate amounts, confer a health benefit to the host such as stimulation of immunity, reduction of serum cholesterol content, growth inhibition of pathogens etc. (Hill *et al.*, 2014). Probiotics are also known to depict anti-allergic, tumoricidal, anti-*Helicobacter*, and anti-inflammatory properties (Lee *et al.*, 2014). The potential probiotics must exhibit resistance to acidic conditions, tolerance to bile, and ability to colonize the gastro-intestinal tract (Saad *et al.*, 2013). Currently, the beneficial aspects of probiotics on human health and nutrition are constantly increasing (Monteagudo-Mera *et al.*, 2012). Fermented foods are important consortia for diversified categories of probiotics, particularly lactobacilli, bacilli, enterococci, streptococci, bifidobacteria, and yeasts as dominating microbial genera (Tamang *et al.*, 2016).

Apart from above mentioned microbiota, staphylococci have also been reported in various fermented foods and created colossal interest among researchers now a days. The genus *Staphylococcus* are non-motile, non-spore forming, facultative anaerobe, and catalase positive cocci which contain 47 validly described species which are generally isolated from skin, skin glands, and mucosa of humans and animals (Götz *et al.*, 2006). Interestingly, staphylococci have been extensively isolated from other sources too such as soil, water, sand, air, plant surfaces, meat, poultry, milk, and dairy products (Götz *et al.*, 2006; Irlinger, 2008). Staphylococci are classified into 2 groups: coagulase-positive staphylococci and coagulase-negative staphylococci (CNS) by assessing their potentiality to produce extracellular coagulase (Stutz *et al.*, 2011). Coagulase is *Staphylococcus aureus* associated protein involved in the coagulation of blood. The secretion of coagulase is examined by the enzymatic conversion of fibrinogen in rabbit plasma to fibrin (Rivera *et al.*, 2007). Coagulase production differentiates *S. aureus* from other staphylococci and thus, categorizing coagulase deficient bacteria under CNS species (Götz *et al.*, 2006).

Coagulase-negative staphylococci indigenous to traditional fermented foods have emerged as the prevalent heterogeneous group of non-lactic acid bacteria divulging cogent characteristics (Borah *et al.*, 2016). Coagulase-negative staphylococci are benign and have been considered as non-pathogenic normal commensal flora, indigenous to fermented food products. The well known dominating CNS in fermented foods include *S. saprophyticus*, *S. xylosus*, *S. caprae*, *S. epidermidis*, *S. carnosus*, *S. vitulinus*, *S. haemolyticus*, *S. warneri*, *S. equorum*, *S. succinus*, *S. piscifermentans*, *S. arlettae*, *S. lugdunensis*, *S. cohnii*, *S. hominis*, *S. kloosii*, *S. capitis*, *S. lentus* etc. (Casaburi *et al.*, 2005; Borah *et al.*, 2016; Tamang *et al.*, 2016). Despite the occasional opportunistic infections causing property of few CNS species in terms of enterotoxins productions and resistivity to antibiotics (Widerstrom *et al.*, 2012), they are widely used in the food processing industries due to their vast functional and technological characteristics viz. aroma, flavour, and colour formation. The extensive utilization of CNS in food industries depends on its ability to reveal safety aspects as determined by distinct biochemical and molecular characterization tests (Jeong *et al.*, 2016). In the past few years, CNS have been successfully isolated from diversiform fermented food items viz. sausages (Casaburi *et al.*, 2005), tuna candy products (Hwang *et al.*, 2010), meat products (Landeta *et al.*, 2013), cheese (Kurekci, 2015), and fermented soybean (Jeong *et al.*, 2016) as starter cultures.

At present, infectious diseases are the huge burden for public health all over the world. Plethora of research strategies is being pursued globally to counter major bacterial infections affecting human health. Tuberculosis (TB) is one of the most serious tropical diseases caused by *Mycobacterium tuberculosis*. It is a severe airborne fatal disease which infects one third of the world's population. It is a global pulmonary health problem and is more common among men than women. It infects all age groups, mostly affects adults. According to the World Health Organization (WHO) survey, there were 8.6 million new active cases of TB and 1.3 million deaths in 2012 (World Health Organization, 2012). There were approximately 9.6 million cases of active TB estimated in 2014 which culminated in 1.5 million deaths. Indeed, TB is an endemic disease in the developing countries and the majority of active TB cases were in the South-East Asia [29 percentage (%)], followed by Africa (27%) and Western Pacific (19%) regions.

More than 95% of deaths occurred in developing countries and India alone accounts for 26% of total TB cases (Rodriguez Plaza *et al.*, 2014). In the mid-1990s, the WHO developed the direct observed therapy strategy to control TB. This strategy was adopted by most of the countries and confirms a short-course of chemotherapy treatment by administering crucial first-line drugs (isoniazid, rifampicin, ethambutol, and pyrazinamide), followed by treatment with isoniazid and rifampicin for a period of 4 months. The emergence of multi-drug resistant (MDR) *M. tuberculosis* and disease recrudesces were one of the consequences of this strategy. Surprisingly, among the newly infected cases of TB, approximately 13% were co-infected with human immunodeficiency virus (HIV) due to the impairment of the immune system of the patient, leading to the delayed diagnosis and treatment of TB (Kwan and Ernst, 2011). This is because HIV infected persons are compromised with their immune systems.

The intracellular pathogen, *M. tuberculosis* primarily infects human pulmonary macrophage. Macrophages are specialized cells of the immune system that engulf and remove the invading microorganisms through phagocytosis process (Filion *et al.*, 2013). In general, during this process, microorganisms other than *M. tuberculosis* are trapped into the phagosomes which fuse with lysosome and forms phagolysosome. Eventually, the digestive process occurring inside the phagolysosomes results into the destruction of invaded microorganisms. However, *M. tuberculosis* after phagocytised escapes from this defence mechanism by infecting macrophages and survive within the adverse environment. *M. tuberculosis* utilizes macrophages for its own replication process. The defensive property of *M. tuberculosis* relies on several survival strategies. Unlike non-pathogenic mycobacterium strains, first of all, the pathogenic *M. tuberculosis* arrests the maturation process of phagosomes and prevents the acidification of phagosomal compartments. It also inhibits the formation of the lysosomes and phagosomes complex. Further, the bacterium impairs the apoptosis of macrophage and suppresses the antimicrobial responses, thus helping the bacterium to escape from the phagosomes (Filion *et al.*, 2013). The bacterium becomes undetectable to innate immune system because major histocompatibility complex class II antigen avoids its presentation. In this manner, *M. tuberculosis* is able to manipulate and survive in the adverse environment of pulmonary or any other parts of the host macrophages. Extensive reports have demonstrated that in spite of the digestive property of macrophages, *M. tuberculosis* has developed multiple adaptive strategies to destruct the phagosomal pathways and survive intracellularly in the host macrophages (Welin *et al.*, 2011). The cell envelop of *M. tuberculosis* constituting diverse lipid contents is a major factor towards its virulence property.

Over the past five decades, only two new anti-tubercular drugs were approved and released (Malothu *et al.*, 2016). Bedaquiline is a first-in-class diarylquinoline compound that showed therapeutic potency against drug-sensitive and drug resistant *M. tuberculosis* with a novel mode of action including the inhibition of bacterial adenosine triphosphate (ATP) synthase (by binding to subunit c of the enzyme), the enzyme used by bacteria to generate energy (Field, 2015). Hards *et al.* (2015) clearly showed the uncoupling process induced by bedaquiline. In a typical *M. tuberculosis* cell, the majority of ATP synthesis is respiratory, driven by the proton-motive force. The binding of bedaquiline to the c-ring most likely perturbs the a-c subunit interface, thereby causing an uncontrolled proton leak uncoupled from ATP synthesis and resulting in a futile proton cycle (Hards *et al.*, 2015). This drug is also known by the trade name of 'Sirturo'. Bedaquiline is used in combination with other TB drugs to treat pulmonary TB in adults with MDR-TB. It should only be used when an effective TB treatment cannot otherwise be provided and other drugs are showing severe toxicity to patients. The use of bedaquiline is avoided for the treatment of extra-pulmonary TB, drug sensitive TB, latent TB infections, and infection caused by mycobacteria other than *M. tuberculosis*. In February 2016, it was announced that bedaquiline is to be made available in India and the drug will be available as part of second line treatment for patients suffering from MDR-TB and extensively drug resistant (XDR)-TB. The drug recently is under clinical trials phases in certain hospitals of the country. This drug was approved based on the phase IIb clinical trial results. However, phase III trials are still ongoing and its final approval is pending. There are issues with the safety concerns of bedaquiline, related to QTc prolongation caused by the drug and the observed and yet unexplained higher mortality rate detected in the group treated with bedaquiline compared to placebo. However, smaller counts of patients showed lower mortality rate. A new phase III trial has begun in order to investigate the safety and efficacy of bedaquiline in combination with short MDR-TB regimens of 9 and 6 months duration, respectively.

Delamanid is another approved anti-tubercular drug, and the first drug of the nitroimidazole class to enter clinical practice (Gualano *et al.*, 2016). It is also known by its trade name of 'Deltyba'. It is currently being developed by the Otsuka pharmaceutical company as a treatment for MDR-TB. The drug is known to inhibit the synthesis of cell wall components of *M. tuberculosis*, particularly methoxy mycolic acid and ketomycolic acid (Gualano *et al.*, 2016). Delamanid is a pro-drug which gets activated by the enzyme deazaflavin dependent nitroreductase. A reactive intermediate metabolite, formed between delamanid and desnitro-imidazooxazole derivative, is considered to play a pivotal role in the blockage of mycolic acid production (Xavier and Lakshmanan, 2014). Similar to bedaquiline, a phase III trial on delamanid is in process. The trial includes the use of this drug in combination with moxifloxacin and HIV-positive patients on antiretroviral therapy. In addition to this, other ongoing trials include assessing the use of delamanid for the treatment of pediatric MDR-TB. Preclinical and clinical phase results showed higher potency, lower risk for drug-drug interactions, and better tolerability of delamanid. It should be noteworthy that both bedaquiline and delamanid should only be prescribed as part of a WHO-recommended regimen for patients with MDR-TB in order to avoid the emergence of drug resistance *M. tuberculosis* (Xavier and Lakshmanan, 2014). It is possible that both the drugs would be given to the same patient in the case of difficult-to-treat patients. One of the major challenges will be to ensure the availability of these drugs to all those in need while keeping in mind the WHO policies.

Cancer is a multi-cellular and multi-genic non-infectious disease which is in fact the colossal public burden globally. According to the recent Global Cancer Statistics, there are approximately 32.6 million cancer patients worldwide, representing it as one of the primary causes of mortality in the world (Torre *et al.*, 2015). Cancer cells show high rate of proliferation due to self-sufficient growth signals and sustained angiogenesis. Further, these cells invade tissues, show metastasis, and reveal resistance towards apoptosis (Feitelson *et al.*, 2015). Lung cancer, also known as lung carcinoma, is a malignant tumor characterized by uncontrolled cell growth in tissues of the lung. Worldwide in 2012, lung cancer occurred in 1.8 million people and resulted in 1.6 million deaths. This makes it the most common cause of cancer-related deaths in men and second most common in women after breast cancer (World Cancer Report, 2014). Small-cell lung cancer and non-small-cell lung cancer are two important types of lung cancer. Approximately 20% of all lung cancers are diagnosed with small-cell lung cancer while 80-85% of all lung cancers are categorized into squamous cell carcinoma, adenocarcinoma, and large cell carcinoma (Herbst *et al.*, 2008). The molecular origin of lung cancer relies on complex interaction between host genetic sensitivity and the environment. The activation of oncogenes as well as the inactivation of tumor suppressor genes initiates the lung cancer. Mutations in these genes are mainly caused by carcinogens that develop cancer (Cooper *et al.*, 2013). Lung cancer treatment is an unmet necessity that can possibly be achieved by identifying novel therapeutic agents from un/less exploited sources.

On the other hand, colon or colorectal cancer is the third most common type of cancer, making up about 10% of all cases. In 2012, there were 1.4 million new cases and 694000 deaths from the disease (World Cancer Report, 2014). Colon cancer generally affects older adults. Colorectal cancer originates as a growth called 'polyp' from the epithelial cells lining of the colon or rectum of the gastrointestinal tract, most often due to the mutations in the 'Wnt' signalling pathway that improve signalling activity. The mutation can be inherited or acquired, and most probably occur in the intestinal crypt stem cell. The *APC* gene (known to produce APC protein) is the most common gene that is mutated in colorectal cancer. In fact, the accumulation of β-catenin protein is prevented by APC protein. In the absence of APC, β-catenin accumulates and not only translocates into the nucleus but also binds to deoxyribonucleic acid (DNA), and stimulates the transcription mechanism of proto-oncogenes (Khalek *et al.*, 2010).

Currently, the lengthy therapies and severe side effects of existing drugs have emphasized the worldwide researchers to search for promising anti-tubercular and anticancer agents. Among disparate therapeutic agents, bacteria associated proteins or peptides have created colossal interest due to their pivotal molecular characteristics and unique mode of actions. Naturally-occurring proteins/peptides often possess diversified attributes and indicate pronounced class of lead components for designing new antibiotics. *Staphylococcus* spp. are well known producers of therapeutic metabolites, including proteins or peptides (Bastos *et al.*, 2009). These bioactive proteins have huge applications in pharmaceutical industries in terms of distinct therapies. Antimicrobial proteins or peptides produced by bacteria exhibit growth inhibitory properties against distinct categories of microorganisms. These ribosomally-synthesized proteins or peptides are produced extensively by gram positive (+) bacteria. Amongst diversified gram positive bacteria, *Staphylococcus* spp. are known to produce distinct classes of antimicrobial proteins or bacteriocins (Bastos *et al.*, 2009).

Bacteria are exposed to plethora of stresses during their life cycle that alter their growth and other metabolic processes. In order to combat the environmental stresses, bacteria adapt to the adverse or harsh conditions by inducing molecular processes. In general, external stimulations can elicit variations in disparate stress-associated genes encoding proteins which are known to resist the lethal conditions (Sawatari and Yokota, 2007). Bacteria receive the signal after sensing any kind of environmental stress, and thus, the adaptive process within the cells begins in order to tolerate or pump out the toxicity. The transcriptional alterations in the bacterium are triggered due to the stress environment and initiate the secretion of new proteins as defensive system (Ismail *et al.*, 2013). The exposure of such unfavourable conditions results into the up- and down-regulation of certain genes, thereby triggering transcriptional alterations in the cells and synthesizing new proteins (Khusro and Sankari, 2015). As a matter of fact, the main purpose of adaptive mechanisms to the stress response is to protect cells against lethal factors and to repair damaged organelles. The bacterial adaptation to stress has fascinated researchers for combating infectious and non-infectious diseases. At present, the over-exploitation of antibiotics is the huge worriment of the worldwide researchers for treating TB and cancer. Currently used drugs have not only serious side-effects towards the treatment of lung and colon cancer but also cause the emergence of drugs resistant *M. tuberculosis*. It certainly necessitates searching new therapeutic agents against TB and cancer with novel mode of actions. The synthesis and isolation of protein from probiotic bacteria under mild stress condition of certain antimicrobials might be an ideal therapeutic strategy towards TB and cancer (lung and colon) treatment.

In spite of the identification of potent proteins or peptides from bacteria in recent years, the high cost for the synthesis of proteins/peptides and expensive experimental protocols at pre-clinical and clinical trial phases are the prime concerns for the researchers. In view of this, computational tools have been implemented to predict the biological attributes of proteins/peptides of interest prior to the trail phases so that lengthy time period and high experimental costs can be minimized and, thus, high accuracy of outcomes can be achieved. *In silico* tools are often used to predict the interaction of receptors with ligand of interest (Wang *et al.*, 2014). Such computational approaches play crucial role in designing the hypothesis that can be investigated before time-consuming and resource-demanding processes. Computational approaches or *in silico* studies provide opportunities to find the potential drug targets from proteome analysis.

The application of computational tools such as molecular dynamics, docking, and modelling are often being used in order to understand the protein complexes involved in various diseases (Huang and Zou, 2010). Molecular docking tools can be implied to analyze the interaction between the ligand and a receptor protein which helps us not only to predict the ligand behaviour in the binding site of target proteins but also elucidate fundamental biochemical mechanisms (Ezat *et al.*, 2014). Among varied molecular docking approaches, protein-protein interaction is considered as one of the most important types of *in silico* docking tool due to its vast therapeutic roles in modern structure-based drug design (Wang *et al.*, 2014). Protein structure is a pivotal pre-requisite to understand the evolutionary and functional relationship. The structural modelling of these proteins can help to determine which of these proteins can function as most effective surface epitope for the drug that can lead to the discovery of novel therapeutic drug (Zinzalla and Thurston, 2009). On the other hand amino acid sequences determine and characterize molecule's functional, physical, and chemical properties. Studying the systematic computational analysis between bioactive protein or peptide structure and its molecular mode of action will lead to design and develop novel drugs with desired anti-tubercular and anticancer activities that may create a new era for the possible treatment of TB and cancer in future.

Over the past few decades, nanotechnology has emerged as remarkable dynamic research area in therapeutics. This branch of science helps synthesize distinct groups of metallic nanoparticles of various shapes and sizes. Nanoparticles consist of a larger surface area than macrosize material due to their dimension (Guisbiers *et al.*, 2012). As a matter of fact, nanoparticles of minute dimension exhibit distinct characteristics as compared to the bulk material, thereby showing contribution towards novel developments in biomedicine and bio-nanotechnology (Albrecht *et al.*, 2006). Nanomaterials enter cells through various mechanisms including endocytosis (non-specific uptake), electroporation, and targeted or mediated uptake (Gao and Xu, 2009).

Gold is one of the least chemically active transition metals. Unlike bulk gold, colloidal gold is highly reactive, thereby showing huge applications (Shah *et al.*, 2014).

Among diversiform classes of nanoparticles used, gold nanoparticles (AuNPs) represent exemplary interest because of intrinsic characteristics. In addition, the intrinsic properties allow various molecules attach on the surface of AuNPs by means of covalent and/or electrostatic bonds (Eustis and El-Sayed, 2006). The AuNPs show strong optical absorption and scattering extending from the visible to near-infrared spectrum. This spectral range is termed as surface plasmon resonance (SPR) band owing to the collective oscillations of the conduction electrons coupled with incident light. Additionally, size and shape dependent optical properties, large surface-to-volume ratio, prominent biocompatibility, and reduced toxicity are unique characteristics of AuNPs which makes them pivotal nanomaterials in bio-nanotechnology. The colour of AuNPs varies from brown, orange, and red to purple in aqueous solutions as the size of the particles ranges between 1 to 100 nanometres (nm), and generally show absorption peak between 500 to 600 nm (Yeh *et al.*, 2012).

Plasmonic traits lead to varied biomedical applications of AuNPs (Dykman and Khlebtsov, 2012). Gold nanoparticles exhibit wide applications in medicine, particularly in drug-delivery, photo-thermal therapy, imaging, sensing, catalysis, and various disease treatments (Yeh *et al.*, 2012). In addition, AuNPs are widely used in genomics, clinical chemistry, and target-based therapy (Vicky *et al.*, 2010). The unique properties and vast applications of AuNPs depend on their size. Small size AuNPs (2-15 nm) play prominent role in immunohistochemistry, microscopy, and biomarkers. Medium size AuNPs (20-60 nm) are used in environmental detection and purification, drug delivery, biomarkers, and chemical sensors. Large size AuNPs (80-250 nm) are used in forensic science, electronic device, manufacture, optical mammography etc. The biocompatibility with human cells, facile synthesis, conjugation with different biomolecules, chemical stability, and tunable geometry suggest the preference of AuNPs over other metallic nanoparticles (Shah *et al.*, 2014).

In spite of the biocompatibility attributes of AuNPs, the conventional reduction methods of its synthesis are not eco-friendly. In the recent years, the synthesis of nanoparticles through various biosynthetic methodologies has gained immense attention in order to avoid the necessity of toxic synthetic chemicals. In fact, the chemical route-based synthesis of nanoparticles is considered to contaminate the colloidal solutions (Iravani *et al.*, 2014). Significant attempts have been undertaken in the past to synthesize nanoparticle via eco-friendly processes. In this regard, bacteria-associated synthesis of nanoparticles has shown promising outcomes (Iravani, 2014). In view of the increasing awareness for significant toxicity of conventional methods-based synthesis of AuNPs using bacteria, alternative protocols for biocompatible AuNPs synthesis is gaining importance. Microwave irradiation method is an emerging technology which has shown significant role in the synthesis of AuNPs. Microwave heating process increases reaction kinetics with rapid heating and improves nanoparticles yields (Das *et al.*, 2012). Additionally, this very method of irradiation reduces the reaction period and improves the nanoparticles content without altering the composition of products. Most importantly, microwave irradiation method causes homogeneous heating of the reaction mixture, leading to an easy nucleation of nanoparticles (Patel *et al.*, 2005).

Synthesizing nanoparticles with desired shapes has been an immense area of interest for nanotechnologists (Sau and Rogach, 2010). Currently, it is observed that the SPR absorption of anisotropic/polygonal AuNPs is tunable throughout the visible to near-infrared region, which suggests its various applications in biomedical science (Zijlstra *et al.*, 2009). In fact, investigation on controlled anisotropic gold nanostructures viz. rods, plates, cubes, cages etc. are of paramount importance in drug delivery technology (Zhu *et al.*, 2011). Among nanoparticles of varied shapes, anisotropic gold nanoplates are unique due to their decreased geometrical symmetry which increases distinctive traits (Millstone *et al.*, 2009). Surprisingly, comparatively less attention has been paid toward the extensive applications of anisotropic gold nanoplates. Gold nanoplates contain two surface plasmon absorption bands, making them auspicious candidate for therapeutic applications (Hong *et al.*, 2012). Additionally, gold nanoplates show anisotropic electrical conductivity, strong electric field, and enhanced catalytic characteristics (Huang *et al.*, 2014). On the other hand, the bioconjugation of nanoparticles with certain bioactive proteins/peptides is emerging as a pronounced approach for achieving enhanced therapeutic characteristics (Pal *et al.*, 2016). In biomedical field, the delivery of therapeutic agents to the targeted cells by AuNPs is considered as a crucial process (Yeh *et al.*, 2012). Bioconjugation of anisotropic gold nanoplates with therapeutic proteins/peptides could set a hallmark in biomedical science, particularly as auspicious anti-tubercular and anticancer agents.

Currently, there has been a growing demand to improve the athletic performance of modern horses (*Equus caballus*) (Berthelot *et al.*, 2015). Horses are monogastric non-ruminant herbivores whose hindgut (cecum and colon) is a fermentative chamber for complex microbiota (Shepherd *et al.*, 2012). Horses' forage-based diets are enriched with fibres. The hindgut bacteria help ferment these fibres. Horses obtain approximately 50% of its daily energy requirements from volatile fatty acids that are the by-products of fibres fermentation process (Vermorel and MartinRosset, 1997). Starch enriched feed causes an alteration in the microbial counts of horse intestine, thereby causing various disorders (Rowe *et al.*, 1994). In general, concentrate is increased and forage is reduced in the feed in order to meet caloric demands (Bailey *et al.*, 2003).

Probiotics present in the large intestine of animals produce volatile fatty acids required for energy (Williams *et al.*, 2001). Production of bioactive metabolites from probiotics inhibits the growth of pathogens and maintains a healthy microbiota in the gastro-intestinal tract (Gu *et al.*, 2008). However, there is still an essentiality to search for pivotal sources in order to provide energy demands, improve intestinal health, and increase the athletic performances of modern horses by increasing the fermentative potential of feeds. In the current scenario, the supplementation of disparate additives such as fibrolytic enzymes and commercial probiotics into the diets is considered prominent strategy to improve the fermentation of feed by estimating increased gas production *in vitro* (Vallejo *et al.*, 2016). Surprisingly, the utilization of coagulase-negative *Staphylococcus* spp. (with probiotic characteristics) as an additive in horse nutrition for improving total gas production is undetermined yet. The supplementation of coagulase-negative *Staphylococcus* spp. as ideal additives in the diets of horses may represent a new strategy for veterinarians towards the enhancement of the fermentation of forages.

In spite of the aforementioned exemplary advantages of fermented foods associated plethora of probiotic bacteria in various areas, there is still dearth of study reporting the valuable roles of CNS in varied fields of biological science. Considering the essentiality to explore different category of probiotic bacteria for filling the gap of research, the present research work was carried out to determine disparate biotechnological applications of CNS strains isolated from traditional fermented foods of Tamil Nadu, India towards the welfare of scientific community and humanities

Review of literature

Fermented foods associated probiotic bacteria

The organoleptic properties (texture, acidity, and flavour) and health beneficial aspects of fermented foods are determined by autochthonous microorganisms (Vogel *et al.*, 2011). Microorganisms may be present as the indigenous microbiota of the fermented food or due to the intentional addition of microbes as starter cultures in food fermentation mechanism (Stevens and Nabors, 2009). Bacteria are dominant in both the naturally fermented foods and foods fermented by the supplementation of starter cultures. Among the distinct bacterial cultures, lactic acid bacteria (LAB) are commonly involved in providing acidity to the fermented foods, while non-LAB are involved in the fermentation of foods, frequently as minor or secondary groups (Alexandraki *et al.*, 2013). Major genera of microbes associated with worldwide fermented foods are categorized as: *Acetobacter* spp., *Arthrobacter* spp., *Bacillus* spp., *Bifidobacterium* spp., *Brachybacterium* spp., *Brevibacterium* spp., *Carnobacterium* spp., *Corynebacterium* spp., *Enterobacter* spp., *Enterococcus* spp., *Gluconacetobacter* spp., *Hafnia* spp., *Halomonas* spp., *Klebsiella* spp., *Kocuria* spp., *Lactobacillus* spp., *Lactococcus* spp., *Leuconostoc* spp., *Macrococcus* spp., *Microbacterium* spp., *Micrococcus* spp., *Oenococcus* spp., *Pediococcus* spp., *Propionibacterium* spp., *Staphylococcus* spp., *Streptococcus* spp., *Streptomyces* spp., *Tetragenococcus* spp., *Vagococcus* spp., *Weisella* spp., and *Zymomonas* spp. (Tamang *et al.*, 2016).

Bacillus spp. have been isolated from alkaline-fermented foods of Asia and Africa (Parkouda *et al.*, 2009). *Bacillus amyloliquefaciens*, *B. coagulans*, *B. circulans*, *B. megaterium*, *B. subtilis*, *B. pumilus*, *B. firmus*, *B. licheniformis*, and *B. thuringiensis* are mostly present in soybean-based fermented foods (Kubo *et al.*, 2011), while *B. cereus* have been isolated by the fermentation of *Prosopis africana* seeds for the production of *okpehe* in Nigeria (Oguntoyinbo *et al.*, 2007). Few strains of *B. subtilis* produce λ-polyglutamic acid (an amino acid polymer). These strains are commonly present in the fermented soybean foods of Asia, providing characteristic sticky texture to the product obtained (Nishito *et al.*, 2010). *Brachybacterium* spp., *Brevibacterium* spp., *Bifidobacterium* spp., and *Propionibacterium* spp. have been isolated from fermented milk products (Bourdichon *et al.*, 2012). *Kocuria* spp., *Micrococcus* spp., and *Staphylococcus* spp. have been isolated from fermented milk products, sausages, meat, and fish items (Wu *et al.*, 2000; Martín *et al.*, 2006). *Klebsiella pneumoniae*, *K.*

pneumoniae subsp. *ozaenae*, *Enterobacter cloacae*, *Haloanaerobium* sp., *Halococcus* sp., *Halobacterium* sp., *Propionibacterium* sp., and *Pseudomonas* sp., are present in many fermented food products (Tamang, 2010). *Hafnia* sp. and *Arthrobacter* sp. are found in the fermented meat items (Bourdichon *et al.*, 2012).

There are about 5000 different varieties of fermented foods and beverages globally. However, only small fractions of these fermented products have been investigated for scientific studies so far in Tamil Nadu, India. Surprisingly, the biological and microbiological bases of the fermentation mechanisms are poorly reported for these foods. Whatever little information is known till date, it often discusses only about the identification, preliminary characterization, and limited therapeutic traits of the autochthonous microbes present in those fermented products. Thus, it emphasizes to analyze thorough understanding about the microbiota associated with food products in terms of classification and their particular characteristics.

Probiotic bacteria from traditional fermented foods of Tamil Nadu

Kumar *et al.* (2010) isolated 25 strains of probiotic bacteria from South Indian traditional fermented foods such as *Kallappam* batter, *Koozh*, and *Mor Kuzhambu*. Among those isolates, *Lactobacillus plantarum* AS1 showed promising antimicrobial trait. Further, results showed lack of illness after feeding *L. plantarum* AS1 to the male Albino Wistar rats. In *L. plantarum* AS1-treated group, the total counts of indigenous microflora of coliforms, yeast, and molds were reduced. On the other hand, the total counts of lactobacilli were increased. The increasing dose of bile salt in the medium retained the normal growth of *L. plantarum* AS1. It also showed resistance towards the artificial simulated gastric juice up to 24 hours (h). *L. plantarum* AS1 showed reduction in the cholesterol content in broth medium by 57.3%. Findings proved *L. plantarum* AS1 as an effectual probiont and also suggested its application as an effective biopreservative in cheese for inhibiting the growth of *Salmonella typhi*.

In another study, the home-made curd associated bacteria were evaluated for probiotic traits. The growth of *Lactobacillus* spp. in curd increased sharply at 12 h. Few strains resisted acidic pH. All the strains showed tolerance towards pancreatin or bile salts for 3 h. All the isolates showed negative results towards haemolytic activity and were found resistant to most of the antibiotics used except imipenem. Most of the strains inhibited the growth of *Salmonella* Typhimurium while 5 strains inhibited growth of *Vibrio cholerae* O139. Seven strains showed adherence to Caco-2 cells but all inhibited *V. cholerae* adherence to Caco-2 cells by 20-100%. Strains inhibited interleukin-8 secretion from HT-29 cells, in response to *V. cholerae* by 50-80%. Two strains stimulated IL-10 and IL-12 messenger ribonucleic acid (mRNA) expression in THP-1 cells (Balamurugan *et al.*, 2014).

Kambu koozh (pearl millet) was used for isolating probiotic bacteria. The morphological, cultural, and biochemical characteristics identified the isolate as *Enterococcus* sp. *Enterococcus* sp. showed resistance towards acidic condition, ranging from 80 (pH 5.0) to 69% (pH 2.0) for 1 h and 68 (pH 5.0) to 52% (pH 2.0) for 2 h. Bile salt resistivity of *Enterococcus* sp. was estimated 69% at 1% weight by volume (w/v) to 51% viability (at 4% w/v) for 24 h. Resistance to digestive enzymes exhibited 78.6 to 35.7% viability [2-10 grams per litre (g/L)] towards pepsin and 68.9 to 13.8% viability (2-10 g/L) towards trypsin for 2 h (Veerapagu and Jeya, 2017).

The regular consumption of Black rice (*Karupu kavuni arisi*) is believed to improve the health. On the other hand, the Brown rice (*Kai kuthal arisi*) constitutes wholesome nutrients and vitamins. Black rice and Brown rice have enormous advantages over white rice because of high nutritional components. Manovina *et al.* (2019) isolated and characterized probiotic microbiota from traditionally fermented black rice and brown rice. The fermented rice associated *Lactobacillus* sp. showed tolerance towards high concentration of bile salt, acidic condition, and high doses of salt.

Panchamirtham is a well known fruit-based traditional fermented product. Uma Maheshwari *et al.* (2018) investigated the diversity of autochthonous probiotic microbiota and characterized them. Among 787 isolates, 7 bacteria were reported to be acid producing based on the reaction of colour changes. This research discussed a wide probiotic diversity associated with fermented fruit mix and demonstrated the impact of kind of raw material used and conditions implied.

Anandharaj *et al.* (2015) evaluated the probiotic characteristics of bacteria isolated from traditional foods such as *Koozh* and *Gherkin* (cucumber). A total of 51 bacterial strains were isolated, among which 4 were identified as *Lactobacillus* spp. and 3 as *Weissella* spp. All *Lactobacillus* and *Weissella* strains resisted low pH and bile salt. Isolate GI9 and FKI21 showed resistivity at pH 2.0 and in the presence of 0.5% w/v bile salt for 3 h. All strains revealed growth inhibitory properties against indicator pathogens and deconjugated bile salt. Maximum deconjugation property was reported in the presence of sodium glycocholate (*P*<0.05). Strain FKI21 exhibited maximum auto-aggregation (79%) and co-aggregation traits with *Escherichia coli* MTCC 1089 (68%). The production of exopolysaccharide from strains varied from 68.39 to 127.12 milligrams per litre (mg/L). Additionally, GI9 [58.08 milligrams per millilitre (mg/mL)] and FKI21 (56.25 mg/mL) showed maximum reduction of cholesterol with bile salts.

Uma Maheshwari *et al.* (2019) isolated potential probiotic bacteria from *Panchamirtham* and identified as *Acinetobacter* sp., *Alcaligens* sp., *Bacillus* sp., *Enterobacter* sp., *Kocuria* sp., *Klebsiella* sp., *Microbacterium* sp., *Ornithinibacillus* sp., *Sphingomonas* sp., *Myroides* sp., *Panteoa* sp., and *Brevundimonas* sp. Seventeen isolates revealed antibacterial activities against human pathogens such as *Listeria monocytogens*, *S. aureus*, *E. coli*, and *Pseudomonas aeruginosa*. In addition, all the isolates showed tolerance towards low pH and bile salt, produced biofilm and exopolysaccharide, and demonstrated lack of haemolytic activity. *B. valezensis* M4S1B1 and *Proteus terrae* M7S2B1 depicted *in vitro* anticancer activities against A549 human lung cancer cells. Results showed that *Enterobacter xiangfangensis* M5S2B6, *B. safensis* M5S2B8, *E. hormaechi* subsp. oharae M6S1B2, *B. valezensis* M4S1B1, and *P. terrae* M7S2B1 had unique properties of ideal probiotics and may be utilized as starter cultures in order to produce *Panchamirtham*

Pearl millet porridge (*Kambu koozh*) was used for the isolation of feruloyl esterase producing bacteria. These bacteria were characterized for its probiotic properties with respect to their biological barrier tolerance. Among 5 feruloyl esterase producers, *L. fermentum* was observed to resist phenol and bile acids and tolerated simulated gastro-intestinal passage conditions. The strain produced enzymes such as β-galactosidase and glutamate decarboxylase. It also reduced cholesterol *in vitro*. Findings suggested the safer utilization of this probiotic strain for the formulation of functional foods (Palaniswamy and Govindaswamy, 2016).

Devagaopalan and Krishnaswamy (2018) analyzed the probiotic characteristics of curd associated bacteria. Based on various biochemical analyses, isolates were identified as *L. fermentum*, *L. casei*, *L. acidophilus*, and *Bifidobacterium longum* which also exhibited reliable probiotic traits. These strains were tested for probiotic characteristics such as resistance towards varied concentrations of bile salt, pH, and sodium chloride (NaCl). These strains fulfilled the important criteria of probiotic bacteria, and suggested further research on therapeutic use of these probiotics.

Ragul *et al.* (2019) determined the safety aspects of bacteria isolated from fermented mango Brine pickle for the selection of ideal probiotic culture. *B. licheniformis* KT921419 and *B. methylotrophicus* KT921422 showed lack of adverse safety traits. Results clearly suggested the safety and stability of these potential probiotic cultures, which can certainly be utilized in food processing industries under adverse environment such as high salt and low pH conditions.

Leuconostoc lactis KC117496 was isolated from naturally fermented *Idli* batter. The strain also showed high production of exopolysaccharide (EPS). Among varied disaccharides (sucrose, maltose, and lactose) and monosaccharides (glucose, galactose, and fructose) used, the combination of sucrose and glucose at 2% w/v showed the highest production of EPS. These characteristics of glucan EPS revealed its pivotal applications in food and pharmaceutical industries (Saravanan *et al.*, 2018).

Adhirasam is a commonly consumed cereal-based, doughnut shaped, and deep fried dessert in the southern states of India. The fermented dough used to prepare *Adhirasam* generally contains rice flour and jaggery. Anisha *et al.* (2015) isolated cultivable bacteria from this fermented dough and identified potent starter cultures for the preparation of *Adhirasam* of high quality. *Bacillus* spp. were found to be the dominant cultivable bacteria present in it. These strains were further utilized as ideal starter cultures and investigated for their potentiality to ferment rice flour with jaggery to prepare *Adhirasam* dough. *Adhirasam* prepared using these starter cultures were highly acceptable by consumers. Also, *Adhirasam* prepared using these starter cultures showed increased organoleptic traits such as texture softness, flavor development, enhanced aroma, and improved taste.

Rice and Dhal (pulses) in the form of batter is usually used after fermentation process and utilized in preparing distinct delicacies in South India. David *et al.* (2013) compared the production of prebiotic lactic acid production as a marker of probiotic trait. Results showed that about 50 h of fermentation at standard conditions favoured the increased probiotic impact, evident by improved lactic acid yield. Among 3 probiotic strains assessed, *L. acidophilus* showed maximum potentiality, followed by *Saccharomyces cerevisiae* and *Streptococcus thermophilus.*

Antimycobacterium activity of probiotics

Probiotic bacteria associated bacteriocins have exhibited potential activities against various species of *Mycobacterium*. Nisin (a bacteriocin) was assessed against

Mycobacterium smegmatis and revealed 97.7±2% of reduction in internal ATP and leakage of intracellular ATP (Montville *et al.*, 1999). Mota-Meira *et al.* (2000) revealed antimycobacterium activities of nisin A and mutacin B-Ny266 (type A lantibiotics) against *M. smegmatis*. Donaghy *et al.* (2005) demonstrated that the cell free supernatant of cheese associated *L. paracasei* inhibited the growth of *Mycobacterium avium* subsp. *paratuberculosis*. Bacteriocin of probiotic bacteria isolated from *Boza* (Turkish beverage) showed antimycobacterium activity. *L. plantarum* ST194BZ associated bacteriocin depicted anti-tubercular activity against *M. tuberculosis* with 69% of reduction in bacterial growth, whereas, *L. paracasei* ST242BZ, *L. plantarum* ST414BZ, and *L. plantarum* ST664BZ exhibited 50% inhibition of bacterial growth. In another report, bacteriocins from *L. plantarum* ST202Ch, *L. plantarum* ST216Ch, *L. sakei* ST153Ch, *L. sakei* ST154Ch, and *Enterococcus faecium* ST211Ch (isolated from Portuguese fermented meat products) showed anti-tubercular activities by reducing the growth of *M. tuberculosis* from 16.1 to 48.6% (Todorov and Dicks, 2006; Todorov *et al.*, 2014). Sosunov *et al.* (2007) demonstrated that *L. salivarius*, *Streptococcus cricetus*, and *E. faecalis* associated bacteriocins had promising dose dependent antimycobacterial activities than that of rifampicin. Carroll *et al.* (2010) depicted the antimycobacterium activities of lacticin 3147 against *M. kansasii* and *M. tuberculosis* H37Ra. Lantibiotics certainly reveal potentiality for future TB treatment. Study showed that nisin and lacticin 3147 arrested the bacterial lipid II moiety and suggested that inherent cell wall alterations did not provide lantibiotic resistance to mycobacteria (Carroll and O'Mahony, 2011). Bacteriocins purified from *Pediococcus pentosaceus* VJ13 exhibited antimycobacterium activity against *M. smegmatis*. Zahir *et al.* (2011) demonstrated that the proteinaceous inhibitory substances produced from *Aerococcus* sp. ZI1 had antimycobacterium properties against *M. smegmatis*. Mariam (2014) depicted antagonistic characteristics of lactobacilli starter cultures against *M. bovis*. Sosunov *et al.* (2007) purified 5 varied kinds of bacteriocins with antimycobacterium traits which was tested further using various models including *in vitro Mycobacterium* cultures, *in vitro* infection of mouse macrophages, and *in vivo* infection of inbred mice. Likewise, *L. plantarum* and its bacteriocin (plantaricin 42) were encapsulated in nano-fibers. Findings suggested that this technique may be incorporated for the potential delivery of antimycobacterium bacteriocins to the specific sites of infections (Heunis *et al.*, 2010).

Anticancer activity of probiotics

Probiotics are considered to prevent tumor growth through maintaining homeostasis mechanism. Substantial research activities showed that probiotics had antiproliferative or proapoptotic characteristics against varied human cancer cells. Lee *et al.* (2004) reported significant anticancer traits of *L. acidophilus*, *L. casei*, and *B. longum* against few cell lines. Previous findings exhibited the antiproliferative traits of the cytoplasmic extracts from *L. rhamnosus* strain GG in human gastric as well as colonic cancer cells (Russo *et al.*, 2007; Orlando *et al.*, 2009; Orlando *et al.*, 2012). *B. adolescentis* SPM0212 showed the inhibition of the proliferation of colon cancer cell lines viz. HT-29, SW 480, and Caco-2 (Kim *et al.*, 2008). Probiotics such as *B. polyfermenticus* (Ma *et al.*, 2010), *L. acidophilus* 606 (Kim *et al.*, 2010), LGG/Bb12 (Borowicki *et al.*, 2011), and LGG/*B. animalis* subsp. *lactis* (Stein *et al.*, 2012) revealed anticancer activities against colon cancer cells. Cousin *et al.* (2012) demonstrated that *Propionibacterium freudenreichii* had the potentiality to improve the cytotoxicity of camptothecin that was implied as a chemotherapeutic agent for gastric cancer. In another *in vitro* study, the anticancer activities of probiotics were demonstrated against colorectal carcinoma cells (Escamilla *et al.*, 2012). Other examined cell types also included cervical cancer cells (Cha *et al.*, 2012), breast cancer cells (Azam *et al.*, 2014), and myeloid leukemia cells (Ghoneum and Gimzewski, 2014).

According to Chiu *et al.* (2010), *L. casei* and *L. rhamnosus* have properties to induce the apoptosis of human monocytic leukemia-cell line. In another study, Choi *et al.* (2006) demonstrated the anticancer impact of *Lactobacillus* spp. on various human cancer cell lines. Peptidoglycans of the cell walls of varied probiotic bacteria, particularly lactobacilli exhibited anticancer traits (Kim *et al.*, 2002). Wang *et al.* (2013) evaluated *in vitro* anticancer activities of *L. plantarum* derived exopolysaccharide against HepG-2, BGC-823, and HT-29 cell lines. Results suggested that the EPS produced by *L. plantarum* might be an alternate for natural anticancer drugs. Knecht *et al.* (2014) reported antiproliferative properties of the cell-free filtrate and the cell-free lyophilized filtrate of *Pediococcus pentosaceus*, *L. plantarum*, and *Weissella confusa* on colorectal adenocarcinoma cells. Lee *et al.* (2004) reported anticancer traits of *Lactococcus lactis* KC24 against gastric carcinoma (AGS), colon carcinoma (HT-29 and LoVo), breast carcinoma (MCF-7), and lung carcinoma (SK-MES-1) cells.

L. lactis KC24 showed anticancer activities against varied cancer cell lines such as lung carcinoma (SK-MES-1), breast carcinoma (AGS and MCF-7), and colon carcinoma (HT-29 and LoVo) using 3-(4,5-dimethylthiazol-2-yl)-2,5-diphenyltetrazolium bromide (MTT) assay (Lee *et al.*, 2015). Another study demonstrated the anticancer and anti-inflammatory activities of *L. lactis* NK34 against various cancer cell lines like DLD-1 (human colon adenocarcinoma cell line), SK-MES-1 (human lung carcinoma cell line), LoVo (human colon adenocarcinoma cell line), HT-29 (human colon adenocarcinoma cell line), AGS (human stomach adenocarcinoma cell line), and MCF-7 (human breast adenocarcinoma cell line). The cytotoxicity of NK34 strain was reported against normal and cancerous cells using MTT assay. In addition, the anti-inflammatory trait of *L. lactis* NK34 exerted a reduction in pro-inflammatory cytokines (Han *et al.*, 2015).

Rajoka *et al.* (2019) demonstrated *in vitro* anticancer activity of *L. kefiri* MSR101 associated EPS against HT-29 cell lines. Results suggested that MSR101 derived EPS had not only potential anticancer trait on HT-29 cancer cells but also up-regulated the expression of Cyto-c, BAX, BAD, caspase3, caspase8, and caspase9. In general, results suggested that the EPS from *L. kefiri* MSR101 may not only be used as functional food product but also considered as a topical medication due to their effectiveness against colon cancer.

Awaisheh *et al.* (2016) screened the anticancer traits of cell extracts of 40 potential probiotic bacteria against 2 colorectal cancer cell lines (Caco-2 and HRT-18), and vero cells using MTT and Trypan Blue assays. Results demonstrated that *L. acidophilus* LA102 and *L. casei* LC232 had promising cytotoxic properties with anti-proliferation characteristics of 37 and 68.5% for LA102, and 48 and 45.7% for LC232 against Caco-2 and HRT-18, respectively.

The anticancer activities of *L. acidophilus* 36YL were tested against 4 human cancer cell lines (AGS, HeLa, MCF-7, and HT-29) and one normal cell line (HUVEC) using cytotoxicity assay and apoptosis analyses (Nami *et al.*, 2014). Results showed satisfactory anticancer activities against 4 tested cancer cell lines and exerted negligible side effects on the normal cell line. Findings revealed that the anticancer characteristics of *L. acidophilus* 36YL strain secretions rely on the induced apoptosis in cancer cells. *L. acidophilus* 36YL strain is considered as a nutraceutical alternative or a topical medication with a potent therapeutic index due to the lack of cytotoxicity towards normal cells but significant toxicity to cancer cells.

Fermented foods associated CNS

Borah *et al.* (2016) isolated and characterized novel indigenous probiotic bacterial strains from traditionally fermented fish and meat products of Assam, India. The most potent probiotic isolate was identified as *Staphylococcus* sp. DBOCP6. The strain was observed non-haemolytic and non-pathogenic in nature based on its sensitivity towards broad and narrow spectrum conventional antibiotics. The isolate exerted antagonistic activity against *E. coli* MTCC 40. The viability of isolate in the presence of lysozyme, bile salt, and varied pHs showed its potentiality to tolerate gastro-intestinal (GI) tract conditions. The isolate also showed significant hydrophobicity and auto-aggregation traits, indicating its potential to adhere to the intestinal wall based on its cell surface characteristics. High thermal death point of the isolate represents its exploitation for further commercial purposes. Findings concluded that strain DBOCP6 could certainly be used as an ideal probiotic candidate for industrial purposes.

Sung *et al.* (2010) isolated and characterized an antagonist for its application as a probiotic agent against *S. aureus*. *S. hominis* MBBL 2-9 exerted desirable probiotic characteristics such as acid resistance, bile tolerance, and adherence to epithelial cell line. The isolate also secreted a bacteriocin with unique molecular mass and significant antimicrobial activity similar to conventional antibiotics. This study represented the first report of bacteriocin-producing *S. hominis* MBBL 2-9 that has potential for its use as a promising probiotic agent against *S. aureus* infection.

Previous study showed the isolation of CNS from Slovak traditional sausages and demonstrated the metabolic characteristics of potent *S. xylosus* and *S. carnosus* strains for the selection of ideal starter cultures towards its applications in the processing of sausages. *S. xylosus* and *S. carnosus* inhibited the growth of *Listeria innocua* and *Pseudomonas* sp. Findings suggested that *S. xylosus* can be utilized as pronounced starter culture in the preparation of sausage (Simonova′ *et al.*, 2006).

Coagulase-negative staphylococci were also isolated from meju and doenjang (traditional Korean fermented soybean foods). None of *S. succinus* strains exerted antibiotic resistance or haemolytic activities. Thirty-three selected strains produced cadaverine, putrescine, and tyramine. The secretion of these 3 biogenic amines may however, be insignificant in view of the increased amounts of tyramine produced by the control (*E. faecalis*). All 33 CNS strains showed growth on tryptic soy agar constituting 21% (w/v) NaCl, revealed acid producing property at 15% (w/v) NaCl, and showed strain-dependent protease and lipase activities. *S. succinus* 14BME1, the potent starter culture produced significant rates of benzeneacetic acid, 2,3-butanediol, trimethylpyrazine, and tetramethylpyrazine through the fermentation of soybean (Jeong *et al.*, 2016).

Mauriello *et al.* (2004) demonstrated the presence of Micrococcaceae in various kinds of fermented sausages of Southern Italy and assessed the technological characteristics of staphylococci strains for evaluating the potentiality of selected strains as starter culture candidates in the processing of dry fermented pork sausages. A total of 96 strains were investigated to determine nitrate reductase, proteolytic, lipolytic, and antioxidant properties as well as their viability at varied temperatures, pHs, and NaCl concentrations. *S. xylosus* strains revealed the desirable technological characteristics that would make them ideal starter cultures for the fermentation of meat products. Additionally, bacteria from other species also exhibited promising technological traits. Results depicted that a variety of *Staphylococcus* sp. based starter cultures can be formulated, considering the desirable technological properties of strains.

Two strains of *S. simulans* (Ssm12 and Ssm21) and 4 strains of *S. carnosus* (SC28, SC31, SC54, and SC55) were studied to determine the technological attributes for their selection as potential starter cultures in order to utilize in the processing of dry fermented sausages. All the strains were able to reduce nitrate to nitrite at different temperature. All the strains showed antioxidative enzymes such as superoxide dismutase and catalase. All strains hydrolysed sarcoplasmic proteins only but not myofibrillar proteins. Results showed that these strains possessed satisfactory technological traits that would make them ideal starter cultures for the fermentation of sausages (Casaburi *et al.*, 2005).

Coagulase-negative staphylococci such as *S. hominis*, *S. vitulinus*, *S. epidermidis*, *S. saprophyticus*, *S. haemolyticus*, *S. xylosus*, *S. lentus*, and *S. warneri* were isolated from 72 cheese samples. As per disc diffusion assay, strains were observed resistant to penicillin (76.5%), erythromycin (35.3%), tetracycline (29.4%), and trimethoprim-sulfamethoxazole (17.6%). However, all CNS strains were observed to be sensitive to vancomycin, streptomycin, linezolid, and gentamycin (Kürekci, 2016).

Thai fermented marine fish associated *S. hominis* KQU-131 secreted a thermo-stable bacteriocin. Structural and genetic analyses showed that the bacteriocin was a variant of nukacin ISK-1, a type-A(II) lantibiotic, and termed the bacteriocin nukacin KQU-131. Three different amino acid residues were observed between nukacin ISK-1 and nukacin KQU-131, 1 residue in the leader peptide and the other 2 in the mature peptide (Wilaipun *et al.*, 2008).

Gold nanoparticle synthesis using probiotics

Over the past few decades, AuNPs have been implemented extensively in biomedicine due to their unique optical, electrical, and photothermal characteristics. Among distinct groups of microbes, prokaryotes have received enormous attention in the synthesis of AuNPs. Bacteria are considered promising alternative to chemical synthesis methods since they have unique potentiality to produce nanoparticles efficiently.

Probiotics can be considered as pronounced candidates for the biosynthesis of distinct categories of nanoparticles (Korbekandi *et al.*, 2012). Probiotic bacteria constitute undesirable electro-kinetic potential, which attracts the cations, and acts as a threshold level of the synthesis mechanism (Jha *et al.*, 2009). Probiotic bacteria have been known to synthesize nanocrystals of gold, silver, and their alloys (Prasad *et al.*, 2007). Additionally, probiotics synthesize plethora of metal nanoparticles or oxide nanoparticles such as Silver, Titanium dioxide, Antimony oxide, Gadolinium oxide, Cadmium sulphide, Selenium, and Zinc oxide. Surprisingly, the synthesis of AuNPs using probiotic bacteria is very limited.

Previously, *L. kimchicus* DCY51T isolated from Korean kimchi was used for synthesizing AuNPs. The synthesized AuNPs were observed to be spherical in shape with varying sizes of 5-30 nm. The biosynthesized AuNPs revealed antioxidant properties by scavenging free radicals. Findings suggested the development of a new class of probiotics mediated and non-toxic carriers in targeted drug delivery treatments, cancer therapy, photothermal therapies, biosensing, and medical imaging (Markus *et al.*, 2016).

Mossallam *et al.* (2014) demonstrated the impact of *L. acidophilus* CH1 associated bacteriocin, with or without AuNPs against intestinal microsporidiosis in immunosuppressed mice. Results showed significant ($P<0.05$) anti-microsporidial effect of bacteriocin. This effect was further studied by conjugating bacteriocin with AuNPs which showed the maximum reduction in the intestinal spore load in bacteriocin/AuNPs-inoculated mice, followed by bacteriocin-inoculated group. Results suggested that *L. acidophilus* CH1-derived bacteriocin can represent a strong safer treatment against intestinal microsporidiosis.

Probiotics in livestock industries

Livestock industries are one of the fastest growing sectors contributing about 40% of the global value of agricultural production (Bruinsma, 2003). Livestock provide a prime source of disposable income for developing countries. Horses are hindgut fermenters and consume diets containing fibrous plant material which is mostly digested in the hindgut (Julliand, 2005). Horse's gastrointestinal microbiome is a complex system with microorganisms that are responsible for protecting the host against pathogens and providing a barrier against food and other antigens (Costa and Weese, 2012). Antibiotics are commonly administered to horses not only for the treatment of various bacterial infections but also improving their growth performances. As a matter of fact, antibiotics medication-based treatments can disrupt the indigenous microbial counts within the gastrointestinal tract of horses as well as the targeted pathogens causing diseases (Gronvold *et al.*, 2010). In spite of enormous benefits to many of increased livestock production, it has raised colossal public health problems. Thus, the uncontrolled use of commercial antibiotics as growth promoters in animal feed has caused global concern. The use of antibiotics has been banned in several countries due to its ability to develop antibiotic resistance microorganisms associated with human and animal infections.

Currently, feed additives are considered potential substitute for antibiotic growth promoters. Probiotics are used widely in farm livestock, as they are associated with reducing clinical disease and increasing growth performances. The most important objectives for using probiotics in animal feed are to maintain and improve the performance of the animals. Several reports have demonstrated the significant effects of probiotics on horses. Oral administration of probiotic yeasts improved digestion, while the oral supplementation of probiotic bacteria improved symptoms of enterocolitis in horses (Desrochers *et al.*, 2005; Jouany *et al.*, 2008). The supplementation of probiotics improved lactobacilli proliferation and reduced faecal pH (Roessler *et al.*, 2012). The metabolic by-products of probiotic bacteria such as lactic acid ($C_3H_6O_3$) and acetic acid (CH_3COOH) may lower the intestinal pH, which helps the inhibition of the growth of pathogenic bacteria (Miyazaki *et al*., 2010). The supplementation of probiotic yeasts in the feeding diets improved digestion and growth performances of horses (de Rezende *et al*., 2012). Agazzi *et al.* (2009) suggested that feeding the horses with probiotic yeasts improved dry and organic matter, neutral detergent fibre, and acid detergent fibre digestibility. Prior reports also revealed the beneficial impact of exogenous lactobacilli and other probiotics in horses towards digestibility and fermentative end products (Desrochers *et al*., 2005; Swyers *et al*., 2008).

Aim and Objectives

Aim:

To assess biotechnological attributes of coagulase-negative staphylococci isolated from traditional fermented foods of Tamil Nadu, India.

Objectives:

i. To isolate and characterize anti-pathogenic bacteria indigenous to traditional fermented foods.
ii. To assess probiotic and technological properties of coagulase-negative *Staphylococcus* spp.
iii. To optimize biomass and anti-tubercular activity of *Staphylococcus hominis* strain MANF2 using statistical tools.
iv. To purify anti-tubercular and anticancer protein from strain MANF2.
v. To predict anti-tubercular and anticancer traits of peptide NMANF2 using *in silico* docking tools.
vi. To synthesize and purify anti-tubercular and anticancer protein in strain MANF2 under mild stress condition of certain antimicrobial agent.
vii. To predict anti-tubercular and anticancer traits of peptide SMANF2 using *in silico* docking tools.
viii. To determine the effect of *Mentha piperita* stress on some functional properties of strain MANF2.
ix. To synthesize anisotropic gold nanoplates using strain MANF2 as reductant and conjugate with purified protein for therapeutic attributes.
x. To estimate *in vitro* gas production and fermentation kinetics in horses using strain MANF2 as ideal feed additive.

Chapter 1

Anti-pathogenic traits, molecular characterization, and sequence analyses of bacteria indigenous to traditional fermented foods

1. Introduction

Fermentation of foods through disparate techniques has been in existence since ancient periods in India. Ethnic people produce fermented foods by utilizing a variety of locally available common substrates. In the recent years, research on fermented foods has been extensively investigated due to tremendous industrial as well as therapeutic demands. However, there are several foods which are traditionally consumed in specific regions of India and deserve scientific attention because of their colossal health benefits. Tamil Nadu (a southern state of India) is traditionally rich in diversified fermented foods. These fermented foods are consumed routinely in the people's diet and play pivotal role in their daily life due to huge functional attributes. In fact, naturally fermented foods are the reservoir of functional microorganisms that transform the chemical components of raw materials during the fermentation of food, thereby enhancing the bioavailability of nutrients, enriching sensory quality of the food, improving food safety, producing antioxidant and antimicrobial compounds, and stimulating the functional properties (Tamang *et al.*, 2016).

Fermented foods associated non-pathogenic microorganisms confer a health benefit to the host. Among those microbiota, *Enterococcus* spp., *Lactobacillus* spp., *Lactococcus* spp., *Leuconostoc* spp., *Pediococcus* spp., *Weissella* spp., *Bacillus* spp., *Bifidobacterium* spp., *Brachybacterium* spp., *Brevibacterium* spp., *Propionibacterium* spp., and *Saccharomyces* spp. were widely reported (Bourdichon *et al.*, 2012; Lv *et al.*, 2013; Tamang, 2015; Aarti *et al.*, 2016; Lima *et al.*, 2017). But the exploitation of wide groups of bacteria in traditional fermented food products of Tamil Nadu, India for their vast therapeutic applications is very limited.

Considering the functional characteristics of traditional foods and necessity for scientific attention, the present chapter was investigated to isolate distinct groups of bacteria from diversified traditional foods of Tamil Nadu, India and to determine their anti-pathogenic properties not only against foodborne and enteric pathogenic bacteria but also *M. tuberculosis*. Further, the potent isolates were identified and characterized through biochemical, molecular, and sequence analyses tools in order to appraise their biotechnological applications.

2. Materials and methods

2.1. Fermented foods used

'*Palayasatham*', 'Buttermilk', 'Curd', '*Idli* and *Dosa* Batter', '*Koozh*', '*Appam* Batter', and '*Paniyaram* Batter' were used as traditional fermented food samples for the isolation of distinct bacteria. Figure 1 shows the traditional method of preparation for each fermented food used in this study.

2.2. Isolation of bacteria

One gram (g) for semi-solid sample) / 1 millilitre (mL; for liquid sample) of traditionally prepared fermented foods was mixed with sterile distilled water, and centrifuged at 2500 relative centrifugal force (*g*) for 10 minutes (min) using centrifuge (Model - REMI: C-24 PLUS) in order to remove heavy particles. The collected supernatant was serially diluted (10^{-1}-10^{-6}) and 1 mL of the suspension was poured onto sterilized De Man, Rogosa and Sharpe (MRS) agar plates. After spreading the suspension, plates were incubated at 30 degree Celsius (°C) in incubator (Model - ORBITEK: LE0102DCBA) for 48 h under aerobic condition. After required period of incubation, the appearance of different colonies on the agar plates was observed. The morphologically dissimilar colonies were selected and streaked on the freshly prepared MRS agar plates. Purified cultures were maintained in 50% (volume by volume: v/v) glycerol stock at -80°C for further experiments.

2.3. Antibacterial activities against foodborne and enteric pathogens-

2.3.1. Cell free neutralized supernatant (CFNS) preparation

Isolates were inoculated into sterilized MRS broth and incubated at 30°C for 48 h. Bacteria were centrifuged at 8000 *g* for 10 min, and the culture supernatant was subjected to membrane filtration [0.22 micrometre (μm)]. The sterilized cell free supernatant was neutralized (pH 7.0) using 1Normal (N) sodium hydroxide (NaOH) in order to exclude the anti-tubercular effect of organic acids in the medium. The CFNS was treated individually with catalase (Sigma, India; 1 mg/mL) and incubated at 37°C for 2 h in order to eliminate the inhibitory effect of hydrogen peroxide (H_2O_2). After catalase treatment, the CFNS obtained was then screened for anti-pathogenic activity.

2.3.2. Antagonistic activities

Foodborne pathogens (*Staphylococcus epidermidis* MTTC 3615, *Staphylococcus aureus* MTCC 96, *Enterococcus faecalis* MTCC 439, and *Micrococcus luteus* MTCC 106) and enteric pathogenic bacteria (*Shigella flexneri* MTCC 1457, *Yersinia enterocolitica* MTCC 840, *Enterobacter aerogenes* MTCC 111, and *Proteus vulgaris* MTCC 1771) used in this study were obtained from Microbial Type Culture Collection (MTCC) and GenBank, Chandigarh, India. All the indicator pathogens were sub-cultured into Tryptone Soya Broth medium. Cultures were incubated at 37°C for 24 h. After required period of incubation, the indicator pathogens were swabbed onto sterile Mueller Hinton Agar plates. The agar media were punched using cork borer, and CFNS [100 microlitres (µL)] of isolates was poured into the respective wells. Streptomycin ($C_{21}H_{39}N_7O_{12}$; 0.4 mg/mL) was used as positive control. The growth inhibitory property of isolates against indicator pathogens was expressed in arbitrary unit/mL (AU/mL) after 24 h of incubation. One AU was defined as the reciprocal of the highest level of dilution resulting in a clear zone of growth inhibition.

2.4. Anti-tubercular activities of potent isolates-

Isolates exhibiting pronounced anti-pathogenic activities against indicator foodborne and enteric pathogens were used for determining anti-tubercular activities against *M. tuberculosis* H37Rv.

2.4.1. Preparation of cell suspension

Cell suspension equivalent to #2 MacFarland standards was prepared by inoculating the log phase culture of reference laboratory strain *M. tuberculosis* H37Rv from Lowenstein Jensen slope into Middlebrook 7H9 broth medium.

2.4.2. Luciferase reporter phase (LRP) assay

Anti-tubercular activities of the CFNS of isolates were determined by adopting LRP assay as described by Sivakumar *et al.* (2007) with slight modifications. Approximately 350 µL of 7H9 broth supplemented with 10% albumin dextrose complex and 0.5% glycerol ($C_3H_8O_3$) were taken in cryovials, and CFNS (100 µL) was added into it. Hundred microliters of *M. tuberculosis* cell suspension were inoculated into all the vials. Sterile double distilled water was used as solvent control. Rifampicin ($C_{43}H_{58}N_4O_{12}$; 1.2 mg/mL) was used as standard drug control. All the vials were incubated at 37^{0}C for 72 h. After required period of incubation, 50 µL of high titre mycobacteriophage phAETRC202 and 40 µL of 0.1 molar (M) calcium chloride ($CaCl_2$)

solution were added into the test as well as control vials. All the vials were incubated at 37^0C for further 4 h. After incubation, 100 μL from each vial were transferred to luminometer (Model - Monolight 2010) cuvette. About 100 μL of D-luciferin [0.3 millimolar (mM) in 0.05M sodium citrate buffer, pH 4.5] was added into it and relative light unit (RLU) was measured in luminometer. All the readings were recorded in triplicate, and the mean values were calculated. The RLU reduction was calculated as follows-

$$\% \text{ RLU reduction} = RLU_{Control} - RLU_{Test} / RLU_{Control} \times 100 \qquad \text{[Equation 1]}$$

Isolates showing RLU reduction by 50% or more when compared to control were considered as demonstrating anti-tubercular activity. The most active isolates were identified using varied biochemical and molecular characterization tools.

2.5. Identification of potent isolates-

2.5.1. Morphological and biochemical characterization

The morphological and biochemical characteristics of potent isolates were carried out using standard Bergey's Manual of Systemic Bacteriology (Sneath, 1994). Gram staining test was performed to differentiate Gram positive (+) and Gram negative (-) isolates. Endospore test was carried out to confirm the sporulating or non-sporulating bacteria. The cellular morphology and colony characteristics of isolates were also examined on agar plates. Biochemical tests viz. indole, methyl red, voges-proskauer, citrate utilization, ortho-nitrophenyl-β-galactoside ($C_{12}H_{15}NO_8$; ONPG), nitrate reductase, arginine, malonate, and catalase were performed aseptically. On the other hand, the potentiality of isolates to ferment various carbohydrates like glucose ($C_6H_{12}O_6$), sucrose ($C_{12}H_{22}O_{11}$), arabinose ($C_5H_{10}O_5$), mannitol ($C_6H_{14}O_6$), trehalose ($C_{12}H_{22}O_{11}$), lactose ($C_{12}H_{22}O_{11}$), and dextrose ($C_6H_{12}O_6$) were also tested.

2.5.2. Molecular characterization-

2.5.2.1. Genomic deoxyribonucleic acid (DNA) isolation

Genomic DNA was isolated using NucleoSpin® DNA isolation kit (Macherey-Nagel) following manufacturer's instructions. Two millilitres of log phase grown culture was taken in a microcentrifuge tube. One hundred and eighty microlitres of T1 buffer and 25 μL of proteinase K were added and incubated at 56^0C in a water bath (VANI SCIENTIFIC & EQUIPMENTS) until it was completely lysed. After lysis, 5 μL of RNase A (100 mg/mL) was added and incubated at room temperature for 5 min. Two hundred microlitres of B3 buffer was added and incubated at 70^0C for 10 min. Two hundred and ten microlitres of 100% ethanol were added and mixed uniformly. The mixture was pipetted into NucleoSpin® Tissue column placed in a 2 mL collection tube and centrifuged at 11000 *g* for 1 min. The NucleoSpin® Tissue column was transferred to a new 2 mL tube and washed with 500 μL of buffer. Washing step was repeated using 600 μL of B5 buffer. After washing, the NucleoSpin® Tissue column was placed in a clean 1.5 mL tube and DNA was eluted out using 50 μL buffer.

2.5.2.2. Agarose gel electrophoresis of genomic DNA

The quality of DNA isolated was checked using agarose gel electrophoresis. One microlitre of 6X gel-loading buffer (0.25% bromophenol blue, 30% sucrose in Tris-Ethylenediaminetetraacetic acid (EDTA: TE) buffer, and pH 8.0) was added to 5μL of DNA. Samples were loaded to 0.8% (w/v) agarose gel prepared in 0.5X Tris/Borate/EDTA (TBE) buffer containing 0.5 μg/mL ethidium bromide. Electrophoresis was performed with 0.5X TBE as electrophoresis buffer at 75 Volt (V) until bromophenol dye front has migrated to the bottom of gel. The gel was visualized in ultraviolet (UV) transilluminator (GeNei™) and the image was captured under UV light using gel documentation system (Bio-Rad).

2.5.2.3. Polymerase chain reaction (PCR) amplification

The PCR amplification reactions were carried out in a 20 μL reaction volume which contained 1X PCR buffer (Tris-hydrochloric acid (Tris-HCl) 100mM, pH 8.3; potassium chloride (KCl) 500mM), 0.2mM each deoxyribonucleotide triphosphate (dNTPs: dATP, dGTP, dCTP, and dTTP), 2.5mM magnesium chloride ($MgCl_2$), 1 unit of AmpliTaq Gold DNA polymerase enzyme, 0.1 mg/mL bovine serum albumin (BSA), 4% dimethyl sulphoxide (DMSO), 5 picomole (pM) of forward and reverse primers, and template DNA. Primers used for amplification process is mentioned below:

Target	Primer	Direction	Sequence (5' → 3')
16S ribosomal ribonucleic acid (rRNA)	16S-RS-F	Forward	CAGGCCTAACACATGCAAGTC
	16S-RS-R	Reverse	GGGCGGWGTGTACAAGGC

The PCR amplification was carried out in a PCR thermal cycler (Model - GeneAmp PCR System 9700, Applied Biosystems). The PCR amplification profile was set as per the conditions mentioned below:

95°C - 5.00 min
95°C - 30 seconds (sec)
60°C - 40 sec } 35 cycles
72°C - 60 sec
72°C - 7.00 min

2.5.2.4. *Agarose gel electrophoresis of amplicon*

The PCR products were checked in 1.2% (w/v) agarose gels prepared in 0.5X TBE buffer containing 0.5 microgram per millilitre (µg/mL) ethidium bromide. One microlitre of 6X gel loading dye was mixed with 5 µL of PCR products, loaded into wells, and electrophoresis was performed at 75V power supply with 0.5X TBE electrophoresis buffer for about 1-2 h, until the bromophenol blue front had migrated to almost the bottom of the gel. The molecular standard used was a 2-log DNA ladder. The gels were visualized in a UV transilluminator and the image was captured under UV light using gel documentation system.

2.5.2.5. *ExoSAP-IT treatment*

ExoSAP-IT (USB) consists of two hydrolytic enzymes, Exonuclease I and Shrimp Alkaline Phosphatase, in a specially formulated buffer for the removal of unwanted primers and dNTPs from a PCR product mixture with no interference in downstream applications. Five microlitres of PCR product were mixed with 2 µL of ExoSAP-IT and incubated at 37°C for 15 min, followed by enzyme inactivation at 80°C for 15 min.

2.5.2.6. *Sequencing using BigDye Terminator v3.1*

Sequencing reaction was done in a PCR thermal cycler using the BigDye Terminator v3.1 Cycle sequencing kit (Applied Biosystems, USA) following manufactures protocol.

The PCR mix consisted of the following components:

PCR Product (ExoSAP treated)	-	10-20 nanograms (ng)
Primer	-	3.2 pM (either Forward or Reverse)
Sequencing Mix	-	0.28 µL
Reaction buffer	-	1.86 µL
Sterile distilled water	-	make up to 10 µL

The sequencing PCR temperature profile consisted of a 1st cycle at 96°C for 2 min, followed by 30 cycles at 96°C for 30 sec, 50°C for 40 sec, and 60°C for 4 min.

2.5.2.7. Post sequencing PCR clean up

The amplicon was taken in fresh vial and 5 μL of 3M sodium acetate solution (pH – 4.6) and 100 μL of absolute ethanol were added into it. The vial was mixed thoroughly and kept at -20°C for 30 min to precipitate the PCR product and centrifuged at 10000 *g* for 5 min. Three hundred microlitres of 70% ethanol (C_2H_5OH) were added to the pellet and centrifuged again at 10000 *g* for 5 min. The pellet was air dried until the ethanol effervescence was removed. The pellet was suspended in 10 μL of sterile distilled water. The cleaned up air dried product was sequenced in ABI 3730 DNA analyzer (Applied Biosystems).

2.5.2.8. 16S rRNA gene sequencing

The sequence quality was checked using Sequence Scanner Software v1 (Applied Biosystems). Sequence alignment and required editing of the obtained sequences were carried out using Geneious Pro v5.6 (Drummond *et al.*, 2012). The 16S rRNA sequences were submitted to Basic Local Alignment Search Tool (BLAST), National Centre for Biotechnology Information (NCBI) (https://blast.ncbi.nlm.nih.gov/Blast.cgi) for similarity search. Novel strains were deposited to GenBank, NCBI (https://www.ncbi.nlm.nih.gov/genbank/submit/) and accession number was assigned for each isolate.

2.6. Coagulase test

Coagulase is an enzyme that coverts fibrinogen of plasma into fibrin, causing coagulation of plasma. The secretion of free coagulase from bacterial source is extracellularly. The detection of free coagulase production from potent strains was carried out using tube test method (Sneath, 1994). Two hundred microlitres of plasma (from sheep blood) were mixed with 1.8 mL of saline in a clean test tube. One millilitre of diluted plasma was mixed with 0.5 mL of active bacterial culture and mixed well. The tube was incubated at room temperature for 2-3 h and observed for clotting by tilting the tube about 90 degrees (°).

2.7. Sequence analyses using bioinformatics tools-

2.7.1. Thermodynamic structure prediction

The minimum free energy (MFE), mountain plot, and entropy of sequences were determined using RNAfold web server (Gruber *et al.*, 2008). Temperature was set at 37°C for evaluating the stability of chemical or biological molecules or entities of the isolate.

2.7.2. Determination of Guanine Cytosine (GC) content

The GC content of the sequences was calculated according to the algorithm of Rosano and Ceccarelli (2009). The GC content (%) was calculated as:

$$\%\ \text{GC content} = \frac{\text{Total number of G and C}}{\text{Total number of A,T,C,and G}} \times 100 \qquad \text{[Equation 2]}$$

2.7.3. Open reading frame (ORF) determination

The ORF of sequences of strains was determined using ORF Finder (https://www.ncbi.nlm.nih.gov/orffinder/). The 16S rRNA sequences of strains in the FASTA format were pasted in the box provided in the tool and ORF was determined.

2.7.4. Phylogenetic tree construction

Phylogenetic relationship of strains was inferred by comparison with the 16S rRNA sequences of close isolates. The variable and incomplete sites at both the 5′ and 3′ ends of the 16S rRNA gene sequences were excluded from the alignment. Regions that could not be aligned unambiguously were excluded from the analysis. Phylogenetic tree was inferred using Neighbor Joining (NJ) algorithm with the Kimura two-parameter model in Molecular Evolutionary Genetics Analysis (MEGA) software version 4.0 (Tamura *et al.*, 2007).

2.8. Statistical analyses

All the experimental sections of the study were carried out in triplicate and data were represented as mean±standard variation (SD). Data were analysed using one way analysis of variance (ANOVA) and values $P \leq 0.05$ were considered significant.

3. Results

3.1. Isolation of bacteria from fermented foods

Distinct groups of bacteria were isolated from '*Palayasatham*', 'Buttermilk', '*Koozh*', '*Idli* and *Dosa* Batter', '*Appam* Batter', '*Paniyaram* Batter', and 'Curd' using spread plate technique. Figure 2 shows growth of distinct colonies of probiotic bacteria on MRS agar medium. Morphological dissimilar colonies were selected and purified by quadrant streaking method (Figure 3). A total of 56 bacterial cultures were isolated from fermented foods used.

3.2. Anti-pathogenic activities of isolates

Anti-pathogenic activities of CFNS of isolates were assessed against foodborne and enteric pathogens using agar well diffusion assay. The zone of inhibition of CFNS of few isolates as well as positive control against foodborne and enteric bacterial pathogens is shown in Figure 4 and Figure 5, respectively.

Table 1A exhibits antagonistic activities of CFNS of bacteria isolated from '*Palayasatham*' against foodborne pathogens. Isolate PLSM1, PLSM3, PLSM5, PLSM7, and PLSM8 revealed significant (P<0.05) antagonistic activities against indicator pathogens in the range of 420.32±20.2-810.52±24.6 AU/mL. Streptomycin showed comparatively higher activities (1300.23±26.3-2300.22±26.3 AU/mL) against the indicator pathogens. The antagonistic activities of CFNS of bacteria isolated from '*Palayasatham*' against enteric bacterial pathogens are shown in Table 1B. Isolate PLSM1, PLSM3, PLSM5, PLSM7, and PLSM8 revealed significant (P<0.05) antagonistic activities against indicator pathogens in the range of 420.24±20.3-680.32±22.3 AU/mL. None of the isolates exhibited growth inhibitory traits against *P. vulgaris*. Streptomycin showed comparatively higher activities (1200.22±25.3-1800.31±22.3 AU/mL) against the indicator pathogens.

The anti-pathogenic activities of CFNS of bacteria isolated from 'Buttermilk' against foodborne bacterial pathogens are shown in Table 2A. Isolate BTM1, BTM2, and BTM6 exhibited antagonistic activities against indicator pathogens, ranging from 400.12±20.4-492.64±24.5 AU/mL. *E. faecalis* and *M. luteus* were found to be resistant to all the isolates. In like manner, enteric pathogens such as *S. flexneri*, *Y. enterocolitica*, and *E. aerogenes* were susceptible to isolate BTM1, BTM2, and BTM6 only. None of the isolates showed activities against *P. vulgaris* (Table 2B). Streptomycin showed comparatively higher activities against all the indicator pathogens.

Table 3A illustrates antagonistic activities of CFNS of bacteria isolated from '*Koozh*' against foodborne bacterial pathogens. All the isolates were found significantly (P<0.05) affective against indicator pathogens used. However, isolate MANF2 exhibited promising antagonistic activities against indicator pathogens in the range of 1220.22±21.3-1600.31±22.3 AU/mL. Likewise, all the isolates revealed significant (P<0.05) activities against enteric pathogens too. Among them, isolate MANF2 showed pronounced activities against the indicator pathogens, ranging from 720.11±21.3-1500.23±22.3 AU/mL (Table 3B). Streptomycin showed comparatively higher activities against all the indicator pathogens.

The antagonistic activities of CFNS of bacteria isolated from '*Idli* and *Dosa* Batter' against foodborne bacterial pathogens are shown in Table 4A. The indicator bacterial pathogens were susceptible to the isolate IDB2, IDB6, and IDB7 with activities of

482.18±22.5-680.44±24.8 AU/mL. None of the isolates were found affective against *M. luteus*. The enteric bacterial pathogens were sensitive to isolate IDB2 and IDB6 only, showing growth inhibitory activities of 420.22±23.5-500.5±22.4 AU/mL. *P. vulgaris* was found resistant to the CFNS of all the isolates (Table 4B). Streptomycin showed comparatively higher activities against all the indicator pathogens.

Table 5A illustrates anti-pathogenic traits of CFNS of bacteria isolated from '*Appam* Batter' against foodborne bacterial pathogens. Isolate APMB1, APMB2, APMB4, and APMB5 showed significant ($P<0.05$) antagonistic activities of 490.28±20.5-710.22±23.5 AU/mL against foodborne pathogens. The indicator pathogenic bacteria were resistant to the CFNS of rest of the isolates. Similarly, the enteric bacterial pathogens were observed susceptible to the isolate APMB1, APMB4, and APMB5 only (Table 5B). Streptomycin showed comparatively higher activities against all the indicator pathogens.

Table 6A exhibits anti-pathogenic activities of CFNS of bacteria isolated from '*Paniyaram* Batter' against foodborne bacterial pathogens. The isolate PYB1, PYB3, PYB5, PYB7, and PYB8 revealed significant ($P<0.05$) growth inhibitory activities against indicator pathogens in the range of 600.42±23.3-980.23±24.5 AU/mL. On the other hand, enteric bacterial pathogens were significantly ($P<0.05$) susceptible to the isolate PYB1, PYB3, PYB5, and PYB6 with arbitrary unit values of 410.23±22.6-1300.24±23.6 AU/mL (Table 6B). Streptomycin showed comparatively higher activities against all the indicator pathogens.

The anti-pathogenic activities of CFNS of bacteria isolated from 'Curd' against foodborne bacterial pathogens are shown in Table 7A. The isolate LXD5 and LXD7 were found affective against *S. aureus* and *E. faecalis* only with arbitrary unit values of 610.32±24.3-720.45±25.3 AU/mL. The indicator pathogens were found resistant to the rest of the isolates. On the other hand, enteric pathogens (*Y. enterocolitica* and *E. aerogenes*) were susceptible to LXD1, LXD3, LXD5, and LXD7 with antagonistic activities range of 480.32±21.3-620.23±22.3 AU/mL. *S. flexneri* and *P. vulgaris* were resistant to the rest of the isolates tested (Table 7B). Streptomycin showed comparatively higher activities against all the indicator pathogens.

3.3. Anti-tubercular activities of potent isolates

Isolates revealing anti-pathogenic activities against foodborne and enteric bacterial pathogens were selected for determining anti-tubercular activities against *M.*

tuberculosis H37Rv. Figure 6 illustrates the stepwise process for the reduction of RLU by luminometer due to the action of CFNS of bacteria. The CFNS of bacteria isolated from '*Palayasatham*', particularly PLSM1, PLSM3, and PLSM5 demonstrated significant ($P<0.05$) RLU reductions of 60.3±0.3, 64.1±0.2, and 52.3±0.5%, respectively with respect to rifampicin (99.9±0.3%). On the other hand, isolate PLSM7 and PLSM8 showed low RLU reductions (<50%), thereby revealing weak anti-tubercular properties (Figure 7a). Similarly, the CFNS of 'Buttermilk' associated isolates (BTM1, BTM2, and BTM6) exhibited weak anti-tubercular activities, showing RLU reductions of 46.3±0.4, 38.7±0.3, and 22.3±0.5%, respectively (Figure 7b).

Bacterial cultures isolated from '*Koozh*' were tested for anti-tubercular properties against *M. tuberculosis* H37Rv. Among those cultures, 6 isolates revealed the strongest anti-tubercular activities. Based on LRP assay, the CFNS of isolate MANF2 exhibited 97.7±0.4% inhibition of *M. tuberculosis* H37Rv growth in terms of RLU reduction, followed by isolate MANF1 (96.1±0.3%), MANF4 (95.8±0.2%), MANF3 (95.7±0.3%), MANF5 (94.1±0.5%), and MANF6 (92.4±0.3%). Isolate MANF7 and MANF8 showed comparatively lower activities with RLU reductions of 70.3±0.2 and 74.3±0.4%, respectively. The anti-tubercular activities of all the isolates varied significantly ($P<0.05$) with respect to rifampicin (Figure 7c).

Figure 7d depicts anti-tubercular activities of CFNS of bacterial cultures isolated from '*Idli* and *Dosa* Batter'. Isolates exhibited significantly ($P<0.05$) low anti-tubercular activities, showing RLU reductions in the order of IDB7 (47.3±0.3%) > IDB6 (42.4±0.3%) > IDB2 (35.5±0.5%). In contrary to this, the CFNS of bacteria isolated from '*Appam* Batter' demonstrated promising anti-tubercular activities in the order of APMB1 (68.3±0.4%) > APMB5 (60.3±0.4%) > APMB2 (58.3±0.5%) > APMB4 (54.2±0.5%). The RLU reductions for all the isolates varied significantly ($P<0.05$) with respect to rifampicin (Figure 7e).

The anti-tubercular potentialities of CFNS of bacteria isolated from '*Paniyaram* Batter' are depicted in Figure 7f. Isolate PYB1, PYB3, PYB5, and PYB6 revealed significant ($P<0.05$) RLU reductions of 54.3±0.2, 56.4±0.5, 66.4±0.3, and 52.4±0.2%, respectively. On the other hand, isolate PYB7 and PYB8 exhibited low RLU reductions of 18.4±0.4 and 32.5±0.3%, respectively, indicating lack of anti-tubercular properties. Likewise, the CFNS of bacteria isolated from 'Curd' showed lack of anti-tubercular traits. Isolate LXD1, LXD3, LXD5, and LXD7 demonstrated significantly ($P<0.05$) low

RLU reductions of 23.3±0.5, 26.4±0.5, 18.4±0.4, and 12.5±0.3%, respectively with respect to rifampicin (Figure 7g).

3.4. Identification of potent isolates

Since, '*Koozh*' associated 6 isolates exhibited pronounced anti-tubercular activities, hence, isolate MANF1, MANF2, MANF3, MANF4, MANF5, and MANF6 were selected for identification through morphological, biochemical, and molecular characterization tools. The colonies of all the isolates were observed to be small, smooth, round, non-sporulating, and creamy white in colour. After Gram staining, cells were stained purple in colour and arranged in clusters, indicating gram (+) in nature (Figure 8). Biochemical tests showed that all isolates were negative towards indole, voges-proskauer. citrate utilization, arginine, malonate, and methyl red tests. On the other hand, isolates were positive towards ONPG, catalase, and nitrate reductase. Additionally, all the isolates were able to ferment various carbohydrates viz. glucose, sucrose, arabinose, mannitol, trehalose, lactose, and dextrose (Table 8).

Genomic DNA of six isolates was isolated, visualized under UV transilluminator, and the image was captured under UV light using gel documentation system (Figure 9a). The amplicon of 1257, 1160, 1170, 1175, 1250, and 1172 base pairs was visualized using gel documentation system (Figure 9b). Further, 16S rRNA sequencing and BLAST, NCBI similarity search results identified the isolates as *Staphylococcus saprophyticus* strain MANF1 (Accession number-MF196973), *Staphylococcus hominis* strain MANF2 (Accession number-MF196974), *Staphylococcus saprophyticus* strain MANF3 (Accession number-MF196975), *Staphylococcus xylosus* strain MANF4 (Accession number-MF196976), *Staphylococcus equorum* strain MANF5 (Accession number-MF196977), and *Staphylococcus equorum* strain MANF6 (Accession number-MF196978). In addition, none of the staphylococci strains coagulated the plasma, thereby indicating lack of free coagulase production from the strains (Figure 10). Thus, all the strains were further categorized as CNS.

3.5. Sequence analyses using bioinformatics tools

The 16S rRNA sequences of strains were used to determine the secondary structure of ribonucleic acid (RNA) using RNAfold web server. The thermodynamic parameter i.e. MFE for strain MANF1, strain MANF2, strain MANF3, strain MANF4, strain MANF5, and strain MANF6 was calculated as -423.3, -392.3, -395.4, -395.9, -423.2, and -395.5 kilocalories per mole (kcal/mol), respectively (Figure 11). Mountain plot and entropy were observed to depict the hierarchical representation of RNA secondary structure (Figure 12). Further, the GC content of sequence for strain MANF1, strain MANF2, strain MANF3, strain MANF4, strain MANF5, and MANF6 was calculated as 51.1, 51.2, 51.4, 51.4, 51.2, and 51.5%, respectively. Figure 13 shows 5 ORFs for strain MANF1 and strain MANF5, while 4 ORFs were observed for strain MANF2, strain MANF3, strain MANF4, and strain MANF6. The evolutionary history of CNS strains was inferred using NJ method. The phylogenetic tree with the sum of branch length of 45.02656873 is shown. The tree is drawn to scale, with branch lengths in the same units as those of the evolutionary distances used to infer the phylogenetic tree. All positions containing gaps and missing data were eliminated (Figure 14).

Table 1A: Antagonistic activities (AU/mL) of bacteria isolated from '*Palayasatham*' against foodborne bacterial pathogens.

Isolates	Indicator bacteria			
	S. epidermidis	*S. aureus*	*E. faecalis*	*M. luteus*
PLSM1	500.34 ± 20.5^{b}	420.32 ± 20.2^{c}	610.32 ± 22.4^{a}	NA
PLSM2	NA	NA	NA	NA
PLSM3	475.32 ± 16.6^{c}	525 ± 18.7^{b}	660.25 ± 20.8^{a}	NA
PLSM4	NA	NA	NA	NA
PLSM5	480.21 ± 22.3^{b}	584.34 ± 18.5^{a}	NA	NA
PLSM6	NA	NA	NA	NA
PLSM7	565.34 ± 21.5^{b}	630.25 ± 18.3^{a}	NA	NA
PLSM8	710.32 ± 22.6^{b}	NA	NA	810.52 ± 24.6^{a}
Streptomycin	1550.18 ± 26.3^{c}	1800.17 ± 22.3^{b}	2300.22 ± 26.3^{a}	1300.23 ± 26.3^{d}

NA - No activity; Values are represented as mean±SD of experiments carried out in triplicate (n = 3).
^{abcd}Values with different superscript letters within the same row are significantly ($P<0.05$) different.

Table 1B: Antagonistic activities (AU/mL) of bacteria isolated from '*Palayasatham*' against enteric bacterial pathogens.

Isolates	Indicator bacteria			
	S. flexneri	*Y. enterocolitica*	*E. aerogenes*	*P. vulgaris*
PLSM1	510.14 ± 22.5^{a}	500.32 ± 21.2^{a}	NA	NA
PLSM2	NA	NA	NA	NA
PLSM3	500.22 ± 18.4^{b}	530 ± 20.7^{a}	540.25 ± 20.4^{a}	NA
PLSM4	NA	NA	NA	NA
PLSM5	420.24 ± 20.3^{b}	564.44 ± 20.5^{a}	NA	NA
PLSM6	NA	NA	NA	NA
PLSM7	420.35 ± 20.8^{b}	500.15 ± 22.3^{a}	426.61 ± 21.5^{b}	NA
PLSM8	680.32 ± 22.3	NA	NA	NA
Streptomycin	1200.33 ± 24.4^{c}	1800.31 ± 22.3^{a}	1300.13 ± 23.4^{b}	1200.22 ± 25.3^{c}

NA - No activity; Values are represented as mean±SD of experiments carried out in triplicate (n = 3).
^{abc}Values with different superscript letters within the same row are significantly ($P<0.05$) different.

Table 2A: Antagonistic activities (AU/mL) of bacteria isolated from 'Buttermilk' against foodborne bacterial pathogens.

Isolates	Indicator bacteria			
	S. epidermidis	*S. aureus*	*E. faecalis*	*M. luteus*
BTM1	425.24±22.5^{a}	400.12±20.4^{b}	NA	NA
BTM2	445.54±20.8^{a}	432.26±20.5^{a}	NA	NA
BTM3	NA	NA	NA	NA
BTM4	NA	NA	NA	NA
BTM5	NA	NA	NA	NA
BTM6	492.64±24.5	NA	NA	NA
BTM7	NA	NA	NA	NA
BTM8	NA	NA	NA	NA
Streptomycin	1550.18±26.3^{c}	1800.17±22.3^{b}	2300.22±26.3^{a}	1300.23±26.3^{d}

NA - No activity; Values are represented as mean±SD of experiments carried out in triplicate (n = 3).
^{abcd}Values with different superscript letters within the same row are significantly (P<0.05) different.

Table 2B: Antagonistic activities (AU/mL) of bacteria isolated from 'Buttermilk' against enteric bacterial pathogens.

Isolates	Indicator bacteria			
	S. flexneri	*Y. enterocolitica*	*E. aerogenes*	*P. vulgaris*
BTM1	480.24±21.5^{a}	468.22±20.2^{b}	NA	NA
BTM2	440.32±23.4^{b}	510.45±24.5^{a}	432.45±22.4^{b}	NA
BTM3	NA	NA	NA	NA
BTM4	NA	NA	NA	NA
BTM5	NA	NA	NA	NA
BTM6	500.25±22.6^{a}	410.44±18.6^{b}	NA	NA
BTM7	NA	NA	NA	NA
BTM8	NA	NA	NA	NA
Streptomycin	1200.33±24.4^{c}	1800.31±22.3^{a}	1300.13±23.4^{b}	1200.22±25.3^{c}

NA - No activity; Values are represented as mean±SD of experiments carried out in triplicate (n = 3).
^{abc}Values with different superscript letters within the same row are significantly (P<0.05) different.

Table 3A: Antagonistic activities (AU/mL) of bacteria isolated from '*Koozh*' against foodborne bacterial pathogens.

Isolates	Indicator bacteria			
	S. epidermidis	*S. aureus*	*E. faecalis*	*M. luteus*
MANF1	800.34±20.8^{c}	823.21±21.8^{c}	1020.22±20.8^{a}	920.15±20.8^{b}
MANF2	1230.32±21.3^{c}	1600.31±22.3^{a}	1520.25±20.3^{b}	1220.22±21.3^{c}
MANF3	930.23±26.3^{a}	860.13±24.3^{b}	920.14±23.3^{a}	860.24±23.3^{b}
MANF4	1120.31±25.8^{b}	1200.32±24.8^{a}	1110.25±24.8^{b}	1130.22±24.8^{b}
MANF5	833.26±22.3^{c}	870.17±22.3^{bc}	900.25±22.3^{b}	1030.19±22.3^{a}
MANF6	900.25±24.3^{a}	800.28±25.3^{b}	860.22±23.3^{b}	970.16±22.3^{a}
MANF7	810.32±24.3^{a}	760.22±20.3^{b}	NA	NA
MANF8	NA	845.54±20.3^{b}	NA	900.32±21.6^{a}
Streptomycin	1550.18±26.3^{c}	1800.17±22.3^{b}	2300.22±26.3^{a}	1300.23±26.3^{d}

NA - No activity; Values are represented as mean±SD of experiments carried out in triplicate (n = 3).
^{abcd}Values with different superscript letters within the same row are significantly (P<0.05) different.

Table 3B: Antagonistic activities (AU/mL) of bacteria isolated from '*Koozh*' against enteric bacterial pathogens.

Isolates	Indicator bacteria			
	S. flexneri	*Y. enterocolitica*	*E. aerogenes*	*P. vulgaris*
MANF1	520.32±21.8^{b}	1110.12±21.8^{a}	520.25±20.8^{b}	500.14±21.8^{b}
MANF2	760.22±22.3^{c}	1500.23±22.3^{a}	820.21±20.3^{b}	720.11±21.3^{c}
MANF3	526.35±26.3^{c}	920.45±24.3^{a}	600.14±22.3^{b}	520.23±23.3^{c}
MANF4	600.14±25.8^{b}	1250.13±24.8^{a}	620.22±24.8^{b}	570.32±24.8^{c}
MANF5	530.15±22.3^{b}	970.43±22.3^{a}	570.34±22.3^{b}	500.14±21.3^{bc}
MANF6	500.27±23.3^{c}	930.22±25.3^{a}	610.14±22.3^{b}	520.15±22.3^{c}
MANF7	610.45±24.2	NA	NA	NA
MANF8	NA	744.23±25.3	NA	NA
Streptomycin	1200.33±24.4^{c}	1800.31±22.3^{a}	1300.13±23.4^{b}	1200.22±25.3^{c}

NA - No activity; Values are represented as mean±SD of experiments carried out in triplicate (n = 3).
^{abc}Values with different superscript letters within the same row are significantly (P<0.05) different.

Table 4A: Antagonistic activities (AU/mL) of bacteria isolated from '*Idli* and *Dosa* Batter' against foodborne bacterial pathogens.

Isolates	Indicator bacteria			
	S. epidermidis	*S. aureus*	*E. faecalis*	*M. luteus*
IDB1	NA	NA	NA	NA
IDB2	560.44±24.4^{b}	482.18±22.5^{c}	610.32±22.5^{a}	NA
IDB3	NA	NA	NA	NA
IDB4	NA	NA	NA	NA
IDB5	NA	NA	NA	NA
IDB6	630.54±22.5^{a}	644.5±25.6^{a}	NA	NA
IDB7	680.44±24.8	NA	NA	NA
IDB8	NA	NA	NA	NA
Streptomycin	1550.18±26.3^{c}	1800.17±22.3^{b}	2300.22±26.3^{a}	1300.23±26.3^{d}

NA - No activity; Values are represented as mean±SD of experiments carried out in triplicate (n = 3).
^{abcd}Values with different superscript letters within the same row are significantly (P<0.05) different.

Table 4B: Antagonistic activities (AU/mL) of bacteria isolated from '*Idli* and *Dosa* Batter' against enteric bacterial pathogens.

Isolates	Indicator bacteria			
	S. flexneri	*Y. enterocolitica*	*E. aerogenes*	*P. vulgaris*
IDB1	NA	NA	NA	NA
IDB2	420.22±23.5^{a}	430.45±23.5^{a}	460.45±20.4^{a}	NA
IDB3	NA	NA	NA	NA
IDB4	NA	NA	NA	NA
IDB5	NA	NA	NA	NA
IDB6	480.15±24.6^{b}	420.44±21.3^{b}	500.5±22.4^{a}	NA
IDB7	NA	NA	NA	NA
IDB8	NA	NA	NA	NA
Streptomycin	1200.33±24.4^{c}	1800.31±22.3^{a}	1300.13±23.4^{b}	1200.22±25.3^{c}

NA - No activity; Values are represented as mean±SD of experiments carried out in triplicate (n = 3).
^{abc}Values with different superscript letters within the same row are significantly (P<0.05) different.

Table 5A: Antagonistic activities (AU/mL) of bacteria isolated from '*Appam* Batter' against foodborne bacterial pathogens.

Isolates	Indicator bacteria			
	S. epidermidis	*S. aureus*	*E. faecalis*	*M. luteus*
APMB1	700.32 ± 25.4^{a}	640.23 ± 24.3^{b}	612.32 ± 22.5^{b}	620.24 ± 22.6^{b}
APMB2	540.41 ± 23.4^{b}	490.28 ± 20.5^{c}	710.22 ± 23.5^{a}	NA
APMB3	NA	NA	NA	NA
APMB4	670.34 ± 24.3^{a}	680.42 ± 21.3^{a}	NA	NA
APMB5	640.44 ± 20.3^{a}	610.32 ± 23.3^{a}	650.34 ± 22.3^{a}	630.34 ± 22.3^{a}
APMB6	NA	NA	NA	NA
APMB7	NA	NA	NA	NA
APMB8	NA	NA	NA	NA
Streptomycin	1550.18 ± 26.3^{c}	1800.17 ± 22.3^{b}	2300.22 ± 26.3^{a}	1300.23 ± 26.3^{d}

NA - No activity; Values are represented as mean±SD of experiments carried out in triplicate (n = 3).
^{abcd}Values with different superscript letters within the same row are significantly ($P<0.05$) different.

Table 5B: Antagonistic activities (AU/mL) of bacteria isolated from '*Appam* Batter' against enteric bacterial pathogens.

Isolates	Indicator bacteria			
	S. flexneri	*Y. enterocolitica*	*E. aerogenes*	*P. vulgaris*
APMB1	480.22 ± 25.3^{a}	400.23 ± 23.3^{ab}	430.22 ± 22.5^{a}	450.23 ± 22.6^{a}
APMB2	NA	NA	NA	NA
APMB3	NA	NA	NA	NA
APMB4	485.24 ± 25.3^{b}	480.44 ± 20.3^{b}	NA	500.45 ± 22.3^{a}
APMB5	475.34 ± 22.3^{a}	430.33 ± 24.3^{a}	470.24 ± 22.5^{a}	450.34 ± 22.6^{a}
APMB6	NA	NA	NA	NA
APMB7	NA	NA	NA	NA
APMB8	NA	NA	NA	NA
Streptomycin	1200.33 ± 24.4^{c}	1800.31 ± 22.3^{a}	1300.13 ± 23.4^{b}	1200.22 ± 25.3^{c}

NA - No activity; Values are represented as mean±SD of experiments carried out in triplicate (n = 3).
^{abc}Values with different superscript letters within the same row are significantly ($P<0.05$) different.

Table 6A: Antagonistic activities (AU/mL) of bacteria isolated from '*Paniyaram* Batter' against foodborne bacterial pathogens.

Isolates	Indicator bacteria			
	S. epidermidis	*S. aureus*	*E. faecalis*	*M. luteus*
PYB1	730.32±22.4^{a}	640.13±22.3^{b}	NA	NA
PYB2	NA	NA	NA	NA
PYB3	810.43±22.6^{b}	910.23±23.5^{a}	NA	920.34±20.4^{a}
PYB4	NA	NA	NA	NA
PYB5	740.54±20.3^{b}	600.42±23.3^{c}	850.34±22.6^{a}	700.34±21.3^{b}
PYB6	NA	NA	NA	NA
PYB7	980.23±24.5^{a}	810.34±25.3^{b}	710.43±23.3^{c}	NA
PYB8	NA	NA	900.34±24.4	NA
Streptomycin	1550.18±26.3^{c}	1800.17±22.3^{b}	2300.22±26.3^{a}	1300.23±26.3^{d}

NA - No activity; Values are represented as mean±SD of experiments carried out in triplicate (n = 3).
^{abcd}Values with different superscript letters within the same row are significantly (P<0.05) different.

Table 6B: Antagonistic activities (AU/mL) of bacteria isolated from '*Paniyaram* Batter' against enteric bacterial pathogens.

Isolates	Indicator bacteria			
	S. flexneri	*Y. enterocolitica*	*E. aerogenes*	*P. vulgaris*
PYB1	420.32±25.3^{b}	513.13±23.3^{a}	NA	410.23±22.6^{b}
PYB2	NA	NA	NA	NA
PYB3	NA	630.25±25.2	NA	NA
PYB4	NA	NA	NA	NA
PYB5	710.24±25.3^{c}	820.23±25.3^{b}	430.34±24.5^{d}	1300.24±23.6^{a}
PYB6	920.34±24.3^{a}	820.23±26^{b}	NA	NA
PYB7	NA	NA	NA	NA
PYB8	NA	NA	NA	NA
Streptomycin	1200.33±24.4^{c}	1800.31±22.3^{a}	1300.13±23.4^{b}	1200.22±25.3^{c}

NA - No activity; Values are represented as mean±SD of experiments carried out in triplicate (n = 3).
^{abc}Values with different superscript letters within the same row are significantly (P<0.05) different.

Table 7A: Antagonistic activities (AU/mL) of bacteria isolated from 'Curd' against foodborne bacterial pathogens.

Isolates	Indicator bacteria			
	S. epidermidis	*S. aureus*	*E. faecalis*	*M. luteus*
LXD1	NA	NA	NA	NA
LXD2	NA	NA	NA	NA
LXD3	NA	NA	NA	NA
LXD4	NA	NA	NA	NA
LXD5	NA	720.32±24.3	NA	NA
LXD6	NA	NA	NA	NA
LXD7	NA	610.32±24.3^{b}	720.45±25.3^{a}	NA
LXD8	NA	NA	NA	NA
Streptomycin	1550.18±26.3^{c}	1800.17±22.3^{b}	2300.22±26.3^{a}	1300.23±26.3^{d}

NA - No activity; Values are represented as mean±SD of experiments carried out in triplicate (n = 3).
^{abcd}Values with different superscript letters within the same row are significantly (P<0.05) different.

Table 7B: Antagonistic activities (AU/mL) of bacteria isolated from 'Curd' against enteric bacterial pathogens.

Isolates	Indicator bacteria			
	S. flexneri	*Y. enterocolitica*	*E. aerogenes*	*P. vulgaris*
LXD1	NA	550.45±23.3^{b}	610.23±25.2^{a}	NA
LXD2	NA	NA	NA	NA
LXD3	NA	480.35±24.2	NA	NA
LXD4	NA	NA	NA	NA
LXD5	NA	620.23±22.3^{a}	530.34±23.5^{b}	NA
LXD6	NA	NA	NA	NA
LXD7	NA	NA	480.32±21.3	NA
LXD8	NA	NA	NA	NA
Streptomycin	1200.33±24.4^{c}	1800.31±22.3^{a}	1300.13±23.4^{b}	1200.22±25.3^{c}

NA - No activity; Values are represented as mean±SD of experiments carried out in triplicate (n = 3).
^{abc}Values with different superscript letters within the same row are significantly (P<0.05) different.

Table 8: Morphological and biochemical properties of six selected isolates.

Tests	Isolates					
	MANF1	**MANF2**	**MANF3**	**MANF4**	**MANF5**	**MANF6**
Colony colour	Cream white	Cream white	Cream white	Cream white	Cream white	Cream white
Colony shape	Small, smooth, and round	Small, smooth, and round	Small, smooth, and round	Small, smooth, and round	Small, smooth, and round	Small, smooth, and round
Gram staining	Gram (+)	Gram (+)	Gram (+)	Gram (+)	Gram (+)	Gram (+)
Endospore test	-	-	-	-	-	-
Indole	-	-	-	-	-	-
Voges-proskauer	-	-	-	-	-	-
Citrate utilization	-	-	-	-	-	-
ONPG	+	+	+	+	+	+
Nitrate reductase	+	+	+	+	+	+
Arginine	-	-	-	-	-	-
Malonate	-	-	-	-	-	-
Catalase	+	+	+	+	+	+
Methyl red	-	-	-	-	-	-
Carbohydrate fermentation						
Glucose	+	+	+	+	+	+
Sucrose	+	+	+	+	+	+
Arabinose	+	+	+	+	+	+
Mannitol	+	+	+	+	+	+
Trehalose	+	+	+	+	+	+
Lactose	+	+	+	+	+	+
Dextrose	+	+	+	+	+	+

Note: '+' = Positive; '-' = Negative

Clean rice was washed with water

↓

Cooked by excess water method

↓

Excess water was drained after cooking

↓

Cooled to room temperature

↓

Cooked rice was soaked with water overnight

↓

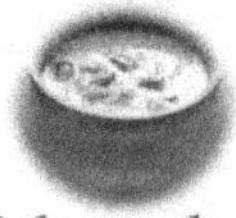

Palayasatham

a

Curd, cumin seeds, and salt were mixed in a bowl

↓

Chilled water was added and mixed well

↓

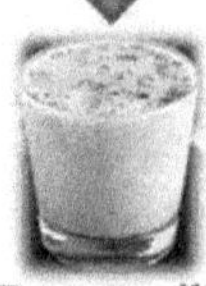

Buttermilk

b

Continued………………

Milk was boiled and allowed to warm

↓

Stalks of chillies were added into half cup of warm milk

↓

Kept aside overnight for the preparation of starter

↓

One tablespoon starter was added into rest of the warm milk

↓

Kept aside overnight undisturbed

↓

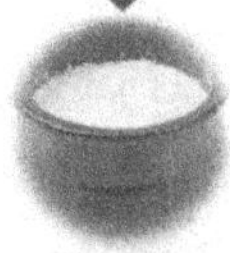

Curd

c

Idli rice and *Urad dal* were soaked in water separately overnight

↓

Soaked *Idli* rice and *Urad dal* were ground into paste

↓

The paste was fermented overnight

↓

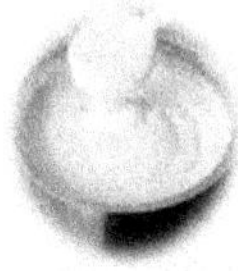

***Idli* and *Dosa* Batter**

d

Continued……………

Finger millet (*Eleusine coracana*) was washed in running water

↓

Millets were ground into flour and stored in sterile polythene bag

↓

Flour (25 g) was mixed with de-ionized water in the ratio of 2:1

↓

The mixture was incubated at room temperature for 12-15 h
(Primary fermentation)

↓

Cooked in earthen pot and incubated at room temperature for further 12-15 h
(Secondary fermentation)

↓

Fortified with broken rice

↓

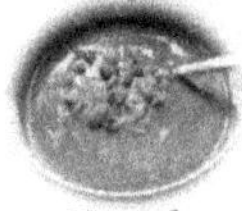

Koozh

e

Rice was washed and soaked in water for 6 h

↓

Water was drained, mixed with coconut, and blended

↓

The paste was kept in air tight container and allowed to ferment overnight

↓

Sugar, salt, baking soda, and water were added

↓

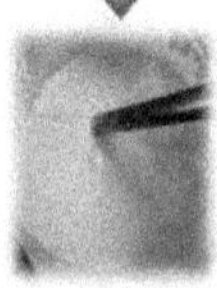

Appam Batter

f

Continued……………

Rice, fenugreek seeds, and urad dal were washed

↓

Mixture was soaked in water for 6-8 h

↓

Mixture was ground to a smooth paste

↓

Salt was added to the paste and fermented overnight

↓

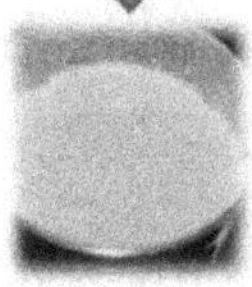

Paniyaram Batter

g

Figure 1: Traditional method of preparation of (a) '*Palayasatham*', (b) 'Buttermilk', (c) 'Curd', (d) '*Idli* and *Dosa* Batter', (e) '*Koozh*', (f) '*Appam* Batter', and (g) '*Paniyaram* Batter'.

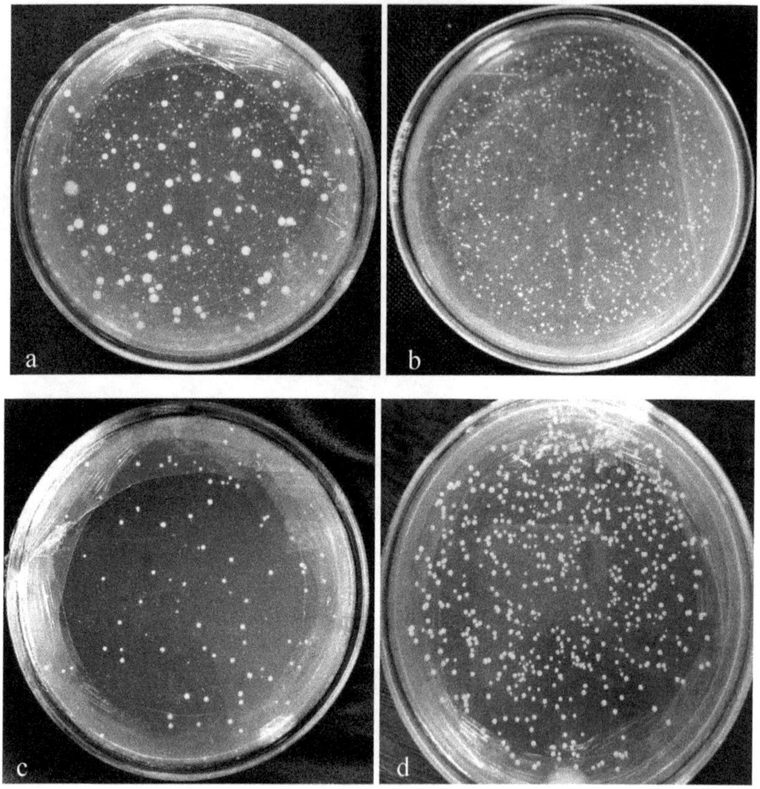

Continued………………

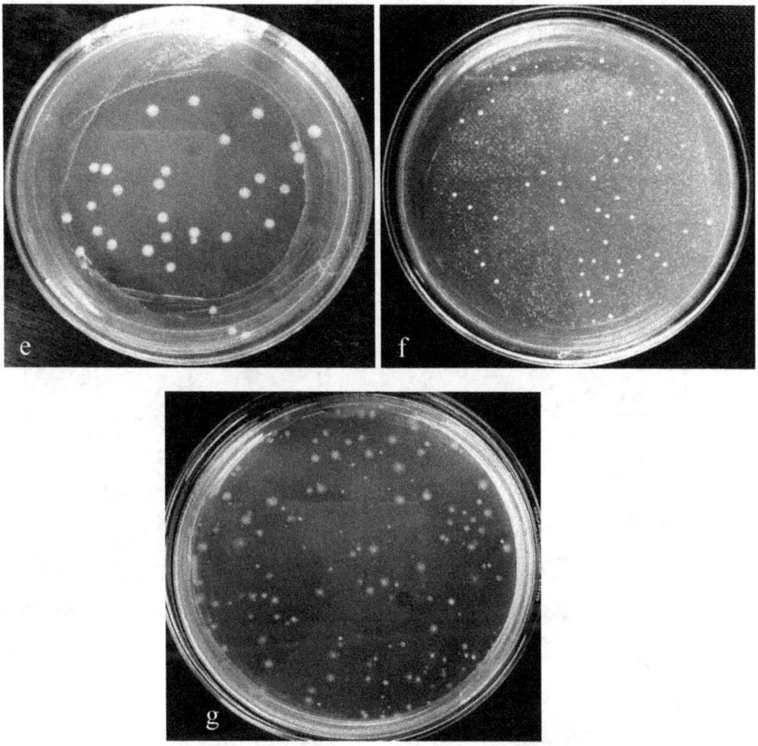

Figure 2: Distinct colonies of bacteria isolated from (a) '*Palayasatham*', (b) 'Buttermilk', (c) '*Koozh*', (d) '*Idli* and *Dosa* Batter', (e) '*Appam* Batter', (f) '*Paniyaram* Batter', and (g) 'Curd' on MRS agar medium.

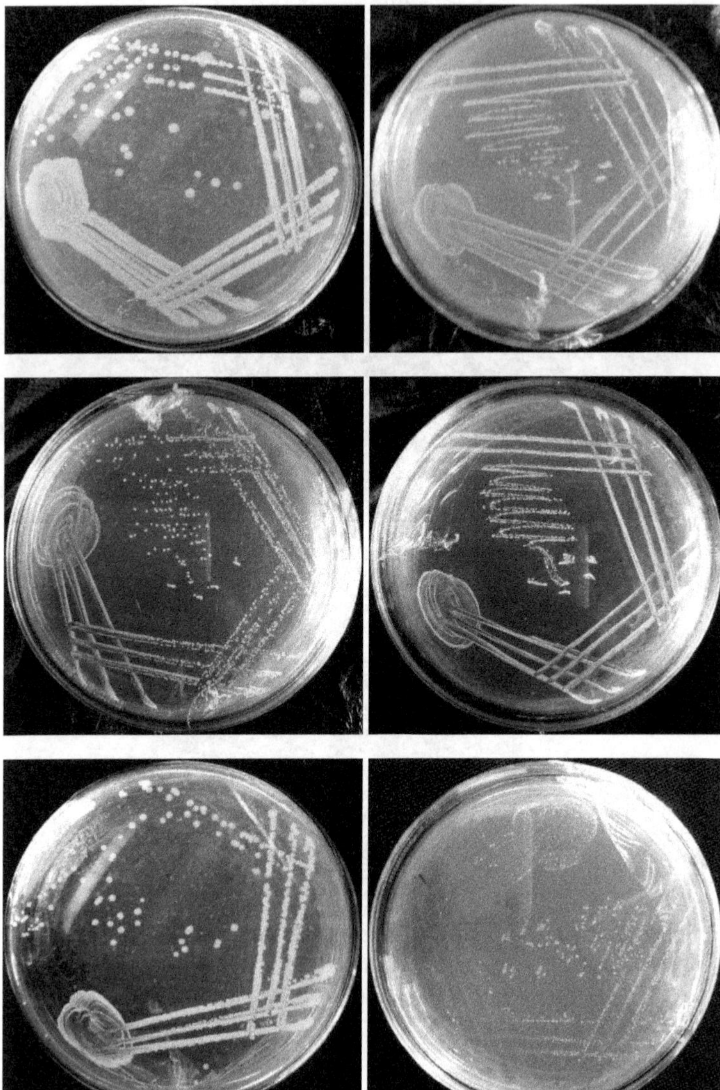

Continued………

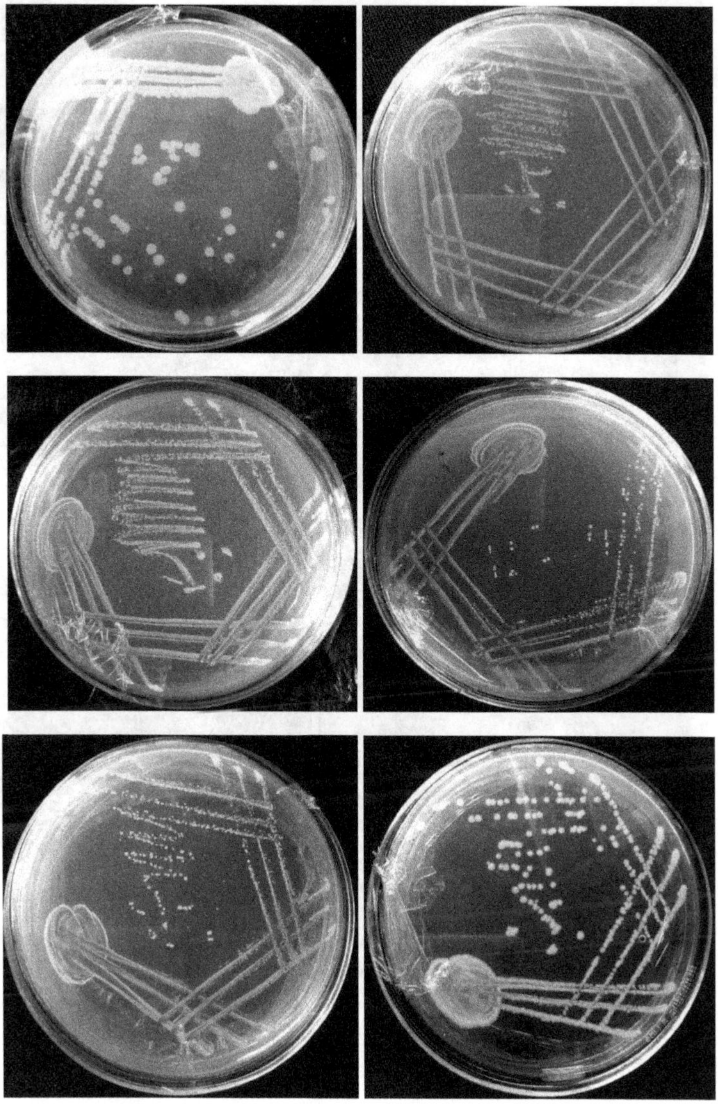

Figure 3: Pure cultures of bacteria streaked on MRS agar medium.

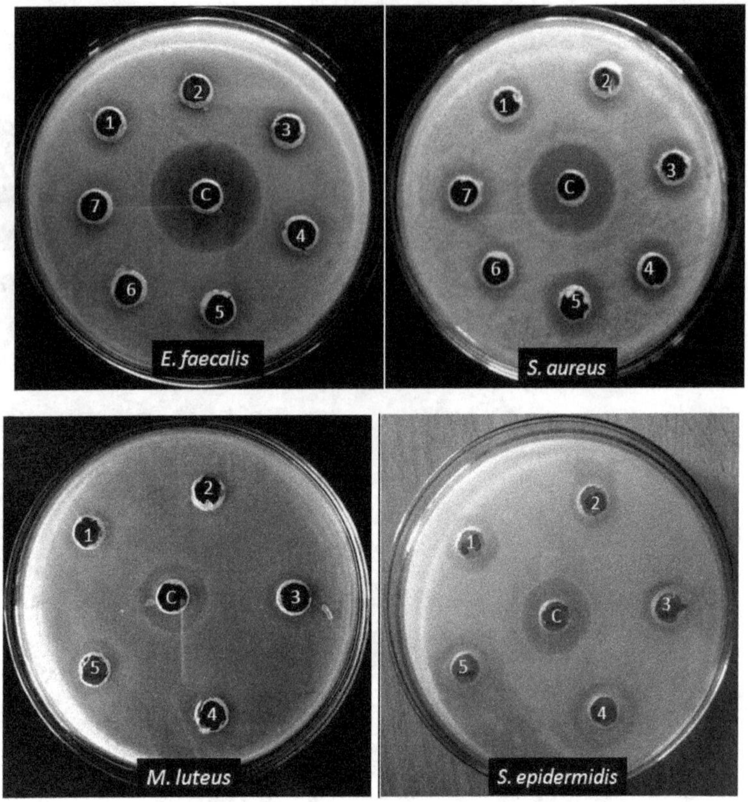

Figure 4: Antagonistic activities of few bacterial isolates against foodborne pathogens using agar well diffusion assay.

[Note: 1, 2, 3, 4, 5, 6, and 7 - Isolates; C - Positive control]

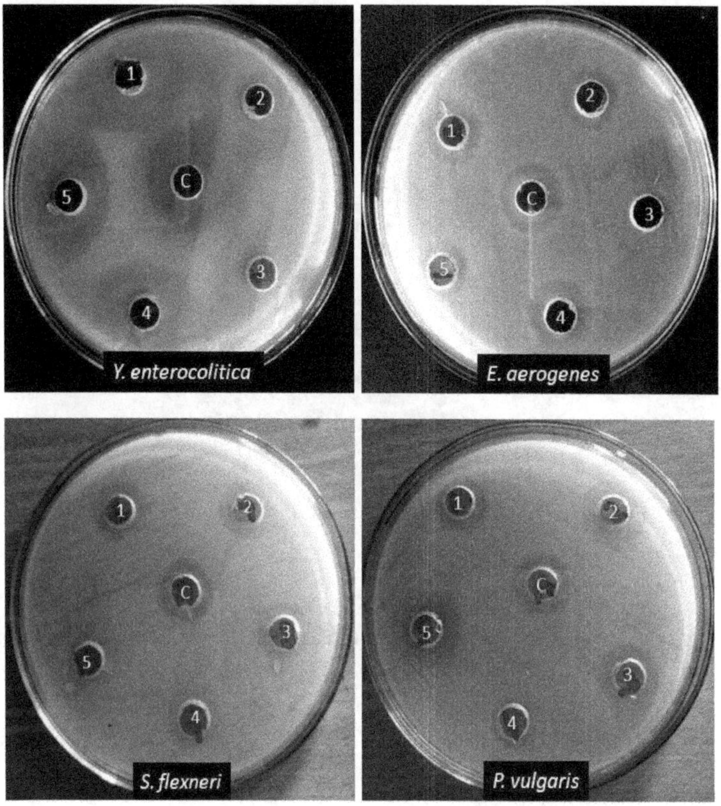

Figure 5: Antagonistic activities of few isolates against enteric pathogens using agar well diffusion assay.

[Note: 1, 2, 3, 4, and 5 - Isolates; C - Positive control]

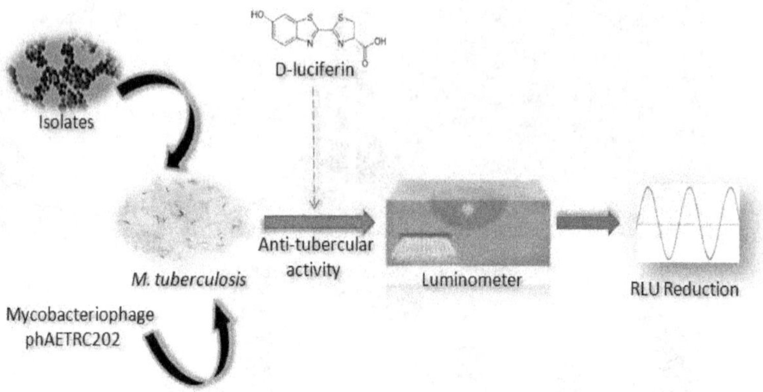

Figure 6: Determination of anti-tubercular activities of CFNS of isolates against *M. tuberculosis* H37Rv using LRP assay.

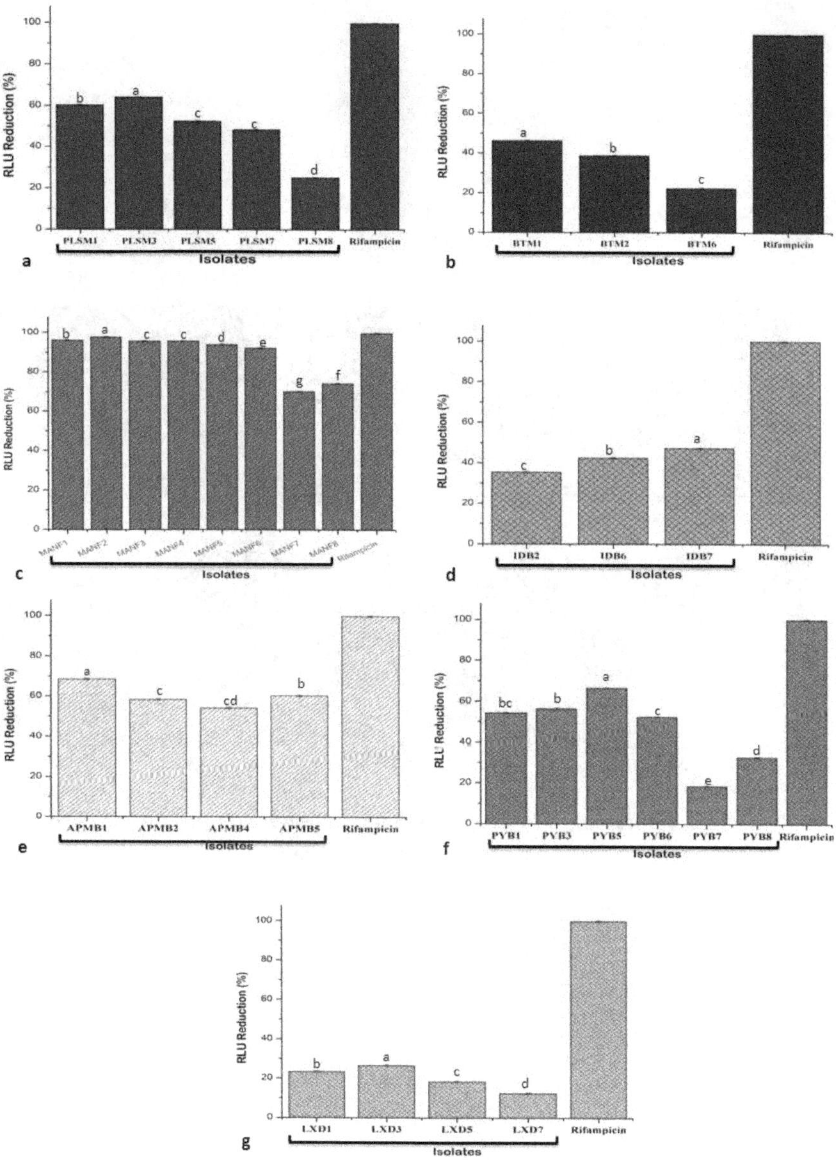

Figure 7: Anti-tubercular activities of potent bacterial cultures isolated from (a) '*Palayasatham*', (b) 'Buttermilk', (c) '*Koozh*', (d) '*Idli* and *Dosa* Batter', (e) '*Appam* Batter', (f) '*Paniyaram* Batter', and (g) 'Curd'.

[Note: Values are represented as mean±SD of experiments carried out in triplicate (n = 3). [abcdefg]Values with different letters are significantly (P<0.05) different.]

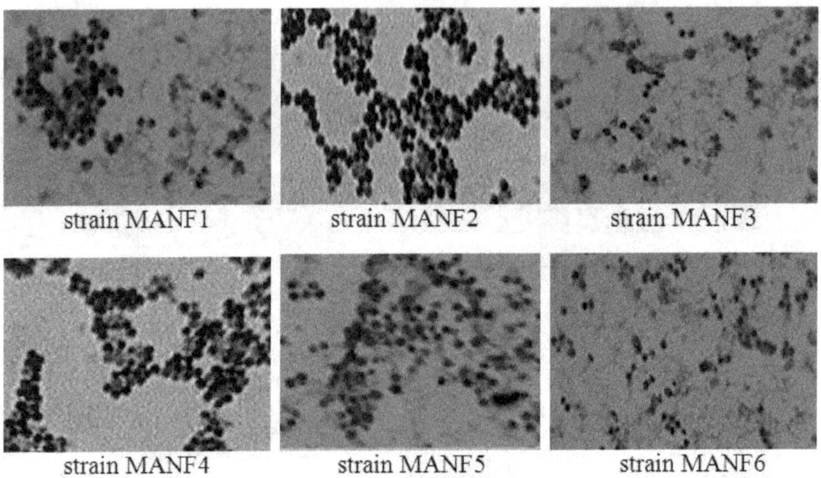

Figure 8: Gram staining of 6 selected isolates. Cells were stained purple in colour and arranged in clusters, indicating gram positive in nature.

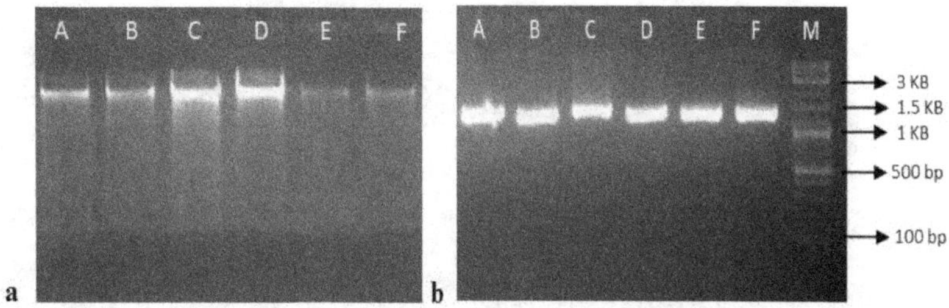

Figure 9: (a) Genomic DNA isolation and (b) PCR amplification of 6 selected isolates.

[Note: A, B, C, D, E, F - Isolate MANF1, MANF2, MANF3, MANF4, MANF5, and MANF6; M - Marker]

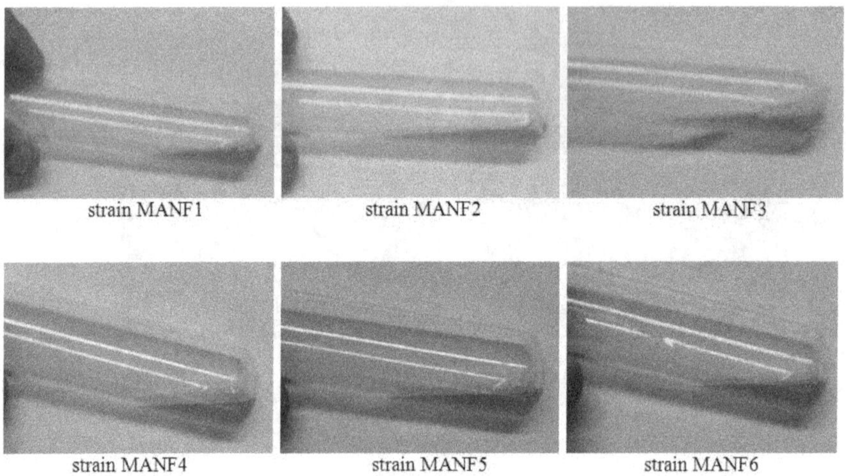

Figure 10: Coagulase test for staphylococci strains. All the strains showed lack of free coagulase production, thus, categorizing the strains under coagulase-negative *Staphylococcus* spp.

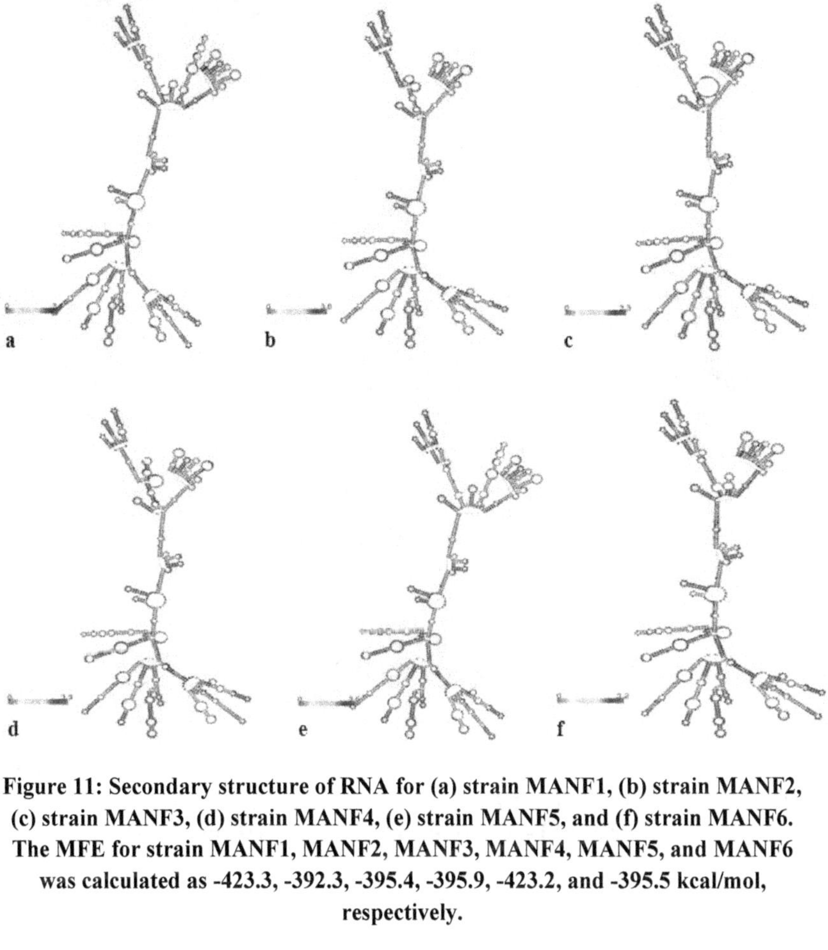

Figure 11: Secondary structure of RNA for (a) strain MANF1, (b) strain MANF2, (c) strain MANF3, (d) strain MANF4, (e) strain MANF5, and (f) strain MANF6. The MFE for strain MANF1, MANF2, MANF3, MANF4, MANF5, and MANF6 was calculated as -423.3, -392.3, -395.4, -395.9, -423.2, and -395.5 kcal/mol, respectively.

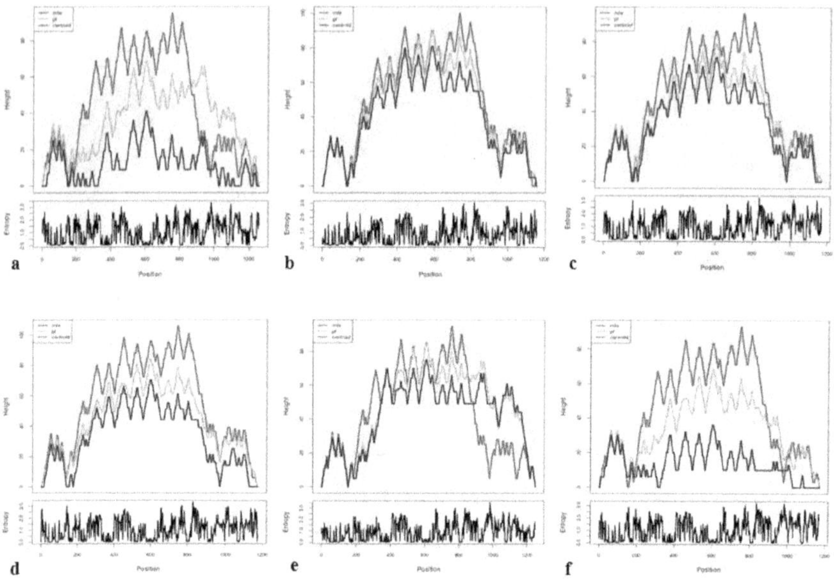

Figure 12: Mountain plot and entropy showing hierarchical representation of RNA secondary structure for (a) strain MANF1, (b) strain MANF2, (c) strain MANF3, (d) strain MANF4, (e) strain MANF5, and (f) strain MANF6.

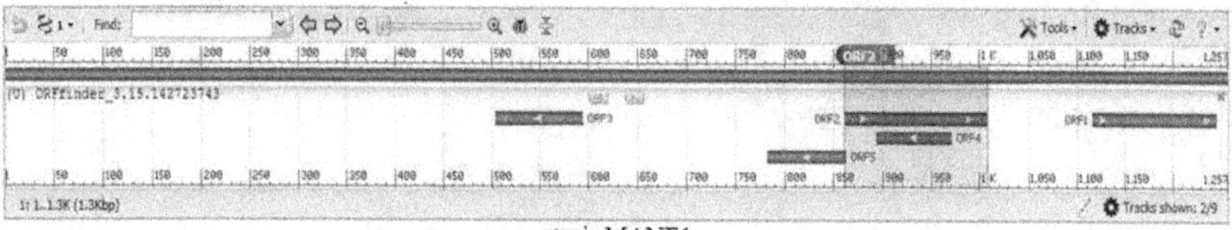

strain MANF1

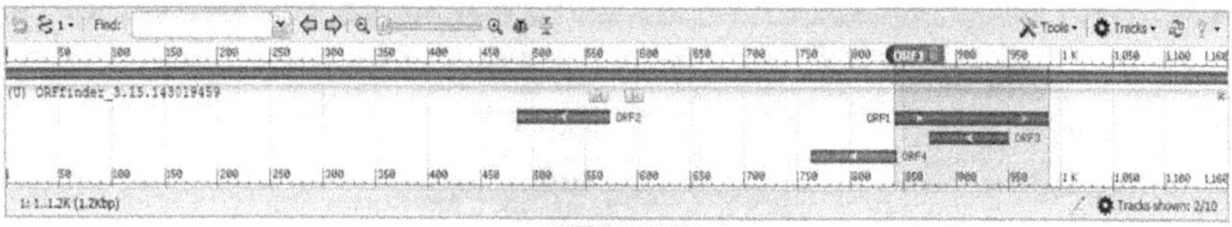

strain MANF2

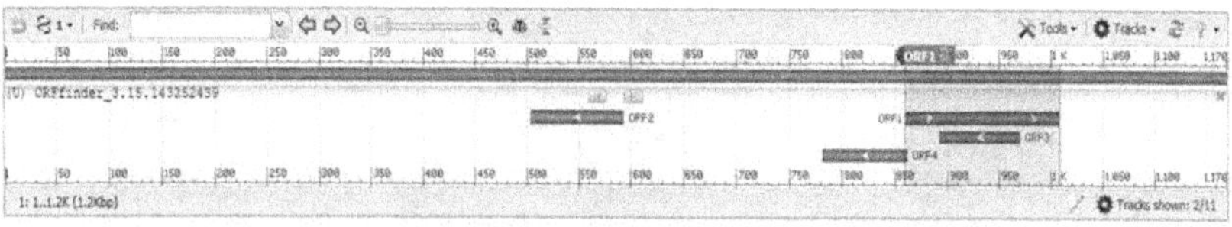

strain MANF3

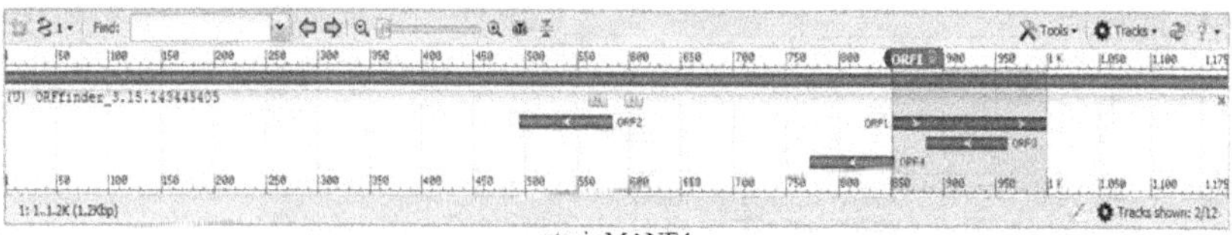

strain MANF4

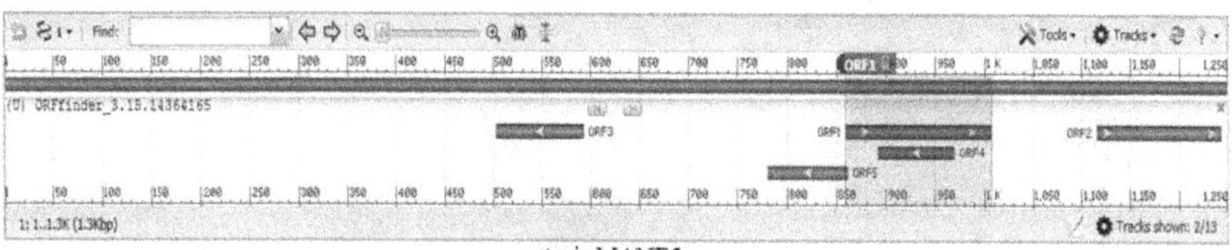

strain MANF5

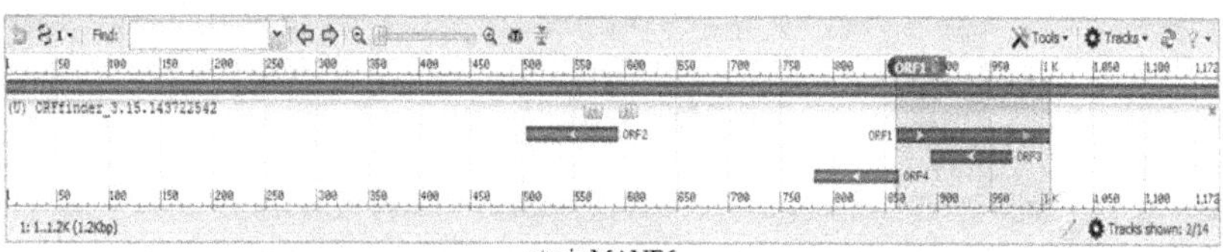

strain MANF6

Figure 13: Distinct ORF regions for CNS strains.

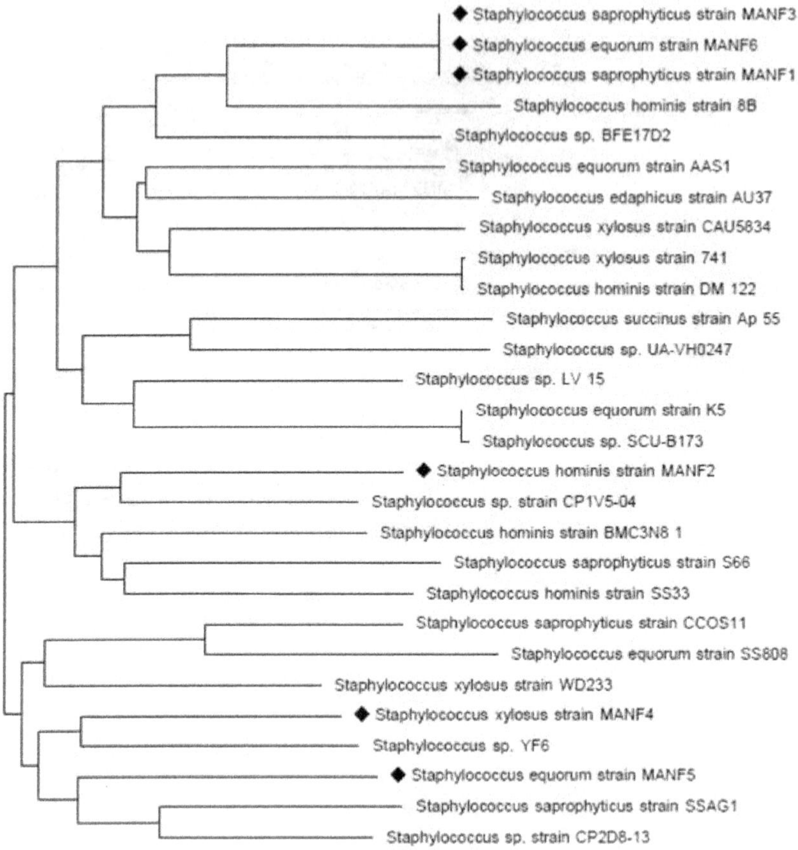

Figure 14: Phylogenetic tree construction for CNS strains with respect to other staphylococci strains.

4. Discussion

The processing of foods through diversified traditional techniques and their pivotal biotechnological attributes has been recognized for many years in India. Traditional fermented foods of India are categorized as 'functional food' due to the presence of a number of functional constituents, especially probiotics and other bioactive components. These functional components of foods are known to deliver disparate biological functions in the human body (Sarkar *et al.*, 2015).

Southern states of India, particularly Tamil Nadu is known for the traditional processing and utilization of fermented foods. As a matter of fact, traditional fermented food items of Tamil Nadu play paramount role in the diet of people due to the vast nutritional significance and functional values, and provide healthy life style. Despite the colossal health beneficial aspects, the information regarding the medicinal traits of microbiota indigenous to those fermented foods is scarce. In view of this, the present research was investigated to assess the anti-pathogenic attributes of bacteria isolated from disparate traditional fermented foods of Tamil Nadu, India.

In the current scenario, severe concerns have been précised regarding the increasing incidences of diseases associated with foodborne pathogens (Gad *et al.*, 2016). In this study, among diversiform groups of bacteria isolated from fermented foods, '*Koozh*' associated CNS strains portrayed noticeable antagonistic activities against a panel of foodborne pathogens. Previous reports had confirmed the inhibitory effects of distinct probiotic bacteria on the viability of foodborne pathogenic bacteria (Yah *et al.*, 2014; Bajpai *et al.*, 2016; Manzoor *et al.*, 2016). Recently, bacteria isolated from Kimchi (Korean fermented food) exhibited growth inhibitory effects against foodborne pathogens (Bajpai *et al.*, 2016). The broad spectrum antagonistic activities of CNS strains against these pathogens might be due to the fact that the presence of discrete metabolites as well as bioactive peptides interacts to antagonize the indicator bacterial growth.

Enteric pathogenic bacteria infect the host in distinctive atmospheric conditions of GI tract, thereby causing diarrhoeal disease. In the present context, CNS strains showed remarkable antagonistic properties against bacteria causing enteric infections. Previous studies evidenced the promising role of bacteria against a range of enteric pathogens (Kanmani *et al.*, 2013; Adeniyi *et al.*, 2015; Gad *et al.*, 2016). Mechanisms by which these bacteria may protect the host from intestinal infections include the production of inhibitory substances, blocking of adhesion sites on the intestinal surface, competition for nutrients, and stimulation of mucosal and systemic immunity (Servin, 2004; Gibson *et al.*, 2005).

The current scenario of anti-tubercular therapies has drawn attention to achieve competent and durable treatment of the emerging problems of TB. Previously, anti-tubercular bacteriocins viz. nisin and lacticin had shown significant growth inhibitory activities against *M. tuberculosis* (Chung *et al.*, 2000; Carroll *et al.*, 2010). In the present study, 6 CNS strains showed promising anti-tubercular activities against *M. tuberculosis* H37Rv, thereby suggesting the potency of '*Koozh*' associated staphylococci in the prevention of extra-intestinal infection, particularly TB. More or less similar observations were also reported by Gavrilova *et al.* (2014) who demonstrated the ability of fermented foods associated bacteria in the suppression of *M. tuberculosis* growth. The growth inhibition of *M. tuberculosis* in the present study might be due to the production of antimicrobial components, particularly bacteriocins by CNS. Findings of the present context clearly testify the prospects of CNS as propitious anti-tubercular agents which may lead to overcome the failure of existing mycobactericidal agents.

Over the past few decades, the use of new molecular tools of systematic bacteriology has greatly affected the bacterial taxonomy. The detection and classification of bacteria through molecular techniques rely particularly on the sequence analysis of 16S rRNA gene. Targeting 16S rRNA gene for sequence analyses is an appropriate genetic marker because 16S rRNA gene is not only universal among bacteria but also conserved and exhibit variations for distinguishing between taxa (Ntushelo *et al.*, 2012). Analyses of 16S rRNA gene sequence using distinct bioinformatics tools allow researchers to determine comparative studies in order to classify specific bacteria. In this chapter, 16S rRNA sequences of CNS strains were used for deducing RNA secondary structure, thermodynamics parameters, GC content, and dendrogram construction using RNAfold web server.

The minimization of free energy reduces the total Gibbs free energy and provides stability to the sequences, and thus, used for predicting RNA secondary structure. Dynamic programs are used through thermodynamic approaches for computing the optimal secondary structure with MFE for RNA sequences (Zuker and Stiegler, 1981). In this study, the energy structure for 6 CNS strains was found to be different. The variations such as shape of the secondary structure, energy value, and plots among CNS strains were determined by the colour of nucleotides. The MFE determines the suitable structure with high stable energy. In general, Gibbs free energy of RNA secondary structure suggests evolutionary stability of the sequences (Sankari and Khusro, 2014). Mountain plot and entropy for each bacterial sequence was drawn for depicting the hierarchical representation of RNA secondary structure. In each plot, helices represent mountains while terminal loops give rise to peaks, as clearly demonstrated previously by Chandra and Shilpa (2018). Further, the GC content of sequences is known to affect the secondary structure of mRNA (Sankari and Khusro, 2014). In this study, the GC content for each bacterial sequences was calculated as >50%, thereby representing the stability of secondary structure. The evolutionary relationships of strains based on 16S rRNA gene sequences have been implemented to categorize isolates into varied species (Chandra and Shilpa, 2018). In this investigation, the phylogenetic tree of 6 CNS strains showed close resemblance with the existing distinct staphylococcal strains.

5. Conclusions

In summary, a total of 56 bacteria were isolated from traditionally prepared distinct fermented foods of Tamil Nadu, India. Among them, 53.57 and 51.78% of isolates revealed antagonistic activities against foodborne and enteric pathogens, respectively. In addition, 58.92% of isolates depicted promising anti-tubercular activities against *M. tuberculosis* H37Rv based on LRP assay. '*Koozh*' associated 6 bacterial strains showed promising anti-tubercular activities with high RLU reductions (92.4±0.3-97.7±0.4%), which were further identified as coagulase-negative *Staphylococcus* spp. as per morphological, biochemical, molecular characterization, and sequence analyses tools.

Chapter 2

Probiotic and technological properties of coagulase-negative *Staphylococcus* spp.

1. Introduction

At present, the consumption of autochthonous probiotics as health beneficial microbiota from fermented foods has contrived prodigious interest globally because of their non-pathogenic, functional, and technological traits. As a matter of fact, probiotics exhibit disparate physiological properties viz. retaining intestinal microbiota balance, inhibition of pathogens, boosting immunity, removal of carcinogen from intestinal tract, intolerance of lactose, and preferment of nutrients availability to host (Parvez *et al.*, 2006).

For being a potent probiotic strain, the isolate should have diversified potentialities such as survival in the acidic environment of GI tract, susceptibility towards conventional antibiotics, antagonism against pathogens, and adhesion to epithelial lining (Pisano *et al.*, 2014). Furthermore, auto-aggregation is a pivotal characteristic of probiotic bacteria which influences the adhesive trait of bacteria towards the intestinal epithelial cells. Likewise, the adhesion of bacteria is dependent on the non-specific physico-chemical bonding of surfaces. In general, the surface hydrophobicity demonstrates the physico-chemical traits of the cell surface of probiotics (Kotzamanidis *et al.*, 2010).

Aside from finding efficient strain with dormant probiotic traits, it is also imperative to consider its distinct technological properties for utilizing as starter cultures. The taste and aroma of fermented foods are attributed to varied biological factors, particularly its microbiota quality. Since, the selection of autochthonous microbiota for starter formulation is an auspicious tool to preserve the exemplary properties of fermented food products; hence, pervasive knowledge on the technological characteristics of certain strain present in the particular fermented food item would be a matter of comprehensive interest (Mauriello *et al.*, 2004).

In recent times, fermented foods associated CNS have emerged as the prevalent heterogeneous group of bacteria revealing probiotic traits (Borah *et al.*, 2016). The CNS are also known to play a major role in the development of sensory properties and colour development of fermented foods by reducing nitrates to nitrite and then to nitrous oxide, preventing rancidity through peroxide decomposition, and producing flavour and aroma compounds through proteolytic as well as lipolytic activities (Sondergaard and Stahnke, 2002). Over the past few years, CNS have been successfully isolated from various fermented food items and studied for their colossal applications. But the measurement of varied functional attributes of '*Koozh*' associated CNS is largely unknown. Hence, the present chapter was investigated to outline the detail probiotic and technological characteristics of CNS isolated from '*Koozh*' in order to appraise their ample applications in pharmaceutical and food industries.

2. Materials and methods

2.1. Bacteria used

Since, the previous chapter demonstrated the pronounced potentialities of '*Koozh*' associated 6 CNS strains as anti-tubercular agents; hence, strain MANF1, strain MANF2, strain MANF3, strain MANF4, strain MANF5, and strain MANF6 were selected further for assessing their probiotic and technological characteristics.

2.2. Probiotic properties of CNS strains-

2.2.1. Low pH tolerance

The acid tolerance properties of strains were evaluated according to the methodology of Ramos *et al.* (2013) with minor modifications. The exponentially phase grown cultures in MRS broth were centrifuged at 6000 *g* at 4°C for 10 min. On the other hand, the pH of the freshly prepared MRS broth media was adjusted from 2.0 to 5.0 using digital pH meter (SIGMA). MRS broth of pH 6.5 was used as control. Bacterial cells were resuspended in MRS broth of diversified pH ranges and incubated at 30°C up to 3 h. Bacterial suspensions were withdrawn and serially diluted in phosphate buffered saline (PBS) after 0, 1, 2, and 3 h. Samples were plated on sterilized MRS agar plates and incubated at 30°C for 48 h. Total cell viablity was estimated by plate count method in terms of log colony forming unit/mL (cfu/mL), and survival of cells was calculated as follows:

$$\text{Cell survival (\%)} = (\log \text{cfu } 3^{rd} \text{ h}/ \log \text{cfu } 0^{th} \text{ h}) \times 100 \qquad \text{[Equation 1]}$$

2.2.2. Resistance to simulated gastric juice

The resistance of strains to simulated gastric juice was assessed according to the methodology of Charteris *et al.* (1998) with slight modification. Simulated gastric juice was prepared using pepsin (3 mg/mL) and sodium chloride (0.5% w/v), and pHs of the solution were adjusted to 2.0. The overnight grown cultures were centrifuged at 8000 *g* for 10 min. Bacterial cells were washed twice with 10 mL of 50mM dipotassium phosphate (K_2HPO_4) solution, and cells were resuspended in 3 mL of dipotassium phosphate solution of the same molarity. Simulated gastric juice (9 mL) was mixed with bacterial cell suspension and incubated at 30°C for 3 h. Bacterial cell suspensions were plated on the sterilized MRS agar plates at constant intervals (0, 1, 2, and 3 h), and the total viable cells were expressed as log cfu/mL after 48 h. Cell survival percentage was calculated according to the equation 1.

2.2.3. Bile salt resistance

The survival of strains in the presence of bile salt was determined following the modified methodology of Kumar *et al.* (2011). Overnight grown bacterial cultures were inoculated into MRS broth supplemented with oxgall (0.5% w/v) and incubated at 30°C. After a time interval of 24 h, aliquots of this suspension were withdrawn, serially diluted using saline, and plated on MRS agar plates. Viable cell colonies were enumerated after 24 h in a comparison with control culture (without oxgall) as per equation 1.

2.2.4. Bile salt hydrolase (BSH) activity

The BSH activities of strains were determined according to the method of Du Toit *et al.* (2003). Strains were grown on MRS agar media supplemented with 0.5% (w/v) sodium salt of taurocholic acid ($C_{26}H_{45}NO_7S$) and 0.3% (w/v) calcium chloride. Plates were incubated at 30°C and the presence of precipitation zone around the bacterial cultures was observed after 48 h in order to determine BSH activity.

2.2.5. Cell surface hydrophobicity

The adherence property of strains to hydrocarbons was analyzed by employing the methodology of Mishra and Prasad (2005) with minor modifications. Strains were grown in MRS broth for 16-18 h, and centrifuged at 8000 *g* for 15 min. Pellets were collected and washed twice with PBS (pH 7.0). Pellets were re-suspended in the same buffer, vortexed, and absorbance of the cell suspension was read at 600 nm (A). Three millilitres of cell suspension were mixed with 1 mL of various hydrocarbons viz. chloroform ($CHCl_3$), toluene (C_7H_8), and ethyl acetate ($C_4H_8O_2$). The mixture was vortexed for 1 min, and incubated at 30°C for 1 h in order to separate the aqueous and organic phase. The aqueous phase was carefully separated and decrease in absorbance was read at 600 nm (A_0). The cell surface hydrophobicity was calculated as follows:

$$\text{Hydrophobicity (\%)} = [(A-A_0)/A] \times 100 \qquad \text{[Equation 2]}$$

2.2.6. Auto-aggregation

Cell auto-aggregation properties of strains were determined according to the methodology of Juarez Tomas *et al.* (2005) with slight modifications. Bacteria were allowed to grow in MRS broth for 16-18 h and pellets were collected after centrifugation at 8000 *g* for 15 min. Cells were washed twice in PBS (pH 7.0) and adjusted to an absorbance of 0.5-0.6 at 600 nm (A). The cell suspension was further incubated at 30°C for 24 h. The upper phase (1 mL) was carefully separated in order to measure the absorbance at 600 nm (A_0). Decrease in absorbance indicates the cell auto-aggregation property and auto-aggregation rate was calculated according to the following formula:

$$\text{Auto-aggregation (\%)} = [(A-A_0)/A] \times 100 \qquad \text{[Equation 3]}$$

2.2.7. Tolerance to phenol

The potentialities of strains to resist phenol (C_6H_6O) solution were determined according to the methodology of Xanthopoulos *et al.* (2000) with slight modification. The overnight grown bacterial cultures were incubated in MRS broth supplemented with 0.5% phenol, and incubated at 30°C for 24 h. After 0 and 24 h of incubation, bacterial suspension was spread on MRS agar plates and cell viability was enumerated in a comparison with control (without phenol) according to the equation 1.

2.2.8. Resistance to lysozyme

The resistivity of strains to lysozyme was assayed according to the method of Zago *et al.* (2011). Strains were allowed to grow for 16-18 h at 30°C and centrifuged at 8000 *g* for 15 min. Pellets were washed twice with PBS (pH 7.0) and re-suspended in Ringer solution containing lysozyme (100 μg/mL). Samples were incubated at 30°C for 2 h and cell viability was calculated in a comparison with control (without lysozyme) according to the equation 1.

2.2.9. Cholesterol lowering property

The *in vitro* cholesterol ($C_{27}H_{46}O$) lowering characteristics of strains were determined according to the method of Sieladie *et al.* (2011). The log phase grown bacterial cultures were inoculated into MRS broth containing 0.4% (w/v) bile salt and 0.01% (v/v) cholesterol. Cultures were incubated at 30°C for 24 h. After required period of incubation, the culture broth was centrifuged at 6000 *g* for 10 min and the supernatant was collected for reading absorbance at 650 nm using spectrophotometer. The decrease in cholesterol level of treatments (A_0) was compared with the control [A;

MRS broth supplemented with 0.4% (w/v) bile salt and 0.01% (v/v) cholesterol] as follows:

$$\text{Cholesterol assimilation (\%)} = [(A-A_0)/A] \times 100 \qquad \text{[Equation 4]}$$

2.2.10. β-galactosidase activity

β-galactosidase activities of strains were assayed according to the method of Hsu *et al.* (2005) with slight modifications. Bacteria were allowed to grow for 24 h and then centrifuged at 8000 *g* for 15 min at 4°C. The pellet was used as enzyme source. The reaction mixture consisted of 1 mL of intracellular enzyme source and 1 mL of 15mM ONPG, prepared in 0.1M sodium phosphate buffer (pH 7.0). The solution was incubated at 30°C for 10 min and the reaction mixture was stopped after adding 2 mL of 0.1M sodium carbonate (Na_2CO_3) solution. Absorbance was read at 420 nm using spectrophotometer. One unit of β-galactosidase activity was defined as the amount of enzyme required for catalyzing the formation of 1 micromole per minute (μmol/min) of o-nitrophenol under the standard assay conditions.

2.2.11. Proteolytic properties of strains

The exponentially phase grown strains were centrifuged at 8000 *g* for 15 min at 4°C and the supernatant was collected. Agar plates consisting of skim milk (1% w/v) were prepared and allowed to cool aseptically. Agar media were punched with sterilized cork borer and bacterial supernatant was poured into it for the diffusion process. Plates were incubated at 30°C for 24 h and assessed for proteolytic activity by observing clear zone of substrate degradation surrounding the wells.

2.2.12. Antibiotics susceptibility assay

The susceptibility profile of strains to conventional antibiotics was determined by disc diffusion method (Bauer *et al.*, 1966). A homogeneous lawn of the exponentially phase grown strains was prepared on MRS agar plates. The standard antibiotic discs (Himedia, India) such as streptomycin (10 μg), penicillin G (10 μg), chloramphenicol (30 μg), kanamycin (30 μg), gentamicin (10 μg), nalidixic acid (30 μg), and rifampicin (30 μg) were placed aseptically over the agar plates and incubated undisturbed at 30°C for 48 h. The diameter of the zone of bacterial growth inhibition was measured after required period of incubation. Results were expressed in terms of susceptible or resistant.

2.3. *Antioxidant activities of strains-*

2.3.1. *2,2-diphenyl-1-picrylhydrazyl (DPPH) scavenging activity*

The DPPH free radical scavenging activities of strains were assayed according to the methodology of Chen *et al.* (2005) with minor modification. One millilitre of DPPH solution (0.05 mM) was added into different concentrations (10-50 μL) of freshly prepared cells (absorbance of 0.5-0.6). The reaction mixture was kept in dark for 30 min at room temperature. The DPPH solution was used as control, while cells along with methanol (CH_3OH) were used as blank during the assay. The DPPH scavenging capacities of strains as well as ascorbic acid (standard) were read at 517 nm and the scavenging potential was estimated as follows:

$$\text{DPPH scavenging capacity (\%)} = [(A_{sample} - A_{blank}) / A_{control}] \times 100 \qquad \text{[Equation 5]}$$

2.3.2. *Resistance to hydrogen peroxide*

The tolerance characteristics of strains to hydrogen peroxide were assayed based on the methodology of Buchmeier *et al.* (1997) with slight modification. One millilitre of overnight grown cultures was inoculated into 100 mL of sterilized MRS broth constituting various concentrations (1.0, 1.5, and 2mM) of hydrogen peroxide, and incubated in orbital shaker at 30°C. Control flask was also maintained without the supplementation of hydrogen peroxide. Cell viability in terms of absorbance was measured at 600 nm using spectrophotometer.

2.3.3. *Hydroxyl radical scavenging assay*

The hydroxyl radical scavenging activities of strains were determined by the method of He *et al.* (2004) with slight modification. Various concentrations (10-50 μL) of overnight grown bacterial cells were inoculated into a reaction mixture constituting 1.0 mL of Brilliant Green (0.5mM), 2.0 mL of ferrous sulphate ($FeSO_4$: 0.5mM), and 1.5 mL of hydrogen peroxide. The reaction mixture was incubated at room temperature for 15 min and absorbance was measured at 624 nm. Ascorbic acid was used as standard. The hydroxyl radical scavenging activity was calculated as follows:

$$\text{Hydroxyl radical scavenging activity (\%)} = [(A_1 - A_0) / (A - A_0)] \times 100 \qquad \text{[Equation 6]}$$

where A_1 is the absorbance of sample, A_0 is the absorbance of the control, and A is the absorbance without the sample and the Fenton reaction system.

2.4. *Technological traits of strains-*

2.4.1. *Fermentation capabilities*

The carbohydrate fermentation potentialities of strains were determined according to the modified methodology of Delgado *et al.* (2015). The exponentially phase grown strains were inoculated into MRS media (without dextrose) constituting 2% (w/v) of diversified carbohydrates viz. glucose ($C_6H_{12}O_6$), lactose ($C_{12}H_{22}O_{11}$), dextrose ($C_6H_{12}O_6$), maltose ($C_{12}H_{22}O_{11}$), fructose ($C_6H_{12}O_6$), and sucrose ($C_{12}H_{22}O_{11}$). Cultures were incubated at 30°C up to 48 h of incubation, and absorbance was read at 600 nm for the corresponding fermentation broth.

2.4.2. *Effect of temperature and sodium chloride*

To determine the growth of strains at various temperatures, strains were grown in MRS broth for 48 h at 10, 20, 30 (control), 37, and 42°C. The effect of various sodium chloride concentrations on the viabilities of strains were analyzed by inoculating the bacteria into the MRS media supplemented with 2, 5, and 10% (w/v) of sodium chloride. Cultures were incubated at 30°C for 48 h. The potentialities of strains to survive at various temperature and salt concentrations were estimated by plate count method in terms of log cfu/mL. The bacterial growth in MRS medium without the supplementation of sodium chloride was considered as control.

2.4.3. *Exopolysaccharide production*

The potentialities of strains to produce EPS were determined according to the methodology of Owusu-Kwarteng *et al.* (2015) with slight modification. The exponentially phase grown strains were streaked aseptically onto sterilized MRS agar media, and incubated at 30°C for 48 h. The inoculation loop method was applied to determine the stickiness of colonies grown. Strains were tentatively considered positive for EPS if the length of slime was above 1.5 millimitres (mm). Further, strains were grown into MRS-sucrose broth media constituting 5% (w/v) sucrose, and then incubated at 30°C for 48 h. After required period of incubation, 2 mL of culture was centrifuged at 8000 *g* for 10 min (4°C). The collected supernatant was mixed with an equal volume of 99% (w/v) ethanol, and an opaque link at the interface was observed for the confirmation of EPS production from the respective strains.

2.4.4. *Amylolytic and lipolytic activities*

The potentialities of strains to produce amylase were determined by growing them overnight into MRS media. Active cultures were centrifuged at 8000 *g* for 10 min, and supernatant (100 μL) of respective strains was poured into the wells of freshly prepared agar medium constituting 1% (w/v) soluble starch. The plates were incubated at room temperature for 48 h. After incubation, plates were covered by spraying with Lugol's iodine to detect starch hydrolysis. The presence of a clear halo zone around the wells indicates the degradation of starch, and therefore the amylolytic property of strains.

Lipolytic activity was determined by pouring the supernatant of log phase grown strains into the wells prepared on trybutyrin agar medium constituting 1% (v/v) trybutyrin. The plates were incubated at room temperature for 48 h, and the lipase activity was determined by observing the clear zone of hydrolysis around the wells.

2.4.5. Biofilm formation

Biofilm formation abilities of strains were determined as per the modified methodology of Bulgasem *et al.* (2015). Hundred microliters of overnight grown cultures were added in 96-wells microtiter plate and incubated for 24 h. After 24 h of incubation, the content of the respective wells was discarded, and the wells were washed gently twice with PBS (pH 7.0). After that, 100 μL of methanol (99% v/v) was added into each well and kept undisturbed for 15 min. Methanol was discarded and the wells were allowed to dry. After air dry, 100 μL of crystal violet stain solution was added into the wells and held for 10-15 min. The stain was discarded after required incubation period and the wells were washed gently with tap water. The wells were allowed to dry and absorbance was read at 620 nm using enzyme-linked immunosorbent assay (ELISA; Thermo Multiskan Ex, USA) reader.

2.4.6. Cell autolysis

Autolysis of cells was measured according to the methodology of Mora *et al.* (2003) with slight modification. Strains were harvested at the exponential phase, washed in potassium phosphate buffer (0.1M, pH 7.0), re-suspended in the same buffer, and incubated at 30°C. The degree of autolysis was expressed as % decrease in absorbance at 630 nm after 6, 12, and 24 h.

2.4.7. Catalase assay

Catalase activities of strains were determined according to the modified methodology of Aebi (1974). Five millilitres of each active culture were centrifuged at 6000 *g* for 10 min, and the resulting pellet was mixed with 1.5 mL of 60mM hydrogen peroxide in 1M sodium phosphate buffer (pH 7.0). The reaction mixture was incubated for 3 min at room temperature and activity was measured spectrophotometrically at 240 nm. Results were expressed in arbitrary units: µmoles of degraded H_2O_2/min/mL of cells with optical density (OD) at 600 nm equal to 1.0.

2.4.8. Nitrate reductase activity

Ten millilitres of sterilized yeast extract-tryptone (YT)-broth medium were supplemented with 250 parts per million (ppm) of potassium nitrate (KNO_3). Further, 100 µL of log phase grown strains were inoculated into the solution and incubated at 30°C for 24 h. Nitrate reductase activities of strains were estimated spectrophotometrically according to the methodology of Gerhardt *et al.* (1994). One hundred microlitres of active culture were added to 250 µL of Griess I [0.5 g of sulphanilic acid ($C_6H_7NO_3S$) in 150 mL of 5N acetic acid (CH_3COOH)], 250 µL of Griess II [0.5 g of naphthylamine ($C_{10}H_9N$) in 50 mL of distilled water and 100 mL of 5N acetic acid], and 2 mL of distilled water. The solution was then vortexed using vortex mixer (Model - WESWOX: WVM-20) and incubated at room temperature for 15 min. Nitrite production from nitrate was determined by reading absorbance at 540 nm using Ultraviolet-Visible (UV-Vis) spectrophotometer (Model - ELICO: SL 210). Relative activity was calculated as the rate: OD_{540} nm/mg dry weight.

2.5. Safety assessment tests-

In vitro haemolytic, DNase, and gelatinase activities of strains were carried out according to the methodology of Yadav *et al.* (2016) as mentioned below:

2.5.1. Haemolytic activity

Overnight grown strains were streaked on sterile agar plates (g/L - casein enzymic hydrolysate 12.0, peptone 4.0, yeast extract 4.0, sodium chloride 5.0, agar 18.0, and pH 7.2) constituting 7% (v/v) sheep blood. The plates were incubated at 37°C for 48 h, and observed for lack of zone of hydrolysis around the culture grown.

2.5.2. DNase activity

The overnight grown bacterial cultures were streaked on the freshly prepared DNase agar medium. Plates were incubated at 37°C for 48 h, and flooded with 1N HCl. The lack of clear zone was observed against the opaque plate.

2.5.3. Gelatinase activity

The overnight grown cultures were streaked on the freshly prepared nutrient gelatin agar plates. The plates were incubated at 25°C for 48 h. After the required period of incubation, the plates were flooded with ammonium sulphate [$(NH_4)_2SO_4$] solution, and observed for lack of clear zones.

2.6. *Statistical analyses*

All the experimental sections of the study were carried out in triplicate and data were represented as mean±SD. Data were analysed using one way ANOVA and values $P \leq 0.05$ were considered significant.

3. Results

3.1. *Probiotic properties-*

3.1.1. *Low pH tolerance*

Table 1 shows the survival potentialities of strains under acidic pH conditions. All the strains consistently showed resistance up to pH 2.0 after 3 h of incubation. However, strain MANF2 depicted fairly high level of tolerance to acidic pH with survival level of 92.2% after exposure to pH 2.0. The survival rates of other strains were in the order of 91.5% (MANF4) > 90.8% (MANF6) > 90.3% (MANF5) > 87.8% (MANF3) > 83.8% (MANF1) at pH 2.0 up to 3 h of incubation. Further reduction in acidic condition (>pH 2.0) caused significant ($P<0.05$) increment in the cell counts (log cfu/mL) as well as survival rate of strains.

3.1.2. *Resistance to simulated gastric juice*

The abilities of strains to tolerate simulated gastric juice are shown in Table 2. All the strains exhibited remarkable resistance to simulated gastric juice up to 3 h of incubation with survival rate of >80%. Strain MANF2 depicted the highest tolerance level with viable counts of 5.55±0.05 log cfu/mL after 3 h of incubation. The resistance property of all strains to simulated gastric juice varied significantly ($P<0.05$) after required period of incubation.

3.1.3. *Bile tolerance and BSH activities*

The potentialities of strains to resist the impact of bile salt after 24 h of incubation are shown in Table 3. All the strains demonstrated resistance to 0.5% (w/v) bile salt, but only strain MANF2 showed high tolerance to bile salt (91%) and yielded viable counts of 5.71±0.02 log cfu/mL after 24 h in a comparison with the control. The bile tolerance abilities of other strains (MANF1 > MANF4 > MANF6 > MANF5 > MANF3) varied significantly ($P<0.05$).

The deconjugation activities of strains are manifested in Table 3. Among 6 strains, strain MANF2 exhibited high BSH activity by showing comparatively larger precipitation around the culture. Other strains demonstrated lower BSH activity after 48 h of incubation.

3.1.4. Adhesion and auto-aggregation properties

The properties of strains to adhere the epithelia were examined *in vitro* by estimating the cell surface hydrophobicity towards chloroform, toluene, and ethyl acetate (Table 4). All the strains depicted varying degree of hydrophobicity towards tested hydrocarbons. Strain MANF2 was found highly hydrophobic to toluene, ethyl acetate, and chloroform with remarkable adhesion activities ($P<0.05$) of 72.0±1.1, 69.6±2.2, and 64.0±1.1%, respectively. Other strains also revealed good surface hydrophobicity towards toluene in the order of MANF5 (63.1±1.2%) > MANF4 (61.9±1.3%) > MANF1 (60.8±1.4%) > MANF6 (58.9±1.5%) > MANF3 (55.0±1.2%). A significant reduction in the degree of hydrophobicity towards ethyl acetate and chloroform was observed for other strains too.

Furthermore, strain MANF2 showed the highest auto-aggregation ability (68.1±1.5%, $P<0.05$) as compared to the other strains showing moderate level of auto-aggregation (44.4±1.2-52.3±1.1%) after 24 h of incubation (Table 4).

3.1.5. Tolerance to phenol and lysozyme

Table 5 shows the influence of phenol and lysozyme on the growth of strains in a comparison with control. All strains revealed diversified degree of sensitivity towards phenol ($P<0.05$). Strain MANF2 showed maximum resistivity towards phenol, estimating viable counts of 6.27±0.01 log cfu/mL with respect to control (6.3±0.05 log cfu/mL). The viabilities of strain MANF1, strain MANF5, and strain MANF6 were slightly inhibited after 24 h of incubation.

On the other hand, all the strains were resistant to lysozyme, where strain MANF2 revealed maximum cell viability of 81.1±1.6%, followed by strain MANF4 (75.3±1.6%), strain MANF6 (73.3±1.2%), strain MANF3 (64.2±1.3%), strain MANF1 (62.5±1.8%), and strain MANF5 (60.0±1.3%).

3.1.6. Cholesterol lowering properties

The abilities of strains to reduce the cholesterol level from the media are illustrated in Figure 1. All the strains revealed varying degree of cholesterol lowering properties ($P<0.05$). Of 6 strains, strain MANF2 depicted the maximal cholesterol lowering property (70±1.3%), followed by strain MANF4 (65.2±1.1%), strain MANF5 (57.6±1.4%), strain MANF3 (56.2±1.2%), strain MANF1 (54.09±1.2%), and strain MANF6 (40.9±1.4%).

3.1.7. *β-galactosidase activities and proteolytic properties*

All the strains were known to produce lower amount of β-galactosidase after 24 h of incubation (Figure 2). Strain MANF2 showed superiority to other tested strains by producing 25.12±0.5 U/mL of β-galactosidase. The production of β-galactosidase from strain MANF2 differed significantly ($P<0.05$) from other strains which estimated the enzyme activities of 21.34±0.4, 19.23±0.5, 17.34±0.4, 17.13±0.3, and 14.14±0.6 U/mL from strain MANF4, strain MANF5, strain MANF6, strain MANF3, and strain MANF1, respectively.

In a like manner, all the strains showed clear zone of proteolysis on skim milk agar plates, thereby suggesting the abilities of strains to produce remarkable amount of protease after 24 h of incubation (Figure 3).

3.1.8. *Antibiotic susceptibility test*

Table 6 illustrates the susceptibility patterns of all six strains to conventional antibiotics. All the strains showed varied degree of sensitivity towards the tested antibiotics except nalidixic acid. High susceptibility of strains was obtained against penicillin G, gentamicin, and rifampicin. Strains were moderately susceptible to chloramphenicol and kanamycin. However, streptomycin showed lower sensitivity towards tested strains.

3.2. *Antioxidant properties*

The DPPH scavenging characteristics of strains are illustrated in Figure 4a. All the strains exhibited significantly ($P<0.05$) different degradation values of DPPH in a dose dependent manner. Strain MANF2 showed maximum radical scavenging activities of 22.14±1.3 to 72.12±1.5%, followed by strain MANF4, strain MANF3, strain MANF5, strain MANF6, and strain MANF1 at 10 to 50 μL of concentration.

Figure 4b shows the viabilities of strains after the supplementation of varied concentrations of hydrogen peroxide in the medium. Results revealed that all the strains could resist hydrogen peroxide at 1.0-2.0mM concentrations, whereas strain MANF2 exhibited maximum tolerance towards diverse concentration of hydrogen peroxide, showing the absorbance value ranging from 2.3±0.05 to 1.72±0.02.

Results for hydroxyl radical scavenging properties of strains are reported in Figure 4c. The study showed the significant variations ($P<0.05$) in the potentialities of strains to scavenge hydroxyl radical. All the strains depicted increased hydroxyl radical scavenging activity with increase in the cell density. The dose dependent scavenging activities of strains were observed in the order of strain MANF2 (20.14±1.4-68.12±1.3%) > strain MANF4 (16.32±1.7-54.34±1.3%) > strain MANF3 (13.12±1.6-52.12±1.3%) > strain MANF1 (14.12±1.2-51.76±1.5%) > strain MANF6 (13.12±1.6-51.36±1.3%) > strain MANF5 (14.14±1.7-50.64±1.3%).

3.3. Technological attributes

Significant differences ($P<0.05$) were observed among CNS strains in terms of utilization of diversified carbohydrates (Figure 5). All strains depicted promising growth in the basal fermentation medium supplemented with lactose, while strain MANF2 showed the maximal fermentation capacity with an OD of 2.6±0.04 after 48 h of incubation period.

Table 7 shows the viabilities of strains at varied temperatures and sodium chloride concentrations. All the strains showed maximum growth at 30°C (6.1±0.01-6.21±0.04 log cfu/mL), followed by 37, 42, 20, and 10°C. On the other hand, all strains sustained maximal viability at 2% (w/v) sodium chloride. However, the growth of strains reduced markedly at 5 and 10% (w/v) sodium chloride.

Exopolysaccharide productions, amylolytic activities, lipolytic activities, and biofilm forming properties of bacteria are shown in Table 8. All the strains showed slime formation or EPS production after specific time period. However, lack of amylase activities and biofilm formation properties was observed for all the strains. On the other hand, strain MANF2, strain MANF4, and MANF6 showed weak lipolytic activities. The lipase activities for strain MANF1, strain MANF3, and strain MANF5 were not detected.

All the strains exhibited good autolytic abilities at 30°C (Table 9). After 6 h of incubation, the autolysis for all the strains was observed within the range of 35.1±1.2-43.3±1.3%. A significant ($P<0.05$) increment in the autolytic capacities of all the strains was recorded after 12 and 24 h of incubation. Strain MANF2 was particularly notable as level of autolysis ranged from 42.1±1.3 to 52.1±1.2% up to 24 h of incubation.

All the strains of *Staphylococcus* spp. studied in the present context exhibited the production of antioxidative enzyme such as catalase (Table 9). The higher values of catalase activities were estimated for strain MANF2 (16.92±1.2 AU), followed by strain MANF4 (11.31±1.4 AU), strain MANF5 (10.76±1.2 AU), strain MANF1 (10.12±1.3 AU), strain MANF6 (9.95±1.3 AU), and strain MANF3 (9.76±1.1 AU).

The reduction of nitrate to nitrite by strains was detected spectrophotometrically and results are shown in Table 9. Significant differences ($P<0.05$) were observed between the activities in terms of nitrite production for all the strains assayed. The higher quantity of nitrite released (12.23±1.2mM nitrite/mg dry weight) was measured for strain MANF2, whereas the nitrite released for other strains were estimated in the order of strain MANF4 (11.34±1.2mM nitrite/mg dry weight) > strain MANF5 (11.12±1.3mM nitrite/mg dry weight) > strain MANF3 (10.45±1.1mM nitrite/mg dry weight) > strain MANF1 (10.14±1.4mM nitrite/mg dry weight) > strain MANF6 (9.72±1.3mM nitrite/mg dry weight).

3.4. Safety aspects

All the strains were examined for their safety aspects by screening *in vitro* haemolytic, DNase, and gelatinase activities. All the isolates exhibited negative results towards haemolytic, DNase, and gelatinase tests, as confirmed by lack of zone surrounding the cultures after 48 h of incubation (Figure 6).

Table 1: Viable cell counts (log cfu/mL) of strains at various pHs.

Strains	pH 2.0					pH 3.0					pH 4.0					pH 5.0					Control (pH 6.5)				
	0 h	1 h	2 h	3 h	CS (%)	0 h	1 h	2 h	3 h	CS (%)	0 h	1 h	2 h	3 h	CS (%)	0 h	1 h	2 h	3 h	CS (%)	0 h	1 h	2 h	3 h	CS (%)
MANF1	5.25±0.01^{a}	5.21±0.02^{a}	5.11±0.02^{b}	4.4±0.04^{c}	83.8	5.32±0.02^{a}	5.3±0.02^{a}	5.25±0.01^{b}	4.9±0.03^{c}	92.1	5.43±0.02^{a}	5.41±0.0[illegible]^{a}	5.36±0.01^{b}	5.02±0.02^{c}	92.4	6.02±0.01^{a}	6.01±0.03^{b}	5.87±0.01^{c}	5.76±0.04^{d}	95.6	6.12±0.02^{a}	6.10±0.04^{a}	6.11±0.01^{a}	6.11±0.03^{a}	100
MANF2	5.65±0.02^{a}	5.6±0.02^{a}	5.46±0.02^{b}	5.25±0.01^{c}	92.2	5.92±0.03^{a}	5.87±0.06^{b}	5.77±0.03^{c}	5.57±0.01^{d}	94.08	6.0±0.01^{a}	5.96±0.01[illegible]	5.90±0.02^{b}	5.85±0.02^{c}	97.5	6.04±0.03^{a}	6.0±0.01^{b}	5.94±0.05^{c}	5.93±0.01^{c}	98.1	6.21±0.05^{a}	6.21±0.03^{a}	6.22±0.01^{a}	6.2±0.012^{a}	100
MANF3	5.12±0.03^{a}	5.1±0.03^{a}	5.06±0.04^{b}	4.5±0.02^{c}	87.8	5.15±0.04^{a}	5.13±0.01^{a}	5.11±0.01^{a}	4.78±0.05^{b}	92.8	5.28±0.03^{a}	5.17±0.01^{b}	5.14±0.01^{b}	5.01±0.03^{c}	94.8	6.0±0.01^{a}	5.92±0.01^{b}	5.91±0.01^{b}	5.77±0.04^{c}	96.1	6.2±0.01^{a}	6.18±0.01^{b}	6.18±0.01^{b}	6.2±0.01^{a}	100
MANF4	5.08±0.03^{a}	5.06±0.04^{a}	5.03±0.05^{a}	4.65±0.04^{b}	91.5	5.09±0.04^{a}	5.09±0.01^{a}	5.01±0.01^{a}	4.8±0.01^{b}	94.06	5.2±0.02^{a}	5.1±0.01^{b}	5.09±0.03^{b}	5.0±0.01^{c}	96.1	6.1±0.02^{a}	6.08±0.01^{b}	6.06±0.06^{b}	5.91±0.01^{c}	97.0	6.1±0.06^{a}	6.1±0.01^{a}	6.12±0.01^{a}	6.09±0.06^{b}	100
MANF5	4.76±0.02^{a}	4.72±0.01^{a}	4.71±0.02^{a}	4.3±0.03^{b}	90.3	4.9±0.03^{a}	4.81±0.06^{b}	4.78±0.04^{c}	4.59±0.01^{d}	93.6	5.14±0.01^{a}	5.08±0.01^{b}	5.03±0.01^{b}	4.9±0.02^{c}	95.3	6.1±0.01^{a}	6.02±0.01^{b}	6.01±0.02^{b}	5.88±0.05^{c}	96.3	6.11±0.01^{a}	6.08±0.05^{b}	6.09±0.01^{b}	6.1±0.01^{a}	100
MANF6	4.79±0.01^{a}	4.76±0.01^{a}	4.75±0.03^{a}	4.35±0.02^{b}	90.8	4.89±0.02^{a}	4.78±0.01^{b}	4.7±0.01^{b}	4.59±0.02^{c}	93.8	4.91±0.03^{a}	4.8±0.02^{b}	4.78±0.0^{c}	4.69±0.02^{d}	95.5	5.9±0.01^{a}	5.84±0.013^{b}	5.8±0.03^{b}	5.7±0.01^{c}	96.6	6.23±0.06^{a}	6.21±0.01^{a}	6.2±0.01^{a}	6.2±0.05^{a}	100

Values represent mean±SD of experiments carried out in triplicate (n = 3). CS (%) = Cell survival percentage.

[a,b,c,d]Means within the same row followed by different superscripts are significantly different (P<0.05).

Table 2: Resistant properties of strains in the presence of simulated gastric juice.

Strains	Exposure time				CS (%)
	0 h	1 h	2 h	3 h	
MANF1	6.17 ± 0.02^{a}	6.13 ± 0.04^{a}	5.78 ± 0.02^{b}	5.2 ± 0.04^{c}	84.27
MANF2	6.27 ± 0.01^{a}	6.23 ± 0.02^{a}	5.89 ± 0.01^{b}	5.55 ± 0.05^{c}	88.51
MANF3	6.2 ± 0.03^{a}	6.17 ± 0.03^{a}	5.75 ± 0.04^{b}	5.14 ± 0.02^{c}	82.91
MANF4	6.21 ± 0.02^{a}	6.18 ± 0.03^{a}	5.82 ± 0.05^{b}	5.26 ± 0.02^{c}	84.72
MANF5	6.12 ± 0.02^{a}	6.07 ± 0.01^{a}	5.76 ± 0.01^{b}	5.18 ± 0.03^{c}	84.61
MANF6	6.05 ± 0.04^{a}	6.0 ± 0.02^{a}	5.78 ± 0.03^{b}	5.12 ± 0.01^{c}	84.62

Values represent mean±SD of experiments carried out in triplicate (n = 3). CS (%) = Cell survival percentage. ^{a,b,c}Means within the same row followed by different superscripts are significantly different ($P<0.05$).

Table 3: Tolerance of strains to bile salt (0.5% w/v) and BSH activity determination.

Strains	Bile salt resistance (log cfu/mL)				BSH activity (Qualitative assay)
	Control (without bile salt)		With bile salt (0.5% w/v)		
	0 h	24 h	0 h	24 h	
MANF1	6.17±0.02^{b}	6.25±0.01^{a}	6.11±0.03^{a}	5.61±0.04^{b}	+
MANF2	6.2±0.03^{b}	6.27±0.02^{a}	6.17±0.03^{a}	5.71±0.02^{b}	++
MANF3	6.14±0.01^{b}	6.21±0.04^{a}	6.07±0.02^{a}	5.33±0.03^{b}	+
MANF4	6.18±0.02^{b}	6.25±0.02^{a}	6.02±0.01^{a}	5.54±0.02^{b}	+
MANF5	6.13±0.02^{b}	6.18±0.03^{a}	6.07±0.02^{a}	5.42±0.01^{b}	+
MANF6	6.07±0.04^{b}	6.15±0.02^{a}	6.02±0.01^{a}	5.4±0.02^{b}	+

Values represent mean±SD of experiments carried out in triplicate (n = 3); '+'= Slight precipitation, '++' = Moderate precipitation. ^{a,b}Means within the same row followed by different superscripts are significantly different (P<0.05).

Table 4: Adhesion and auto-aggregation properties of strains.

Strains	% Hydrophobicity			% Auto-aggregation
	Chloroform	Toluene	Ethyl acetate	
MANF1	52.1±1.2^{c}	60.8±1.4^{a}	56.5±1.2^{b}	47.6±2.4^{d}
MANF2	64.0±1.1^{c}	72.0±1.1^{a}	69.6±2.2^{b}	68.1±1.5^{a}
MANF3	40.0±2.2^{c}	55.0±1.2^{a}	45.0±1.2^{b}	44.4±1.2^{e}
MANF4	38.0±1.3^{c}	61.9±1.3^{a}	52.3±1.4^{b}	50.3±1.1^{c}
MANF5	36.8±1.2^{c}	63.1±1.2^{a}	52.6±1.2^{b}	52.3±1.2^{b}
MANF6	33.3±1.2^{c}	58.9±1.5^{a}	53.8±2.3^{b}	45.4±1.6^{d}

Values represent mean±SD of experiments carried out in triplicate (n = 3). ^{a,b,c,d,e}Means within the same row and column followed by different superscripts are significantly different (P<0.05).

Table 5: Tolerance of strains to phenol and lysozyme.

Strains	Phenol tolerance				Lysozyme resistance (% cell viability)
	Control		With phenol		
	0 h	24 h	0 h	24 h	
MANF1	6.12±0.02^{b}	6.27±0.02^{a}	6.10±0.01^{a}	6.07±0.01^{b}	62.5±1.8^{c}
MANF2	6.17±0.01^{b}	6.3±0.05^{a}	6.18±0.03^{b}	6.27±0.01^{a}	81.1±1.6^{a}
MANF3	6.14±0.03^{b}	6.25±0.02^{a}	6.16±0.02^{b}	6.18±0.02^{a}	64.2±1.3^{c}
MANF4	6.11±0.02^{b}	6.3±0.01^{a}	6.13±0.02^{b}	6.23±0.04^{a}	75.3±1.6^{b}
MANF5	6.09±0.04^{b}	6.28±0.03^{a}	6.07±0.04^{a}	5.97±0.05^{b}	60.0±1.3^{cd}
MANF6	6.07±0.02^{b}	6.25±0.02^{a}	6.06±0.01^{a}	5.92±0.03^{b}	73.3±1.2^{b}

Values represent mean±SD of experiments carried out in triplicate (n = 3). ^{a,b,c,d}Means within the same row and column followed by different superscripts are significantly different (P<0.05).

Table 6: Antibiotic sensitivity pattern of strains.

Strains	Antibiotics						
	Streptomycin	Penicillin G	Chloramphenicol	Kanamycin	Gentamicin	Nalidixic acid	Rifampicin
MANF1	S (+)	S (+++)	S (++)	S (++)	S (+++)	R	S (+++)
MANF2	S (+)	S (+++)	S (++)	S (++)	S(+++)	R	S (+++)
MANF3	S (+)	S (+++)	S (++)	S (++)	S (+++)	R	S (+++)
MANF4	S (+)	S (+++)	S (++)	S (++)	S (+++)	R	S (+++)
MANF5	S (+)	S (+++)	S (++)	S (++)	S (+++)	R	S (+++)
MANF6	S (+)	S (+++)	S (++)	S (++)	S (+++)	R	S (+++)

Experiments were carried out in triplicate (n = 3); S = Sensitive to antibiotic, R = Resistant to antibiotic, '+++' = Highly sensitive, '++' = Moderately Sensitive, '+' = Sensitive.

Table 7: Viable cell counts (log cfu/mL) of strains at various temperature and NaCl concentrations.

Strains	Temperature (°C)					NaCl (% w/v)		
	10	**20**	**30**	**37**	**42**	**2**	**5**	**10**
MANF1	2.8±0.02^{e}	4.0±0.01^{d}	6.1±0.01^{a}	6.04±0.02^{b}	5.41±0.02^{c}	5.3±0.01^{a}	4.3±0.02^{b}	2.8±0.03^{c}
MANF2	2.6±0.04^{e}	4.2±0.02^{d}	6.2±0.02^{a}	6.1±0.03^{b}	5.4±0.01^{c}	5.4±0.03^{a}	4.2±0.05^{b}	2.7±0.02^{c}
MANF3	2.5±0.02^{e}	4.1±0.04^{d}	6.1±0.03^{a}	6.0±0.02^{b}	5.32±0.06^{c}	5.1±0.03^{a}	4.2±0.02^{b}	2.5±0.02^{c}
MANF4	2.3±0.05^{e}	3.7±0.03^{d}	6.2±0.02^{a}	6.0±0.04^{b}	5.12±0.02^{c}	5.2±0.02^{a}	4.1±0.04^{b}	2.2±0,04^{c}
MANF5	2.0±0.02^{e}	3.8+0.02^{d}	6.21±0.04^{a}	6.13±0.05^{b}	5.0±0.03^{c}	4.9±0.02^{a}	3.9±0.02^{b}	2.0±0.02^{c}
MANF6	2.2±0.01^{d}	3.4±0.04^{c}	6.13±0.02^{a}	6.1±0.02^{a}	5.13±0.02^{b}	4.8±0.01^{a}	3.6±0.03^{b}	2.2±0.03^{c}

Values represent mean±SD of experiments carried out in triplicate (n = 3). ^{a,b,c,d,e}Means within the same row followed by different superscripts are significantly different (*P*<0.05).

Table 8: Exopolysaccharides production, amylase activity, lipolytic activity, and biofilm formation tests of strains.

Strains	Exopolysaccharides production	Amylolytic activity	Lipolytic activity	Biofilm
MANF1	+	-	-	-
MANF2	+	-	+	-
MANF3	+	-	-	-
MANF4	+	-	+	-
MANF5	+	-	-	-
MANF6	+	-	+	-

'+' = Mild production of exopolysaccharides and lipase; '-' = Absence of amylase, lipase activity, and biofilm formation.

Table 9: Autolysis capacity, catalase activity, and nitrate reductase activity ofstrains.

Strains	Autolysis (%)			Catalase activity (AU)	Nitrate reductase activity (mM nitrite/mg dry weight)
	6 h	12 h	24 h		
MANF1	35.1±1.2[c]	37.3±1.3[b]	39.4±1.3[a]	10.12±1.3[c]	10.14±1.4[c]
MANF2	42.1±1.3[c]	44.5±1.4[b]	52.1±1.2[a]	16.92±1.2[a]	12.23±1.2[a]
MANF3	40.1±1.3[c]	42.1±1.2[b]	45.1±1.2[a]	9.76±1.1[d]	10.45±1.1[c]
MANF4	41.3±1.2[c]	44.4±1.3[b]	50.2±1.2[a]	11.31±1.4[b]	11.34±1.2[b]
MANF5	43.3±1.3[c]	46.6±1.1[b]	48.8±1.3[a]	10.76±1.2[c]	11.12±1.3[b]
MANF6	38.8±1.4[c]	40.1±1.4[b]	43.3±1.2[a]	9.95±1.3[d]	9.72±1.3[d]

Cell autolysis (%): [a,b,c]Means within the same row followed by different superscripts are significantly different ($P<0.05$).

Catalase activity: µmoles of degraded H_2O_2/min/mL of cells with optical density (OD_{600} nm) = 1.0; Nitrate reductase: mM nitrite×mg^{-1} dry weight; Values represent mean±SD of experiments carried out in triplicate (n = 3); [a,b,c,d]Means within the same column followed by different superscripts are significantly different ($P<0.05$).

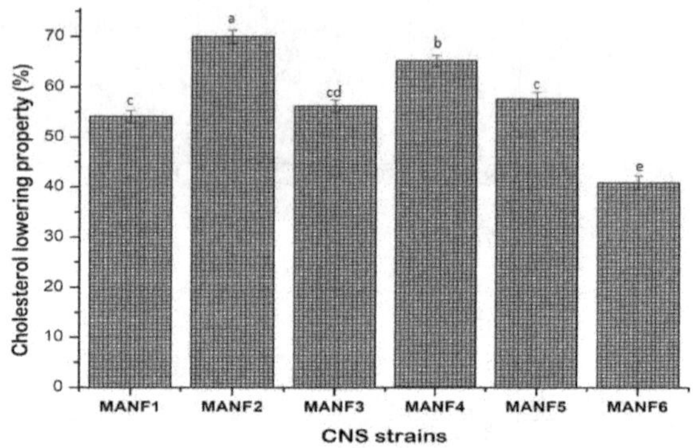

Figure 1: Cholesterol lowering traits of CNS strains.

[Note: Values are represented as mean±SD of experiments carried out in triplicate (n = 3). [abcde]Values with different letters are significantly ($P<0.05$) different.]

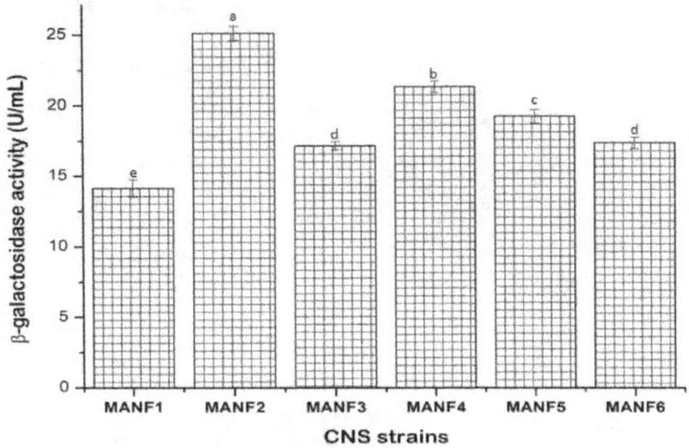

Figure 2: β-galactosidase activities of CNS strains.

[Note: Values are represented as mean±SD of experiments carried out in triplicate (n = 3). [abcde]Values with different letters are significantly ($P<0.05$) different.]

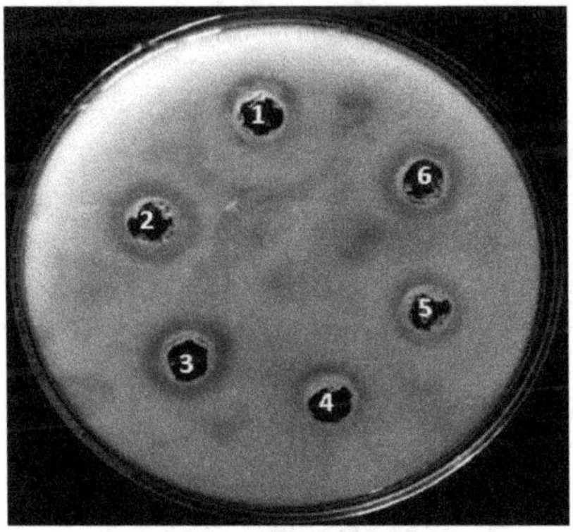

Figure 3: Proteolytic activities of strains on skim milk agar plates.

[Note: 1 - strain MANF1, 2 - strain MANF2, 3 - strain MANF3, 4 - strain MANF4, 5 - strain MANF5, and 6 - strain MANF6]

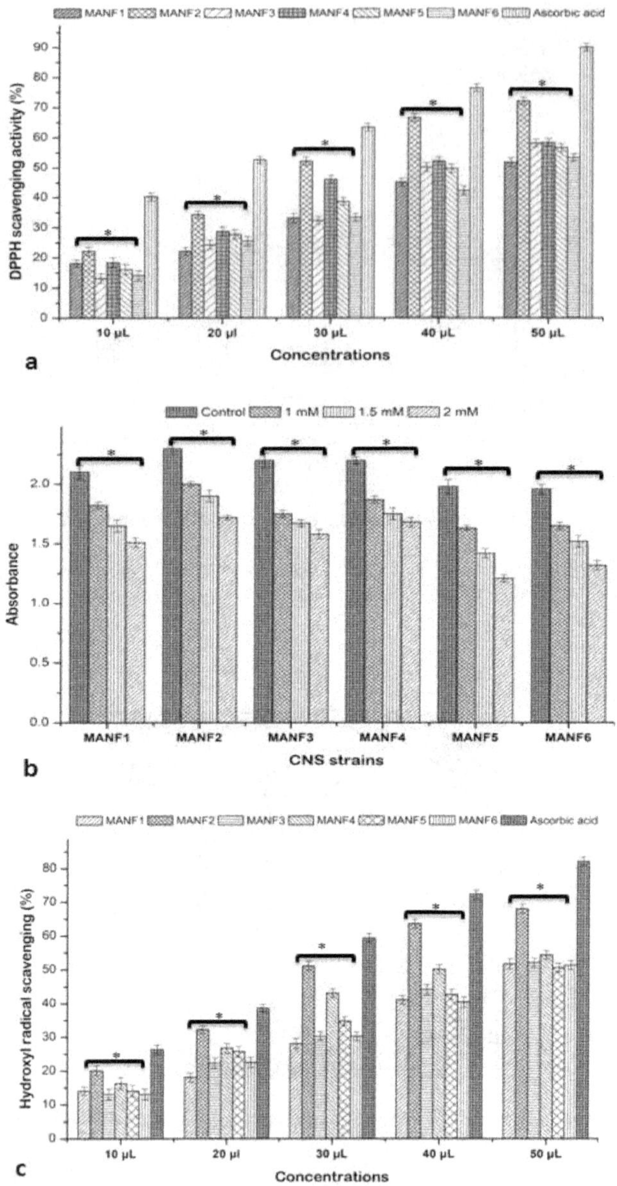

Figure 4: (a) DPPH scavenging, (b) H_2O_2 tolerance, and (c) hydroxyl radical scavenging properties of strains at varied concentrations.

[Note: Values are represented as mean±SD of experiments carried out in triplicate (n = 3).
*Values are significantly (*P*<0.05) different.]

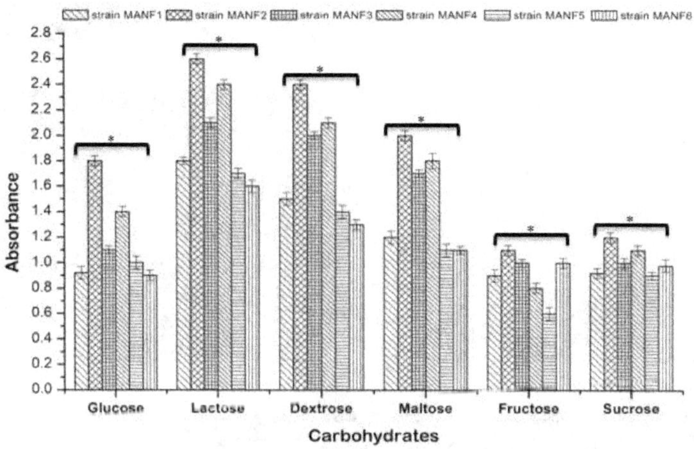

Figure 5: Carbohydrate fermentation potentialities of CNS strains.

[Note: Values are represented as mean±SD of experiments carried out in triplicate (n = 3). *Values are significantly ($P<0.05$) different.]

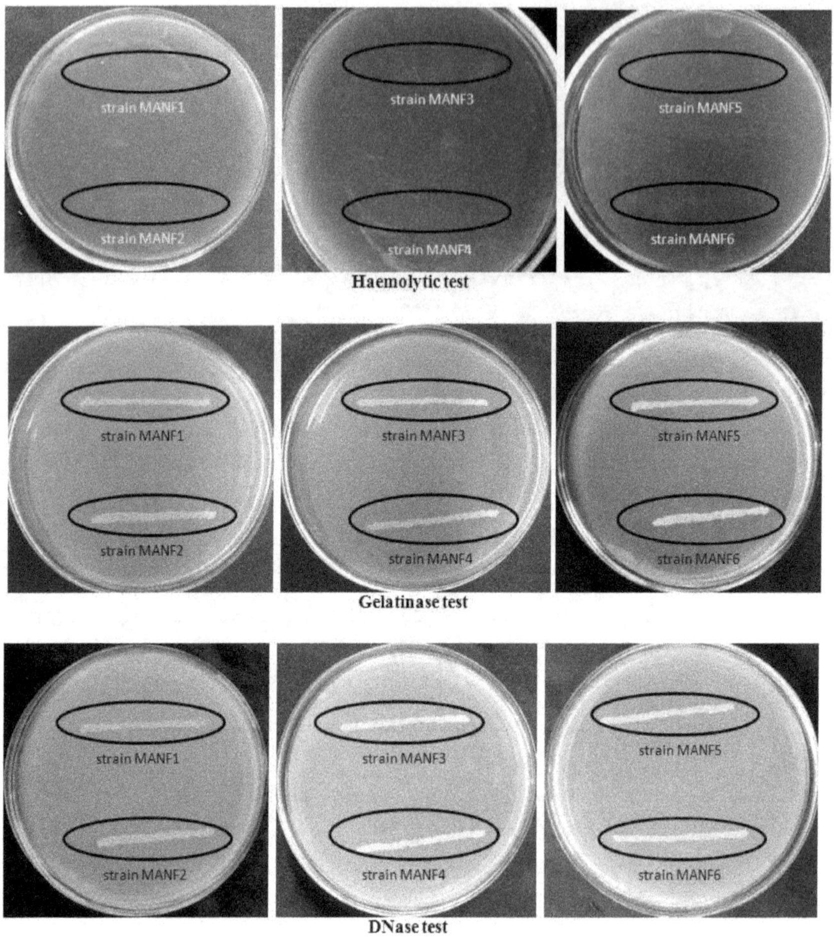

Figure 6: *In vitro* safety assessment tests of CNS strains. None of the strains exhibited haemolytic, gelatinase, and DNase activities, thereby showing lack of zone of hydrolysis around the culture.

4. Discussion

Recently reported several studies demonstrated the probiotic characteristics of lactobacilli from diverse fermented food items (Ramos *et al.*, 2013; Zheng *et al.*, 2013; Shehata *et al.*, 2016). But the integrity of CNS in terms of probiotic characteristics is sparse. The dexterity of bacteria to tolerate acidic environment of GI tract is one of the required probiotic properties. In fact, the bacteria must tolerate through the stomach as well as upper region of the intestinal tract before reaching the distal part of the intestinal tract and manifesting their effect (Bao *et al.*, 2010). In the present context, all the strains were able to survive up to pH 2.0 for 3 h of incubation with varying levels of viability. Similar findings were observed by Borah *et al.* (2016) who also reported the viability of staphylococci up to pH 2.0. In contradictory to this, our findings exhibited superiority to Kim *et al.* (2007) who demonstrated the lower viabilities of the probiotic isolates at acidic pH.

The resistance properties of CNS towards simulated gastric juice are another paramount probiotic parameter enabling the strains to survive in the high acidic condition for a longer period. Our results were in complete agreement with those obtained from previous study in which *S. succinus* survived in the presence of simulated gastric juice (Sathyabama *et al.*, 2012). In general, the acid tolerance characteristics of bacteria up to 2-3 h (time needed to cross the barrier) would be of immense interest for the formulation of the probiotic cultures and it would also be required to ensure persistence in the human upper GI tract as well as fermented products.

Strains should also be resistant to bile salts due to the occasional occurrence of duodeno-gastric biliary reflux. Tolerance to bile salts is a prerequisite for colonization and metabolic activity of bacteria in small intestine of the host (Havenaar *et al.*, 1992). Generally, bile salts are produced due to the catabolism of cholesterol whose physiological concentration in human ranges from 0.3-0.5%. It plays a fundamental role in the specific and non-specific defence mechanisms of the gut (Dunne *et al.*, 2001). In the present investigation, all the strains were resistant to bile salt with considerable variability in their cell viabilities that will help these strains to reach small intestine and colon, and thus enabling them to balance the intestinal microbiota. Similar results were reported by Simonova *et al.* (2006) who observed good tolerance of staphylococci towards bile salt. The bile resistant abilities of strains would most probably be due to the expression of bile-tolerance associated proteins in bacterial cells (Hamon *et al.*, 2011).

The bile salt detoxifying properties of bacteria are often considered another imperative criterion for the selection of potent probiotics. The BSH catalyses the deconjugation of bile salt to liberate free primary bile acids, thereby rendering the probiotic bacteria to resist the bile salts (Noriega *et al.*, 2006). In this study, all the strains exhibited BSH activities, and inferred that isolates may help in their intestinal colonization. The BSH activities of bacteria more or less similar to our studies were previously reported by Yadav *et al.* (2016) as well. However, Sung *et al.* (2010) did not observe the BSH activity in *S. hominis*, despite showing resistance to bile salt. In general, BSH protects bacteria from the toxicity of conjugated bile salts in the GI tract.

The abilities of probiotics to adhere to epithelia are studied *in vitro* by evaluating the cells surface hydrophobicity. In our study, all the strains revealed a variable degree of hydrophobiity, whereas strain MANF2 showed the strongest hydrophobicity to toluene, followed by ethyl acetate and chloroform. Borah *et al.* (2016) also reported the remarkable hydrophobicity of *Staphylococcus* sp. in toluene. Adhesion in the GI tract of the host is believed to be a critical feature required for the delivery of their health benefits, and in fact, it is a prerequisite for colonization (Zheng *et al.*, 2013). As the hydrophobicity of the cell increases, the level of adhesion also increases (Rijnaarts *et al.*, 1993). The high cell surface hydrophobicity of the strain could indicate its capability to attach to the epithelial cell lining of the intestine and resist the movement of digested food materials (Chauviere *et al.*, 1992).

Auto-aggregation of probiotic strains appears to be decisive for adhesion to epithelial cells. Cell aggregation represents the interaction of cellular constituents viz. proteins, soluble proteins, carbohydrates, and lipoteichoic acid. According to Patel *et al.* (2009), cell surface hydrophobicity and auto-aggregation properties of probiotics are directly correlated, as determined by present study too. *Staphylococcus* spp. showed reasonably higher auto-aggregation, thereby suggesting its specific binding capabilities in the GI (Borah *et al.*, 2016). The bacteria with auto-aggregation abilities form adhere to the mucosal surfaces of the host and thus employ their functions (Grześkowiak *et al.*, 2012). The presence of bioactive proteins in the bacterial supernatant as well as on its surface are often considered for the auto aggregation properties of bacteria (Reniero *et al.*, 1991).

During the digestive mechanisms, toxic or bacteriostatic metabolites such as phenols are often produced due to the deamination of amino acids in the gut (Suskovic *et al.*, 1997). It is very important for the bacterium to resist the availability of phenols in the gut, if the particular strain needs to be categorized under probiotic. In our study, strain MANF2 showed high resistivity towards phenol in terms of cell viability even after 24 h of incubation. Our reports were found to be in complete agreement with the findings of Sathyabama *et al.* (2012) who demonstrated the viability of staphylococci in the presence of phenol at two different concentrations. In like manner, the present study exhibited the tolerance ability of all the strains against lysozyme. In fact, the resistivity towards lysozyme indicates the adaptive characteristics of bacteria against mouth saliva after ingestion process. Borah *et al.* (2016) also reported the significant level of *Staphylococcus* sp. viability in the presence of lysozyme.

In this study, all the strains showed significant level of hypocholesteromic effect *in vitro*. In fact, hypercholesterolemia (a high concentration of cholesterol in the blood of humans) is considered as a risk factor for coronary heart disease, type 2 diabetes mellitus, and other metabolic syndromes. The current findings clearly demonstrated the significant cholesterol removal ability of CNS from the culture media, thereby suggesting the therapeutic application of these strains in the prevention of hypercholesterolemia. In the line of our study, previous reports also exhibited *in vitro* cholesterol level reduction ability of probiotic bacteria (Wang *et al.*, 2012; Miremadi *et al.*, 2014). In contradictory to this, Zheng *et al.* (2013) reported *in vivo* cholesterol lowering effect of probiotics in Sprague-Dawley rats. The possible mechanism for how probiotic bacteria reduced the cholesterol level may be due to the potentialities of isolates to deconjugate bile into free radicals and excretion in the faeces, causing reduced concentration of cholesterol in the body (Zheng *et al.*, 2013; Yadav *et al.*, 2016).

Strains of the present study exhibited slight production of β-galactosidase and moderate level of proteolytic activities. The lactose hydrolysing ability of these CNS might be essential for minimizing the effect of lactase insufficiency. The presence of β-galactosidase is associated with the ability to break down lactose in the upper intestinal region, which is in turn utilized by the indigenous microbiota (De Vrese *et al.*, 2001). On the other hand, the proteolytic enzymes have been considered to hydrolyze the milk protein, inducing the peptidases and free amino groups. The probiotics solely depend upon the proteolytic mechanism due to lower level of amino groups and peptidases

(Manisseri and Gudipati, 2012). Most importantly, the proteolytic properties of probiotics are known to enhance the organoleptic quality of food products.

The antibiotic sensitivity of CNS is crucial in order to be used as probiotics because probiotic bacteria may act as potential reservoir of antibiotic resistance genes and which can be transferred to GI tract. In this study, all the strains were found to be susceptible to most of the tested antibiotics, except nalidixic acid. Our study coincides with the report of Borah *et al.* (2016) who observed the susceptibility of *Staphylococcus* sp. to both the broad and narrow spectrum antibiotics, thereby suggesting the non-pathogenicity of isolate. Moreover, similar to our findings, Yadav *et al.* (2016) observed the resistivity of probiotic isolates against nalidixic acid, and susceptibility towards other conventional antibiotics.

Antioxidants play a pivotal role in preventing the cellular damage caused by hydrogen atom transfer and electron transfer. In the present study, all the CNS strains exhibited DPPH scavenging properties in a dose dependent manner, whereas strain MANF2 reduced DPPH with higher scavenging rate. The concentration dependent DPPH free radical scavenging activities of bacteria might be due to the presence of surface active compounds involved in antioxidant activities. All the strains were also able to tolerate the tested concentrations of hydrogen peroxide, and thereby depicted potent antioxidant activities. Similar findings were observed by Lee *et al.* (2005) who also reported the resistivity of probiotic bacteria against particular concentrations of hydrogen peroxide. Additionally, strains of the present study demonstrated the significant hydroxyl radical scavenging activities in a dose dependent manner. In general, hydroxyl radicals are responsible for the oxidative damage of biomolecules, and these originate mainly from the Fenton reaction in the presence of transition metal ions (Kao and Chen, 2006). Our study clearly indicates the chelation of these ions, thereby exhibiting the scavenging of hydroxyl radicals.

Staphylococcus spp. are usually used as starters cultures for fermented foods. Among starters, only few data are available in the literature on technological properties of CNS and little attention has been paid to their contribution in food fermentation (Sondergaard and Stahnke, 2002). Previously, Casaburi *et al.* (2005) and Mauriello *et al.* (2004) studied some of the technological characteristics of CNS such as *S. carnosus* and *S. simulans* strains. In the present investigation, CNS viz. *S. saprophyticus*, *S. hominis*, *S. xylosus*, and *S. equorum* strains were evaluated for their technological attributes and showed beneficial activities that would make them eligible as a good starter cultures for fermented food preparation.

The abilities to ferment various carbohydrates are one of the most substantial technological traits of probiotic bacteria. The present study showed significant differences among CNS strains in terms of their utilization of carbohydrates. All the strains revealed better growth in the fermentation medium constituting lactose. Similar findings were observed by Delgado *et al.* (2015) who reported that most of the lactobacilli strains grew well in the presence of lactose as sole carbon source. In general, CNS are known to contribute in the sensory quality of the fermented foods via the catabolism of carbohydrates (Jeong *et al.*, 2016).

The growth characteristics of CNS strains were found to be affected at various incubation temperatures. In this context, all staphylococci strains grew well at 30^{0}C. In contrast, CNS strains such as *S. carnosus* and *S. simulans* showed viability at 15 and 20^{0}C, temperature usually used for meat fermentation (Casaburi *et al.*, 2005). Salt tolerance is another overriding technological requirement for the starter cultures. All the CNS strains sustained 2% (w/v) sodium chloride concentration with high cell viability, whereas the viability reduced at higher concentration of sodium chloride. These results are not astonishing because '*Koozh*' is prepared with low salt content. In contradictory to our results, Mauriello *et al.* (2004) observed better growth of CNS in the presence of 10 and 15% of sodium chloride.

The potentialities of probiotic bacteria to produce EPS are the key technological property. Technologically, the physicochemical characteristics of EPS, such as viscosity have motivated their applications in food industries, for example, biothickeners (Patel *et al.*, 2012). Therefore, EPS produced by the selected starter cultures will influence the texture and rheological properties of the food which are important attributes associated with the consumption of traditional fermented food items. In the present study, all the CNS strains tested showed EPS production. Previously, the production of EPS has been reported to protect the producing microorganisms against dehydration and other harsh conditions such as acid and bile (Fanning *et al.*, 2012), and may also contribute to the aggregation properties of probiotic bacteria (Owusu-Kwarteng *et al.*, 2015).

All the CNS strains isolated from '*Koozh*' showed lack of amylolytic activities. In general, high prevalence of amylase producing probiotic bacteria has not been reported. However, few lactobacilli strains isolated from fermented maize products have been reported as amylase producers (Sanni *et al.*, 2002). Amylolytic bacteria from traditional fermented foods could be of economic interest because of their abilities to ferment starchy components. Additionally, they may symbolize the ability to decrease the viscosity of bulky, starchy, and weaning porridges which may improve the density of nutrients (Owusu-Kwarteng *et al.*, 2015).

Lipase activities of CNS are known to contribute in the flavour and texture quality of the fermented food products. In this investigation, strain MANF2, strain MANF4, and strain MANF6 showed the existence of weak lipolytic activities, whereas other CNS strains exhibited no lipase activities. This is in agreement with previous study that characterizes few strains of *S. saprophyticus*, *S. succinus*, and *S. xylosus* having moderate lipase activities (Jeong *et al.*, 2016).

The unique properties of bacteria to form biofilm are not a characteristic connected to virulence directly, but it is undesirable in the context of food hygiene and safety because it enhances pathogenicity and antibiotic resistance in bacteria (Bizzini *et al.*, 2006). In the context of biofilm formation abilities, none of the CNS strains of the present study formed biofilm. Generally, the biofilm formation characteristics of strains may not be appropriate for their applications as starter candidates. According to the reports of Jeong *et al.* (2016), biofilm formation of CNS is strain-specific, regardless of species.

Autolysis is another most crucial feature for the utilization of CNS strains as starter/adjunct cultures. The potentialities of strains to lyse and subsequently release intracellular enzymes are a desirable trait because they have an impact on flavour and aroma during fermentation process (Piraino *et al.*, 2008). In general, all the bacteriocinogenic strains present high autolytic activities which may accelerate flavour and texture development.

All the strains of *Staphylococcus* spp. studied in this context showed catalase activities. According to the reports of Mauriello *et al.* (2004), *S. lentus*, *S. equorum*, *S. warneri*, and *S. saprophyticus* strains exhibited the lowest to the highest levels of catalase productions, thereby suggesting antioxidant activities as strain dependent process. In addition to this, Casaburi *et al.* (2005) found staphylococci strains with a cell-bound catalase activity.

Nitrate reductase activities are considered to be the most decisive property of staphylococci to be used as starter cultures for fermented food production (Weber,

1994). Previous finding reported that staphylococcal strains viz. *S. xylosus*, *S. equorum*, and *S. lentus* were able to reduce nitrate to nitrite (Mauriello *et al.*, 2004). Results obtained in our study showed complete agreement with the findings of Casaburi *et al.* (2005) who observed that several strains of CNS were able to reduce nitrates to nitrites.

Isolates were further screened for their safety assessment, and interestingly, none of the strains demonstrated the *in vitro* haemolytic, DNase, and gelatinase activities, thereby exhibiting the safer utilization of these strains. Similar observations towards safety assessment tests of fermented fish associated *Staphylococcus* sp. were reported by Um *et al.* (1996). The safety assessment results have therefore been suggested as a selection criterion for CNS starter strains in food industries (Marty *et al.*, 2012).

5. Conclusions

Results obtained in this chapter concluded the good probiotic attributes of all 6 CNS strains, particularly strain MANF2 by exhibiting vast array of desirable characteristics. Moreover, the findings suggested the application of these strains as starter culture while formulating probiotics derived food items. The study also revealed good technological characteristics of these 6 strains and possible development of functional food preparations. Most importantly, the negative results obtained from haemolytic, DNase, and gelatinase tests revealed the non-pathogenicity and safety aspect of these strains.

Chapter 3

Statistical optimization of distinct parameters and purification of anti-tubercular and anticancer protein from *S. hominis* strain MANF2

1. Introduction

Antimicrobial proteins or peptides produced by *Staphylococcus* spp. are creating immense interest among worldwide researchers. Plethora of studies have described the production, purification, and characterization of staphylococcal proteins (Hale and Hinsdil, 1973; Navartana *et al.*, 1998; Iqbal *et al.*, 2001; Nascimento *et al.*, 2005; Sung *et al.*, 2010). As a matter of fact, proteins or peptides produced by staphylococci show growth inhibitory activities not only against *Staphylococcus* spp. but also against other microorganisms (De-Oliveira *et al.*, 1998). Previously, staphylococcal peptides were investigated for their antagonistic attributes against *Micrococcus luteus* (Saeed *et al.*, 2004), *Corynebacterium fimi* (Nascimento *et al.*, 2005), *S. aureus* (Sung *et al.*, 2010; Kim *et al.*, 2010; Wladyka *et al.*, 2015), and *Listeria monocytogenes* (Matikevičienė *et al.*, 2017). Surprisingly, there is dearth of investigation determining the purification of anti-tubercular protein from *Staphylococcus* sp. Likewise, proteins from varied group of bacteria have revealed selective toxicity toward disparate cancer cells viz. breast cancer, lung cancer, colon cancer, and bone cancer (Kaur and Kaur, 2015). In spite of the promising anticancer traits of gram positive bacteria, the exploitation of *Staphylococcus* sp. associated proteins/peptides as anticancer agents is undetermined yet. Considering this, a significant attempt was undertaken in this chapter to purify anti-tubercular and anticancer protein from strain MANF2.

The non-toxicity characteristics and high antagonistic activities make the proteins/peptides promising therapeutic agents in pharmaceutical industries (Pei *et al.*, 2018). Therefore, it is essential to enhance their yield from the producing organisms. To improve further the activity, the optimization of growth medium constituents and other abiotic factors would undoubtedly be a decisive approach. Despite the extreme applications of one factor at a time (OFAT) method in the enhancement of bioactive metabolites production from bacterial sources (Khusro and Aarti, 2015), this conventional tool is being ruled out now a days due to a time consuming and laborious approach (Aarti *et al.*, 2017). In order to avoid such cumbersome methodology, the statistical optimization tools such as Taguchi orthogonal array (OA) and Box-Behnken

Design (BBD) are being opted for investigating the influence of controlled variables on multivariate system. Taguchi methodology determines the relationship between specific factors and operations conditions, thereby resulting in valid output (Roy, 2001). Moreover, this tool is considered to improve the reliability at low cost with respect to other statistical tools by extracting sufficient quantitative information through few experimental trials. On the other hand, BBD is one of the most effective statistical optimization approaches to explain the combined impact of variables in the fermentation process.

Considering the quest for new therapeutic agents with enhanced bioactivity, the present chapter was aimed not only to improve the activity through Taguchi methodology and BBD design but also to purify and characterize anti-tubercular as well as anticancer protein from strain MANF2.

2. Materials and methods

2.1. Bacterium of interest and growth parameters

Strain MANF2 was sub-cultured at 30°C for 48 h in 250 mL Erlenmeyer flasks constituting 50 mL of MRS broth medium for further experimental studies.

2.2. Media optimization

Strain MANF2 was inoculated into varied sterile production media such as Nutrient broth, Mueller Hinton broth, Luria Bertani broth, MRS broth, Peptone broth, Mannitol Salt broth, and Brain Heart Infusion broth for comparing anti-tubercular attributes. Flasks were incubated at 30°C for 48 h in an orbital shaker at 120 revolutions per minute (rpm). The CFNS was collected and the anti-tubercular activities as well as biomass yield were determined.

2.3. Anti-tubercular activity

The anti-tubercular activity of CFNS of strain MANF2 was determined following LRP assay as described in chapter 1.

2.4. Biomass estimation

The bacterial biomass was determined according to the methodology of Khusro *et al.* (2017). Strain MANF2 was inoculated into sterilized production media and incubated for 48 h at 30°C. The culture was centrifuged at 8000 *g* for 10 min and the supernatant was discarded. The bacterial pellets were dried at 95°C until constant weight and the biomass (mg/mL) was estimated.

2.5. Optimization of parameters by OFAT method

The anti-tubercular activity and biomass yield were optimized using diversiform non-nutritional constituents (pH, temperature, agitation speed, and inoculum volume), medium components (carbon sources, nitrogen sources, and metal ions), and various supplements after working out a series of experiments. The anti-tubercular activity and biomass of strain MANF2 were estimated by adjusting the pH (4.0, 5.0, 6.0, 6.5, 7.0, and 8.0) of the promising production medium using 1N HCl and 1N NaOH. Further, the anti-tubercular activity as well as biomass of strain MANF2 was optimized by altering the incubation temperature (25-50°C), agitation speed (100-150 rpm), and inoculum volume (7.31-54.82 log cfu/mL) at the optimized pH of the medium. Likewise, various carbon sources [1.0% w/v: maltose ($C_{12}H_{22}O_{11}$), fructose ($C_6H_{12}O_6$), sucrose, dextrose, lactose, glucose, and xylose ($C_5H_{10}O_5$)], nitrogen sources [0.5% w/v: yeast extract, ammonium acetate ($NH_4CH_3CO_2$), ammonium citrate ($C_6H_{11}NO_7$), ammonium chloride (NH_4Cl), ammonium nitrate (NH_4NO_3), ammonium sulphate, and sodium nitrate ($NaNO_3$)], and metal ions [0.01% w/v: magnesium sulphate ($MgSO_4$), zinc sulphate ($ZnSO_4$), calcium chloride, copper sulphate ($CuSO_4$), and ferric chloride ($FeCl_3$)] were substituted in the production medium. In addition to this, various supplements such as Tween20 ($C_{58}H_{114}O_{26}$), Tween40 ($C_{44}H_{54}N_7O_8P$), Tween80 ($C_{64}H_{124}O_{26}$), and glycerol at 1.0% v/v were incorporated in the medium for further optimization process. An appropriate control medium was also maintained wherever applicable. The anti-tubercular activity was estimated according to the methodology discussed in chapter 1. The biomass yield was determined as described above.

2.6. Taguchi OA experimental design

Based on the primary screening of several parameters through OFAT tool, a total of 8 factors (pH, temperature, dextrose, yeast extract, ammonium chloride, magnesium sulphate, calcium chloride, and glycerol) were selected further for optimization using Taguchi approach. The minimum and maximum ranges of each selected variable are shown in Table 1. Taguchi OA was performed not only to reduce experimental errors but also improve the efficiency of experiments. A standard OA layout of L18 ($2^2 \times 3^6$) generating 18 runs was constructed at two coded levels for pH and temperature, and three coded levels for dextrose, yeast extract, ammonium chloride, magnesium sulphate, calcium chloride, and glycerol (Table 2).

In Taguchi OA approach, the deviation of a characteristic from its target value is the measurement of quality. A loss function $L(y)$ for the deviation is calculated as mentioned below:

$$L(y) = k\,(y-m)^2 \qquad \text{[Equation 1]}$$

where, k = proportionality constant; m = targeted value; y = observed value obtained for each trial. However, in terms of "bigger and better quality" characteristics, the loss function can be represented according to the formula given below:

$$L(y) = k\,(1/y^2) \qquad \text{[Equation 2]}$$

Likewise, the expected loss function can be expressed by the equation as mentioned below:

$$E[L(y)] = kE\,(1/y^2) \qquad \text{[Equation 3]}$$

where, $E\,(1/y^2)$ can be calculated from 'n' samples as follows:

$$\sum_{i=1}^{n}\left(\frac{1}{y2}\right)/n \qquad \text{[Equation 4]}$$

The submerged fermentation was carried out by varying the composition of medium and altering the non-nutritional parameters as described in Table 2. The most significant variables enhancing the anti-tubercular activity and biomass yield were selected for further optimization using BBD of response surface methodology (RSM).

2.7. Optimization by BBD

Five variables (pH, temperature, yeast extract, magnesium sulphate, and glycerol affecting significantly the anti-tubercular activity and biomass yield were optimized adopting BBD at three different levels (-1, 0, +1). The coded values -1 and +1 indicate low and high levels of the variables studied. All variables were set at a central coded value of zero. Box-Behnken design is an optimization method for a small number of variables that estimates best fit parameters of the quadratic models. It detects not only the lack of fit of the model, but also constructs a sequential design for RSM. According to the present experimental design, the total number of treatment combinations is $2^k + 2k + n$, where "k" is the number of independent variables and "n" is the number of repetition of experiments at the central point.

The dependent variables i.e. anti-tubercular activity and biomass were represented as Y and Z, respectively. The impacts of factors to the respective responses were analyzed using a second-order polynomial equation as mentioned below:

$$Y, Z = \beta_0 + \beta_1 A + \beta_2 B + \beta_3 C + \beta_4 D + \beta_5 E + \beta_{11} A^2 + \beta_{22} B^2 + \beta_{33} C^2 + \beta_{44} D^2 + \beta_{55} E^2 + \beta_{12} AB + \beta_{13} AC + \beta_{14} AD + \beta_{15} AE + \beta_{23} BC + \beta_{24} BD + \beta_{25} BE + \beta_{34} CD + \beta_{35} CE + \beta_{45} DE$$

[Equation 5]

where, Y, Z = Dependent variables; β_0 = Intercept; β_1, β_2, β_3, β_4, and β_5 = Linear coefficients; β_{11}, β_{22}, β_{33}, β_{44}, and β_{55} = Squared coefficients; β_{12}, β_{13}, β_{14}, β_{23}, β_{24}, β_{25}, β_{34}, β_{35}, and β_{45} = Interaction coefficients; A, B, C, D, E, A^2, B^2, C^2, D^2, E^2, AB, AC, AD, AE, BC, BD, BE, CD, CE, and DE = Levels of independent variables.

The goodness of fit of the polynomial equation was expressed by coefficient of determination (R^2) and its statistical significance level was checked by F test, maintaining the desirability at maximum.

2.8. Experiment validation

The statistical optimization was validated by carrying out the experiments using optimized parameters under submerged fermentation. The subsequent estimation of anti-tubercular activity and biomass yield was performed based on the methodology as described above.

2.9. Purification of protein-

2.9.1. Medium preparation

One litre (L) of MRS medium was prepared using statistically optimized parameters and autoclaved. The log phase grown culture of strain MANF2 was inoculated into cooled MRS medium aseptically and incubated at 30^{0}C for 48 h.

2.9.2. Ammonium sulphate precipitation

The bacterial culture was centrifuged at 8000 *g* for 15 min at 4^{0}C. The supernatant was collected, neutralized, and precipitated with varied saturation levels (40, 50, 60, 70, and 80%) of ammonium sulphate. As per the saturation level, ammonium sulphate was weighed and powdered using mortar and pestle (Model - LAB.MOR.31219351). The powdered ammonium sulphate was added in small amount into the supernatant and stirred for 4 h at 4^{0}C using magnetic stirrer. Further, samples were incubated at 4^{0}C in refrigerator for the complete precipitation of protein. The precipitated protein samples were collected after centrifugation at 10000 *g* for 15 min at 4^{0}C. The resulting pellets were re-suspended in sodium phosphate buffer (1M, pH 7.0) for the determination of total protein content using Bradford assay (Bradford, 1976).

2.9.3. Estimation of protein

Bradford reagent preparation - Hundred milligrams of Coomassie Brilliant Blue (CBB) G250 were dissolved in 50 mL of ethanol. Further, 100 mL of orthophosphoric acid (H_3PO_4) were added into it and the volume was made up to 1 L. The solution was filtered using Whatman filter paper 1 in dark and stored at 4^0C in dark bottle for further use.

Bovine serum albumin (BSA) standard preparation - The standard stock solution of BSA was prepared by dissolving 50 mg of BSA into 50 mL of autoclaved distilled water. The BSA stock solution was further diluted in autoclaved distilled water for standard curve analysis.

Protein content of ammonium sulphate precipitated samples was estimated according to the methodology of Bradford (1976) using BSA as standard. Hundred microlitres of samples were pipetted out in clean tubes and volumes were made up to 1 mL using autoclaved distilled water. Five millilitres of Bradford reagent were added into each tube and mixed thoroughly. One millilitre of autoclaved distilled water + 5 mL of Bradford reagent were used as blank. Absorbance of samples was read at 595 nm using UV-Vis spectrophotometer. Protein content of samples was estimated against the standard curve of BSA. The saturation level exhibiting maximum protein content was used for dialysis.

2.9.4. Dialysis-

2.9.4.1. Pre-treatment of dialysis membrane

Dialysis membrane (1.0 kDa cut-off) was pre-treated using freshly prepared 10mM EDTA, 2% (w/v) sodium bicarbonate ($NaHCO_3$), distilled water (65^0C), and distilled water (room temperature). The dialysis membrane was dipped into the solutions in the sequential order of distilled water (65^0C) for 5 min, 10mM EDTA for 5 min, 2% (w/v) sodium bicarbonate for 5 min, and distilled water (room temperature) for 5-10 min. The pre-treated dialysis membrane was used for dialysis process.

2.9.4.2. Dialysis of sample

One end of the pre-treated dialysis membrane was tied with thread and filled with ammonium sulphate precipitated sample. About 1 mL of sodium phosphate buffer (1M, pH 7.0) was added again into the sample and tied another end of the membrane with thread. The sample was mixed by gentle hand press. The sample containing membrane was dipped into approximately 1 L of sodium phosphate buffer (1M, pH 7.0) and kept under slow stirring at cold condition for 2-3 h. The buffer was changed every 2-3 h and continued the process for 4 cycles under cold condition. Total protein content of dialysed sample was estimated according to Bradford assay (Bradford, 1976) as discussed earlier and used for further process.

2.9.5. Diethylaminoethyl (DEAE) -Cellulose column chromatography

DEAE-Cellulose (1.5 g) was soaked in 0.1M (pH 7.0) sodium phosphate buffer. The column was washed using distilled water and then with the buffer. The column was packed with pre-soaked DEAE-cellulose and excess buffer was eluted. The dialyzed sample was loaded into the column. After 30 min, sample was eluted using the same buffer at the flow rate of 0.5 mL/min. The gradient elution was carried out using 0.2, 0.3, 0.4, 0.5M sodium chloride in the same buffer. Fractions were collected and tested for anti-tubercular activities according to the methodology mentioned in chapter 1. Fractions showing maximum anti-tubercular activities were pooled together for determining total protein content (Bradford, 1976) and electrophoresed using sodium dodecyl sulphate-polyacrylamide gel electrophoresis (SDS-PAGE; Model - VMR0007) for the determination of molecular mass.

2.9.6. Molecular mass determination

The purity and molecular mass of the most active fractions were determined using SDS-PAGE with 4% stacking gel and 12% separating gel.

Preparation of separating gel (10 mL)-

Acrylamide (C_3H_5NO):	3.3 mL
Separating buffer (pH 8.8):	2.5 mL
Distilled water:	4 mL
Sodium dodecyl sulfate (SDS) (10%):	100 μL
Ammonium per sulphate (APS) (10%):	100 μL
Tetramethylethylenediamine (TEMED):	5 μL

Preparation of stacking gel (10 mL)-

Acrylamide:	670 μL
Stacking buffer (pH 8.8):	500 μL
Distilled water:	2.7 mL
SDS (10%):	40 μL
APS (10%):	40 μL
TEMED:	4 μL

Clean notched and rectangular glass plates were assembled and kept in vertical position by placing them in a gel casting stand. The separating gel mixture was prepared and poured into the glass plates uniformly without any leakage. After polymerization of the separating gel, the stacking gel so prepared was poured over it and the comb was inserted gently. This setup was kept for few minutes to allow the gel to polymerize completely. The comb was then carefully removed and wells formed in the gel were rinsed with distilled water completely. Protein samples (50 µL) were mixed with 50 µL of sample solubilising buffer (1:1) and the mixture was heated at 95^0C in water bath for 10 min.

Preparation of solubilising buffer-

Sucrose:	20 g
SDS:	10 g
Stacking buffer:	22.5 mL
Distilled water:	60 mL
Mercaptoethanol (C_2H_6OS):	10 mL
Bromophenol blue:	20 mg

Protein samples along with standard protein marker were then loaded into the respective wells. The gel was electrophoresed at 50-100V for 3-4 h in order to allow the samples run completely into the gel. After electrophoresis, the gel was placed in CBB staining solution for 1 h and washed thoroughly with distilled water.

Preparation of CBB staining solution-

Methanol:	125 mL
Acetic acid:	25 mL
Distilled water:	100 mL
CBB G250:	0.05 g

The stained gel was then placed in destaining solution. Destaining solution was prepared as mentioned below:

Preparation of destaining solution-

Methanol:	125 mL
Acetic acid:	25 mL
Distilled water:	100 mL

Destaining solution was changed every 30 min and the destaining was continued till the bands were clearly observed. Protein band was observed and its molecular mass was calculated based on the relative mobility of the standard marker [14.3-66 kilodalton (kDa)].

2.10. Mass spectrometry and N- terminal amino acid sequencing

After SDS-PAGE, the protein band of interest was excised from the gel and kept in 50% (v/v) methanol. Matrix-Assisted Laser Desorption/Ionization-Time of Flight mass spectrometry (MALDI-TOF MS/MS) was used to determine the molecular mass of the purified protein. The protein was digested using trypsin at 37°C for 12 h. An equal volume of α-Cyano-4-hydroxycinnamic acid (CHCA; $C_{10}H_7NO_3$) solution [(10 mg/mL CHCA in 70% acetonitrile (C_2H_3N), 0.03% trifluoro acetic acid ($C_2HF_3O_2$)] was added to the trypsinized protein. MALDI-TOF spectrum depicts the fragmentation of protein into various peptides. The peptide mass fingerprinting (PMF) was carried out to examine the sequence of the peptide fragments of protein. Mass spectra were recorded in the range of 100-2250 mass by charge (m/z). The *N*- amino acid sequence was compared with the sequence available in BLAST, NCBI algorithm (http://www.ncbi.nlm.nih.gov/) with the MASCOT search program (http://matrixscience.com).

2.11. Anti-tubercular activity of purified protein

M. tuberculosis H37Rv was grown in the presence of various concentrations (10-50 μg/mL) of purified protein and the anti-tubercular activity was estimated according to the methodology as mentioned in chapter 1. Rifampicin was used as positive control.

2.12. Characterization of protein-

2.12.1. Effect of pH

pH of the purified protein (1 mg/mL) was adjusted from 3.0 to 8.0 using 1N HCl and 1N NaOH. Samples were incubated at 37°C for 3 h and residual anti-tubercular activities were calculated against the control (pH 6.5).

2.12. 2. Effect of temperature

To investigate the thermal effect on residual anti-tubercular activities, purified protein (1 mg/mL) at optimum pH level was incubated at 40°C for 2 h, 60°C for 1 h, 80°C 30 min, 100°C for 20 min, and 121°C for 15 min. The protein sample without heat treatment was considered as control.

2.12.3. Effect of enzymes

Enzymes (1 mg/mL; pepsin - pH 3.0, trypsin - pH 7.5, protease K - pH 7.5, and α-amylase - pH 7.5) were mixed with purified protein at optimal pH and temperature. The mixture was incubated for 1 h and then subsequently heated at 100^0C for 5 min in order to inactivate the enzymes. Residual anti-tubercular activities were calculated according to the methodology mentioned earlier. The purified protein without the addition of enzymes was used as control.

2.13. Anticancer activity of purified protein-

2.13.1. Cell culture

Human lung cancer cells (A549) and human colon cancer cells (HT-29) were purchased from the National Centre for Cell Sciences, Pune, India. Cells were maintained in Dulbecco's modified eagles medium (DMEM) supplemented with 2mM L-glutamine and balanced salt solution (BSS) adjusted to contain 1.5 g/L sodium carbonate, 0.1mM non-essential amino acids, 1mM sodium pyruvate ($C_3H_3NaO_3$), 2mM L-glutamine, 1.5 g/L glucose, 10mM [4-(2-hydroxyethyl)-1-piperazineethane sulfonic acid: HEPES] and 10% fetal bovine serum (GIBCO, USA). Penicillin and streptomycin (100 IU/100μg) were adjusted to 1 mL/L. Cells were maintained at 37^0C with 5% carbon dioxide (CO_2) in a humidified CO_2 incubator.

2.13.2. In vitro cytotoxicity

Anticancer activities of purified protein (10-50 μg/mL) were evaluated using MTT assay (Mosmann, 1983). Cancer cells were grown (1×10^4 cells/well) in a 96-well plate for 48 h into 75% confluence. The medium was replaced with fresh medium containing protein sample, and cells were further incubated for 48 h. The culture medium was removed, MTT solution (100 μL) was added to each well, and incubated at 37^0C for 4 h. After removal of the supernatant, 50 μL of DMSO was added to each of the wells and incubated for 10 min to solubilise the formazan crystals. The absorbance was measured at 620 nm using an ELISA multi-well plate reader. Doxorubicin ($C_{27}H_{29}NO_{11}$) was used as positive control. The absorbance value was used to calculate the percentage of viability using the following formula:

$$\%\ \text{viability} = \frac{\text{Absorbance of sample}}{\text{Absorbance of control}} \times 100 \qquad \text{[Equation 6]}$$

The minimum concentration of protein required for 50% inhibition of cell viability (IC_{50}) was calculated using linear regression curve statistics (https://www.graphpad.com/quickcalcs/linear1/).

2.14. Fourier-transform infrared (FT-IR) spectroscopy

Three milligrams (mg) of purified protein were mixed with 300 mg of potassium bromide (KBr: FT-IR grade) and pressed into a pellet in a hydraulic press by applying 500 kilograms per cubic metre (kg/m^3) pressure. The pellet was put into the sample holder and FT-IR spectra were recorded ranging 4000-450 per centimetre (cm^{-1}) using FT-IR spectrometer [Model - IRAffinity- 1(SHIMADZU)].

2.15. Statistical analyses and softwares used

Experiments were demonstrated in triplicate and values were expressed in terms of mean±SD. The design of experiments (DOE) and statistical optimization process were interpreted using Qualitek-4 (Automatic Design and Analysis of Taguchi Experiment; Nutek Inc. USA) and Design Expert Version 11.0.0 (Stat-Ease Inc., Minneapolis, Minnesota, USA) software. Data were validated using ANOVA and values $P \leq 0.05$ were considered statistically significant.

3. Results

3.1. Media optimization

Among diversified media tested for the anti-tubercular activity, strain MANF2 revealed significant ($P<0.05$) RLU reduction of 92.5±1.2% in MRS broth, followed by Mannitol salt broth (82.6±1.4%), Brain Heart infusion (72.6±1.2%), Mueller Hinton broth (51.4±1.3%), Nutrient broth (48.7±1.4%), Luria Bertani broth (42.3±1.5%), and Peptone broth (35.3±1.3%). In like manner, the bacterial biomass was significantly ($P<0.05$) influenced in the order of MRS broth (2.3±0.05 mg/mL) > Mannitol salt broth (2±0.04 mg/mL) > Brain Heart infusion (1.8±0.04 mg/mL) > Mueller Hinton broth (1.5±0.05 mg/mL) > Nutrient broth (1.3±0.04 mg/mL) > Luria Bertani broth (1.2±0.04 mg/mL) > Peptone broth (1.02±0.03 mg/mL) (Figure 1).

3.2. Optimization by OFAT method

pHs of MRS medium showed pivotal influence on the anti-tubercular activity and biomass yield of strain MANF2. The strain depicted maximum RLU reduction and biomass yield of 92.5±1.3% and 2.3±0.05 mg/mL, respectively at pH 6.5. A slight reduction in the activity and biomass of strain MANF2 were estimated at pH 6.0 and 7.0, followed by drastic influence at further acidic and alkaline pHs (Figure 2a).

The anti-tubercular activity and biomass of strain MANF2 were significantly ($P<0.05$) influenced by altering incubation temperature. Maximum anti-tubercular activity (92.6±1.3%) and biomass yield (2.33±0.05 mg/mL) were reported at 30^0C.

Further increment in the incubation temperature revealed significant ($P<0.05$) reduction in the anti-tubercular activity and biomass productivity (Figure 2b).

The agitation speed and inoculums volume were observed to be less effective in terms of improving the activity and biomass yield from strain MANF2. However, the maximum activity (92.6±1.3%) and biomass production (2.3±0.05 mg/mL) were estimated at 120 rpm (Figure 2c) but the effect was found to be non-significant ($P>0.05$). Similarly, 18.27 log cfu/mL inoculums volume showed increased anti-tubercular activity (92.58±1.4%) and biomass yield (2.33±1.4 mg/mL) with no significant differences (Figure 2d).

The impact of diversified nutritional components on the anti-tubercular activity and biomass productivity revealed that dextrose and yeast extract were the most effective carbon and nitrogen sources, respectively (Figure 2e and f). A significant ($P<0.05$) RLU reduction of 92.6±1.4 and 92.63±1.4% was estimated in the presence of dextrose and yeast extract, respectively. Likewise, the biomass yield was significantly ($P<0.05$) influenced in the presence of dextrose (2.38±0.03 mg/mL) and yeast extract (2.38±0.04 mg/mL).

Metal ions influenced significantly ($P<0.05$) the anti-tubercular activity and biomass of strain MANF2. Maximum activity (92.67±1.5%) and biomass productivity (2.4±0.05 mg/mL) were obtained in the presence of calcium chloride (Figure 2g). On the other hand, the supplementation of glycerol into the medium significantly ($P<0.05$) improved the activity (94.6±1.3%) and biomass (4.5±0.04 mg/mL) of strain MANF2. Other supplements viz. Tween20, Tween40, and Tween80 revealed comparatively lower anti-tubercular activity and biomass yield (Figure 2h).

3.3. Taguchi OA experimental design

The OFAT based optimization illustrated the significant ($P<0.05$) effect of pH, temperature, dextrose, yeast extract, ammonium chloride, magnesium sulphate, calcium chloride, and glycerol on anti-tubercular activity as well as biomass of strain MANF2. Hence, these 8 controlled variables were further optimized by Taguchi OA design at different ranges in 18 runs for improving the response variables. The outcomes of the experiments revealed that the maximum anti-tubercular activity (96.6±1.4%) and biomass productions (6.5±0.5 mg/mL) were obtained in Run 5 when the non-nutritional and nutritional conditions were as follows: pH 6.5, temperature 30^{0}C, dextrose 1% w/v, yeast extract 0.1% w/v, ammonium chloride 0.1% w/v, magnesium sulphate 0.025%

w/v, calcium chloride 0.05%, and glycerol 1.5% v/v. The experimental values were observed to be close to the predicted values of respective responses (Table 2).

ANOVA was used not only to assess the competence and fitness of the model but also determine how much variation that each variable has contributed for improving respective responses through Taguchi OA design. Table 3 analyses the factors significantly influencing the anti-tubercular activity of strain MANF2. The model *F*-value of 16.54 implies that the model is significant. There is only a 0.03% chance that an *F*-value this large could occur due to noise. $P \leq 0.05$ indicates model terms are significant. In this case A, B, D, F, and H are significant model terms. The R^2 value of 0.949 specifies that 94.9% of the total variation in the anti-tubercular activity is ascribed to the predictor variables. The "Pred R^2" of 0.7365 is in reasonable agreement with the "Adj R^2" of 0.8916. "Adeq Precision" measures the signal to noise ratio. A ratio of 13.412 indicates an adequate signal. The model shows standard deviation, mean, coefficient of variation (C.V.), and prediction residual sum of squares (PRESS) values of 4.65, 68.38, 6.8%, and 893.9, respectively.

ANOVA for significant effect of input variables on the biomass of strain MANF2 is illustrated in Table 4. The model *F*-value of 17.95 implies that the model is significant. There is only a 0.02% chance that an *F*-value this large could occur due to noise. $P \leq 0.05$ indicates model terms are significant. In this case A, B, D, F, and H are significant model terms. The R^2 value of 0.9528 specifies that 95.2% of the total variation in the biomass yield is ascribed to the predictor variables. The "Pred R^2" of 0.7519 is in reasonable agreement with the "Adj R^2" of 0.8997. "Adeq Precision" measures the signal to noise ratio. A ratio greater than 4 is desirable, and thus, a ratio of 13.9798 indicates an adequate signal. The model shows standard deviation, mean, C.V., and PRESS values of 0.3055, 4.56, 6.7%, and 3.93, respectively.

3.4. Optimization by BBD

The influence of five effective variables (pH, temperature, yeast extract, magnesium sulphate, and glycerol) on anti-tubercular activity and biomass production was investigated and optimized using BBD of RSM at three different levels (Table 5). Run no. 7 showed maximum anti-tubercular activity and biomass yield of 98.7±1.3% and 8.3±0.05 mg/mL, respectively in the fermentation medium of pH 6.5 constituting yeast extract 0.5% w/v, magnesium sulphate 0.1% w/v, and glycerol 1.5% v/v, being incubated at 30°C (Table 6). The BBD optimization estimated plausible enhancement in the anti-tubercular activity and approximately 4 fold improvement in the biomass of strain MANF2 with respect to traditional OFAT method. It was reported that the observed values for anti-tubercular activity and biomass production were in good agreement with predicted response values (Table 6), thereby representing closeness to the diagonal lines (Figure 3).

ANOVA was determined for validating as well as evaluating the significance of the quadratic regression model, and the results for anti-tubercular activity using BBD have been depicted in Table 7. The Model F-value of 103.67 implies that the model is significant. Values of "Prob > F" < 0.05 indicate model terms are significant. In this case C, D, E, AC, AD, AE, BC, BE, CE, DE, A^2, B^2, D^2, and E^2 were observed to be statistically significant ($P<0.05$). The R^2 value (0.9881) of this model was close to the "Adj R^2" value (0.9786). The "Pred R^2" of 0.9547 is in reasonable agreement with the "Adj R^2" value. "Adeq Precision" measures the signal to noise ratio. In the present model, a ratio of 40.692 indicates an adequate signal. The Lack of Fit F-value of 2.95 implies the Lack of Fit is not significant relative to the pure error. Non-significant lack of fit is good. Thus, this model can be used to navigate the design space. The model equation for the anti-tubercular activity can be written as given below:

$$\text{Anti-tubercular activity } (Y) = 90.27 + 0.2875A - 0.6813B + 2.79C + 4.53D - 3.78E + 0.00AB + 3.85AC + 2.77AD + 2.83AE + 4.35BC - 0.35BD - 6.93BE + 1.52CD - 3.00CE - 2.83DE - 16.77A^2 - 16.88B^2 - 1.21C^2 - 1.60D^2 - 13.63E^2 \quad \text{[Equation 7]}$$

Table 8 illustrates the ANOVA results for biomass of strain MANF2 using BBD. The Model F-value of 82.00 implies that the model is significant. Values of "Prob > F" < 0.05 indicate model terms are significant. In this case, C, D, E, AC, AD, AE, BC, BE, CE, DE, A^2, B^2, D^2, and E^2 were too observed statistically significant ($P<0.05$). The R^2 value (0.9850) of this model was close to the "Adj R^2" value (0.9730). The "Pred R^2" of 0.9430 is in reasonable agreement with the "Adj R^2" value. "Adeq Precision" measures the signal to noise ratio. In the present model, a ratio of 36.5918 indicates an adequate signal. The Lack of Fit F-value of 2.90 implies the Lack of Fit is not significant relative to the pure error. Non-significant lack of fit is good. Thus, this model can be used to navigate the design space. The model equation for the biomass production can be written as given below:

Biomass (Z) = 7.53 + 0.0312A – 0.05B + 0.2375C + 0.375D – 0.3188E + 0.00AB + 0.325AC + 0.25AD + 0.25AE +0.35BC - 0.05BD - 0.6BE + 0.15CD - 0.225CE - 0.25DE - 1.39A^2 - 1.42B^2 - 0.1C^2 - 0.1333D^2 - 1.14E^2 [Equation 8]

The three dimensional (3D) response surface plots revealed the interdependent interaction between two variables for anti-tubercular activity (Figure 4). The anti-tubercular activity was determined by interacting pH and temperature (Figure 4a), pH and yeast extract (Figure 4b), pH and magnesium sulphate (Figure 4c), pH and glycerol (Figure 4d), temperature and yeast extract (Figure 4e), temperature and magnesium sulphate (Figure 4f), temperature and glycerol (Figure 4g), yeast extract and magnesium sulphate (Figure 4h), yeast extract and glycerol (Figure 4i), and magnesium sulphate and glycerol (Figure 4j). Further, perturbation graph also showed that yeast extract, magnesium sulphate, and glycerol significantly ($P \leq 0.05$) enhanced the anti-tubercular activity (Figure 5). Residuals versus (vs.) Factor or the probability plot of actual and predicted values of response are shown in Figure 6a. The normal probability plot compared the distribution of the residuals to a normal distribution (the straight line). The inside look provides "S-shaped" pattern, which represents that an appropriate analysis can be achieved by response transformation. Residuals vs. Run for anti-tubercular activities are clearly illustrated in Figure 6b, indicating the highest response at Run no. 7. The influence of variables is illustrated in the cube plot which depicts varied predictions for distinct values of response (Figure 7).

Likewise, yeast extract, magnesium sulphate, and glycerol were also observed to enhance the biomass yield significantly, as represented by 2D counter plot (Figure 8). The perturbation graph also showed that yeast extract, magnesium sulphate, and glycerol significantly ($P \leq 0.05$) enhanced the biomass yield (Figure 9). Residuals vs. Factor or the probability plot of actual and predicted values of response are shown in Figure 10a. The normal probability plot compared the distribution of the residuals to a normal distribution (the straight line). The inside look provides "S-shaped" pattern, which represents that an appropriate analysis can be achieved by response transformation. Residuals vs. Run for biomass yield is clearly illustrated in Figure 10b, indicating the highest yield at Run no. 7. The influence of variables is illustrated in the cube plot which depicts varied predictions for distinct values of response (Figure 11).

The optimized variables selected through BBD were further used for the authentication experiment based on the methodology described earlier. The observed response values were estimated to be very much close to the predicted response values, thereby indicating the validation of model towards the enhancement of anti-tubercular activity and biomass of strain MANF2.

3.5. Purification of protein

The anti-tubercular protein was purified using standard protein purification techniques including ammonium sulphate precipitation, dialysis, and DEAE–Cellulose column chromatography. Initially, ammonium sulphate at varied saturation levels (40–80%) was implied to precipitate the protein. Total protein content was estimated based on regression curve equation (Y = -0.122+0.001X) obtained (Figure 12) Proteins precipitated at 60% saturation showed relatively higher total protein content (1922.3±9.3 mg/L) than that of other saturations (Figure 13). The protein precipitated with 60% saturation was used for dialysis which revealed total protein content of 188.3 mg with 75.1% recovery and purification fold of 9.58 (Table 9). The dialysed product was further purified using DEAE-Cellulose column chromatography. After column chromatography, the yield and purification fold of protein were estimated to be 69.4% and 507.31, respectively (Table 9). A total of 16 fractions (2 mL) were collected from the elution process and tested for anti-tubercular activities as well as total protein content determination. Among all the fractions tested, fraction 7 showed maximum protein content and activity. This fraction was lyophilized and used for molecular mass determination.

3.6. Molecular mass determination

The molecular mass of the purified protein was observed using SDS-PAGE which showed a single homogeneous band corresponding to the molecular mass of approximately 8 kDa based on relative mobility (Figure 14).

3.7. Mass spectrometry and N- terminal amino acid sequencing

Figure 15 shows MALDI-TOF MS/MS spectrum of purified protein. The nominal mass of the purified protein was found to be 7712.3 dalton (Da) as obtained from PMF analysis. Each peak in the spectrum represents peptides present in the tryptic digest of purified protein. The size of the peptide ion varies from m/z 101.15 to 1922.12. The most abundant peptide ion is m/z 1922.12. Identification of protein using database which contains theoretical tryptic digests of all known proteins revealed the sequence homology (95%) with 1-336 amino acids of Glyceraldehyde-3-phosphate dehydrogenase from *Staphylococcus* sp. The amino acid sequence of the most abundant peptide (*m/z* = 1922.12) in the purified protein was identified as: 'Lys-Ala-Ile-Gly-Leu-Val-Ile-Pro-Glu-Ile-Asp-Gly-Lys-Leu-Asp-Gly-Gly-Ala-Gln-Arg-Val' (KAIGLVIPEIDGKLDGGAQRV).

3.8. Anti-tubercular activity of protein

The anti-tubercular activities of purified protein were estimated to be increased in a concentration dependent manner (10-50 μg/mL) ranging from RLU reductions of 34.6±0.3 to 71.4±0.4% with respect to the standard (75.5±0.5 to 99.9±0.5%) (Figure 16).

3.9. Characterization of protein

The impact of pH, temperature, and enzymes on the residual anti-tubercular activities of purified protein is shown in Table 10. The anti-tubercular activities of protein varied significantly ($P<0.05$) at various pHs. The protein retained its activity at pH 6.0 and 7.0 with residual activities of 94.6±0.5 and 96.8±0.4%. The residual anti-tubercular activities of protein were reduced at acidic and alkaline pHs.

The heat treatment on purified protein revealed significant ($P<0.05$) variations in residual anti-tubercular activities. The protein retained maximum residual activity of 96.5±0.4% at 40^{0}C for 2 h. The residual anti-tubercular activities were drastically reduced (8.6±0.4%) at high temperature (121^{0}C for 15 min).

The anti-tubercular activities of purified protein were lost completely after treatment with pepsin, trypsin, and protease K. On the other hand, the protein was found resistant to α-amylase, showing residual activity of 98.2±0.5%.

3.10. Anticancer activity of purified protein

The anticancer activities of protein against A549 cell line are shown in Figure 17. After treatment with purified protein at various doses, cell shrinkage followed by rounding of cells and reduction in cell counts occur. The viabilities of A549 cells were estimated (96.6±0.3-46.3±0.4%) to be reduced significantly ($P<0.05$) with increase in the protein concentrations. A similar morphological alteration was observed in HT-29 cells after treatment with purified protein (Figure 18). The viabilities of HT-29 cell lines were also estimated (98.6±0.3-49.5±0.4%) to be reduced significantly ($P<0.05$) with increase in the protein concentrations. The purified protein revealed comparatively higher anticancer activity against A549 cells with respect to HT-29 cells. The IC_{50} values of purified protein against A549 and HT-29 cells were calculated as 46.6 and

48.9 μg/mL, respectively. In contrary to this, doxorubicin exhibited pronounced anticancer activities with IC_{50} values of 7.4 and 9.6 μg/mL against A549 and HT-29 cells, respectively.

3.11. Fourier transform infra-red spectroscopy

The FT-IR spectrum of the purified protein is shown in Figure 19. The high absorption bands at 3448.6, 1637.48, 1401.69, and 1085.87 cm^{-1} indicate the presence of strong N-H stretch, C-N bond of Amide I, N-H bond, and C-N bond, respectively.

Table 1: Selected variables in Taguchi OA design and assigned levels for anti-tubercular activity as well as biomass yield.

Factors	Code	Unit	Level 1	Level 2	Level 3
pH	A	-	6.0	6.5	-
Temperature	B	°C	30	35	-
Dextrose	C	% w/v	0.5	1.0	1.5
Yeast extract	D	% w/v	0.1	0.3	0.5
Ammonium chloride	E	% w/v	0.1	0.25	0.5
Magnesium sulphate	F	% w/v	0.01	0.025	0.05
Calcium chloride	G	% w/v	0.01	0.025	0.05
Glycerol	H	% v/v	0.5	1.0	1.5

Table 2: L18 ($2^2 \times 3^6$) Taguchi OA design experiments for anti-tubercular activity and biomass yield.

Run	A	B	C	D	E	F	G	H	Anti-tubercular activity (% RLU reduction)	Biomass (mg/mL)
1	1	1	1	1	1	1	1	1	48.8	3.2
2	1	2	2	1	2	3	2	1	55.4	3.7
3	2	2	3	1	2	2	1	2	54.6	3.6
4	1	1	3	3	2	3	3	3	52.1	3.5
5	2	1	2	1	1	2	3	3	96.6	6.5
6	2	2	1	1	3	3	3	2	50.4	3.3
7	1	2	2	3	1	3	1	2	58.4	3.9
8	2	2	2	2	2	1	1	3	76.6	5.1
9	1	2	3	2	1	1	3	2	73.6	4.9
10	2	1	1	3	2	1	2	2	92.4	6.2
11	1	2	1	3	3	2	1	3	74.5	5.0
12	2	1	3	2	3	3	1	1	86.4	5.8
13	2	2	2	3	3	1	3	1	62.8	4.2
14	1	1	2	2	3	2	2	2	64.5	4.3
15	1	2	3	1	3	1	2	3	66.4	4.4
16	2	2	1	2	1	3	2	3	76.5	5.1
17	1	2	1	2	2	2	3	1	68.4	4.6
18	2	2	3	3	1	2	2	1	72.4	4.8

Table 3: Analysis of variance of Taguchi OA design for main significant factors towards anti-tubercular activity.

Source	Sum of Squares	df	Mean Square	*F*-value	*P*-value	
Model	3219.22	9	357.69	16.54	0.0003	Significant
A-A	631.31	1	631.31	29.20	0.0006	
B-B	233.07	1	233.07	10.78	0.0111	
D-D	455.23	2	227.62	10.53	0.0057	
F-F	250.30	2	125.15	5.79	0.0279	
H-H	262.99	2	131.49	6.08	0.0248	
Residual	172.97	8	21.62			
Cor Total	3392.19	17				

R^2 = 0.949; Adjusted R^2 = 0.8916; Predicted R^2 = 0.7365; Adeq precision = 13.4119; C.V.% = 6.8; Std. Dev. = 4.65; Mean = 68.38; PRESS = 893.9; df = degree of freedom ; $P \leq 0.05$ = Significant

Table 4: Analysis of variance of Taguchi OA design for main significant factors towards biomass yield.

Source	Sum of Squares	df	Mean Square	*F*-value	*P*-value	
Model	15.08	9	1.68	17.95	0.0002	Significant
A-A	2.80	1	2.80	30.01	0.0006	
B-B	1.14	1	1.14	12.19	0.0082	
D-D	2.18	2	1.09	11.68	0.0042	
F-F	1.12	2	0.5606	6.01	0.0255	
H-H	1.25	2	0.6239	6.68	0.0196	
Residual	0.7467	8	0.0933			
Cor Total	15.82	17				

$R^2 = 0.9528$; Adjusted $R^2 = 0.8997$; Predicted $R^2 = 0.7519$; Adeq precision = 13.9798; C.V.% = 6.7; Std. Dev. = 0.3055; Mean = 4.56; PRESS = 3.93; df = degree of freedom; $P \leq 0.05$ = Significant

Table 5: Experimental range, level, and code of independent variables for BBD design.

Variables	Code	Unit	Range and Levels		
			-1	**0**	**+1**
pH	A	-	6	6.5	7
Temperature	B	^0C	28	30	32
Yeast extract	C	% w/v	0.05	0.1	0.5
Magnesium sulphate	D	% w/v	0.025	0.05	0.1
Glycerol	E	% v/v	1.0	1.5	2.0

Table 6: Box-Behnken design for optimizing anti-tubercular activity and biomass production.

Run order	A	B	C	D	E	Anti-tubercular activity (% RLU reduction)		Biomass (mg/mL)	
						Experimental	Predicted	Experimental	Predicted
1	0	+1	0	0	+1	47.3	48.37	3.9	4.01
2	0	-1	0	+1	0	77.6	77.35	6.5	6.46
3	0	0	+1	0	-1	85.3	85.0	7.1	7.07
4	0	0	0	+1	-1	84.4	86.18	7.0	7.2
5	0	0	-1	0	-1	76.3	73.41	6.4	6.15
6	0	0	0	0	0	91.3	90.27	7.6	7.53
7	0	0	+1	+1	0	98.7	96.3	8.3	8.06
8	0	+1	0	0	-1	70.4	69.78	5.9	5.84
9	+1	0	+1	0	0	78.4	79.21	6.5	6.64
10	0	-1	0	0	+1	60.4	63.58	5.0	5.31
11	-1	0	-1	0	0	70.3	73.05	5.9	6.1
12	+1	0	0	0	+1	60.6	59.19	5.1	4.96
13	-1	0	0	+1	0	73.4	73.36	6.1	6.12
14	+1	+1	0	0	0	57.3	56.22	4.8	4.71
15	0	0	0	0	0	89.3	90.27	7.5	7.53
16	0	0	-1	0	+1	73.4	71.85	6.1	5.96
17	0	0	0	0	0	91.8	90.27	7.7	7.53
18	0	0	+1	-1	0	84.4	84.19	7.0	7.01
19	0	0	-1	-1	0	80.7	81.65	6.7	6.84
20	0	+1	+1	0	0	78.8	78.63	6.6	6.55
21	-1	0	0	-1	0	70.3	69.85	5.9	5.85
22	0	0	-1	+1	0	88.9	87.67	7.4	7.29
23	+1	0	0	+1	0	78.6	79.49	6.6	6.66
24	-1	0	0	0	-1	66.6	66.18	5.6	5.54
25	+1	0	0	-1	0	64.4	64.88	5.4	5.41
26	-1	+1	0	0	0	55.6	55.64	4.6	4.64
27	-1	0	0	0	+1	55.1	52.97	4.6	4.4
28	0	+1	0	+1	0	74.5	75.29	6.2	6.26
29	+1	0	0	0	-1	60.8	61.11	5.1	5.12
30	0	-1	-1	0	0	74.5	74.41	6.2	6.18
31	0	0	0	0	0	89.8	90.27	7.5	7.53

32	0	0	0	+1	+1	72.5	72.96	6.0	6.06
33	0	0	0	0	0	90.3	90.27	7.5	7.53
34	0	-1	0	-1	0	68.5	67.59	5.7	5.61
35	+1	0	-1	0	0	63.7	65.92	5.3	5.51
36	0	+1	0	-1	0	66.8	66.93	5.6	5.61
37	-1	-1	0	0	0	58.1	57.01	4.8	4.74
38	0	0	0	0	0	89.1	90.27	7.4	7.53
39	0	0	+1	0	+1	70.4	71.43	5.9	5.99
40	0	+1	-1	0	0	64.5	64.35	5.4	5.38
41	+1	-1	0	0	0	59.8	57.58	5.0	4.81
42	0	-1	+1	0	0	71.4	71.3	6.0	5.95
43	0	-1	0	0	-1	55.8	57.29	4.6	4.74
44	0	0	0	-1	+1	70.2	69.55	5.9	5.81
45	0	0	0	-1	-1	70.8	71.46	5.9	5.95
46	-1	0	+1	0	0	69.6	70.94	5.8	5.92

Table 7: Analysis of variance for optimizing anti-tubercular activity using BBD.

Source	Sum of Squares	df	Mean Square	*F*-value	*P*-value	
Model	6303.53	20	315.18	103.67	< 0.0001	significant
A-A	1.32	1	1.32	0.4350	0.5156	
B-B	7.43	1	7.43	2.44	0.1307	
C-C	124.88	1	124.88	41.08	< 0.0001	
D-D	328.52	1	328.52	108.06	< 0.0001	
E-E	228.77	1	228.77	75.25	< 0.0001	
AB	9.095E-13	1	9.095E-13	2.992E-13	1.0000	
AC	59.29	1	59.29	19.50	0.0002	
AD	30.80	1	30.80	10.13	0.0039	
AE	31.92	1	31.92	10.50	0.0034	
BC	75.69	1	75.69	24.90	< 0.0001	
BD	0.4900	1	0.4900	0.1612	0.6915	
BE	191.82	1	191.82	63.10	< 0.0001	
CD	9.30	1	9.30	3.06	0.0925	
CE	36.00	1	36.00	11.84	0.0020	
DE	31.92	1	31.92	10.50	0.0034	
A^2	2455.25	1	2455.25	807.63	< 0.0001	
B^2	2487.07	1	2487.07	818.10	< 0.0001	
C^2	12.87	1	12.87	4.23	0.0502	
D^2	22.28	1	22.28	7.33	0.0120	
E^2	1621.62	1	1621.62	533.42	< 0.0001	
Residual	76.00	25	3.04			
Lack of Fit	70.07	20	3.50	2.95	0.1166	not significant
Pure Error	5.93	5	1.19			
Cor Total	6379.53	45				

$R^2 = 0.9881$; Adjusted $R^2 = 0.9786$; Predicted $R^2 = 0.9547$; C.V.% = 2.39; Adeq precision = 40.6916; df = degree of freedom; Highly significant = $P \leq 0.0001$; Significant = $P \leq 0.05$; Non- significant = $P > 0.05$

Table 8: Analysis of variance for optimizing biomass yield using BBD.

Source	Sum of Squares	df	Mean Square	*F*-value	*P*-value	
Model	44.15	20	2.21	82.00	< 0.0001	significant
A-A	0.0156	1	0.0156	0.5805	0.4532	
B-B	0.0400	1	0.0400	1.49	0.2342	
C-C	0.9025	1	0.9025	33.53	< 0.0001	
D-D	2.25	1	2.25	83.59	< 0.0001	
E-E	1.63	1	1.63	60.39	< 0.0001	
AB	7.105E-15	1	7.105E-15	2.640E-13	1.0000	
AC	0.4225	1	0.4225	15.70	0.0005	
AD	0.2500	1	0.2500	9.29	0.0054	
AE	0.2500	1	0.2500	9.29	0.0054	
BC	0.4900	1	0.4900	18.20	0.0002	
BD	0.0100	1	0.0100	0.3715	0.5477	
BE	1.44	1	1.44	53.50	< 0.0001	
CD	0.0900	1	0.0900	3.34	0.0794	
CE	0.2025	1	0.2025	7.52	0.0111	
DE	0.2500	1	0.2500	9.29	0.0054	
A^2	16.90	1	16.90	627.95	< 0.0001	
B^2	17.52	1	17.52	650.72	< 0.0001	
C^2	0.0873	1	0.0873	3.24	0.0838	
D^2	0.1552	1	0.1552	5.76	0.0241	
E^2	11.38	1	11.38	422.61	< 0.0001	
Residual	0.6729	25	0.0269			
Lack of Fit	0.6196	20	0.0310	2.90	0.1202	not significant
Pure Error	0.0533	5	0.0107			
Cor Total	44.82	45				

R^2 = 0.9850; Adjusted R^2 = 0.9730; Predicted R^2 = 0.9430; C.V.% = 2.7; Adeq precision = 36.5918; df = degree of freedom; Highly significant = $P \leq 0.0001$; Significant = $P \leq 0.05$; Non- significant = $P > 0.05$

Table 9: Purification of protein from strain MANF2.

Purification step	Volume (mL)	RLU (%)	Total protein (mg)	Specific activity	Purification fold	Yield (%)
CFNS	1000	98.7	2432.4	0.041	1	100
Ammonium sulphate precipitation	1000	82.3	1922.3	0.042	1.02	83.4
Dialysis	10	74.1	188.3	0.393	9.58	75.1
DEAE – Cellulose column chromatography	2	68.4	3.3	20.8	507.31	69.4

Table 10: Effect of pH, temperature, and enzymes on residual anti-tubercular activity of protein.

Treatment	Residual activity (%)
pH	
Control	100±0.5^{a}
3	41.3±0.4^{f}
4	48.6±0.4^{e}
5	53.5±0.5^{d}
6	94.6±0.5^{c}
7	96.8±0.4^{b}
8	52.6±0.4^{d}
Temperature	
Control	100±0.5^{a}
40°C, 2 h	96.5±0.4^{b}
60°C, 1 h	51.3±0.4^{c}
80°C, 30 min	28.5±0.5^{d}
100°C, 20 min	12.3±0.5^{e}
121°C, 15 min	8.6±0.4^{f}
Enzymes	
Control	100±0.5^{a}
Pepsin	0.00±0.00
Trypsin	0.00±0.00
Protease K	0.00±0.00
α-amylase	98.2±0.5^{b}

Values represent mean±SD of experiments carried out in triplicate (n = 3).

^{a,b,c,d,e,f}Means followed by different superscripts are significantly different (*P*<0.05).

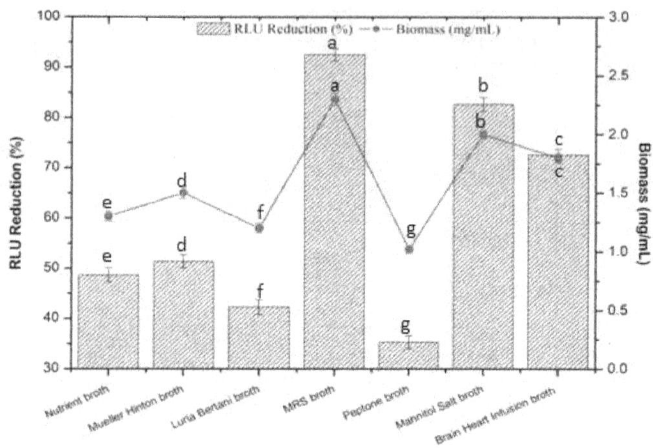

Figure 1: Anti-tubercular activity and biomass yield of strain MANF2 in the presence of various media.

[Note: Values are represented as mean±SD of experiments carried out in triplicate (n = 3). [abcdefg]Values with different letters are significantly (P<0.05) different.]

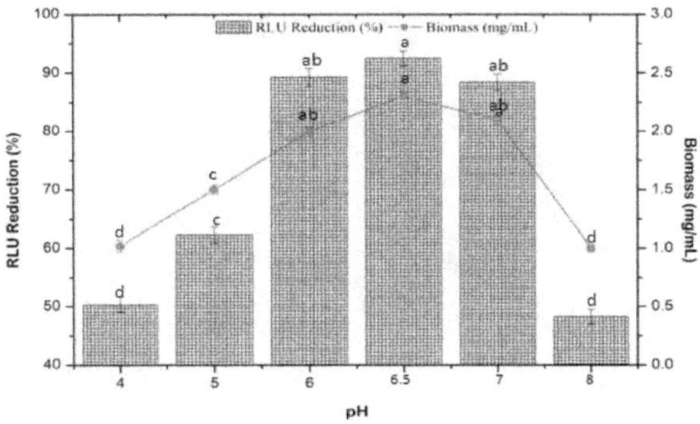

a

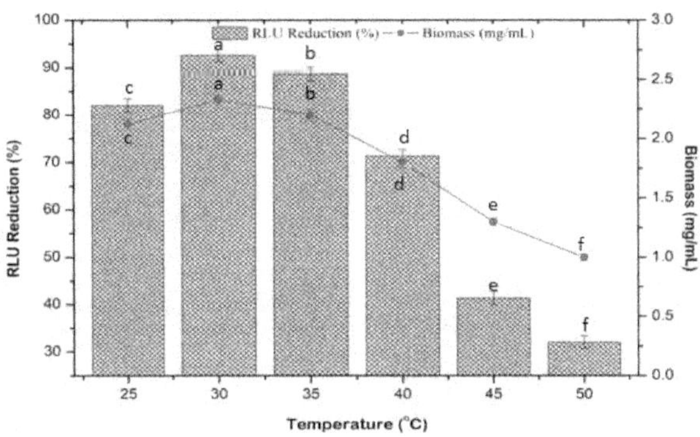

b

Continued……………

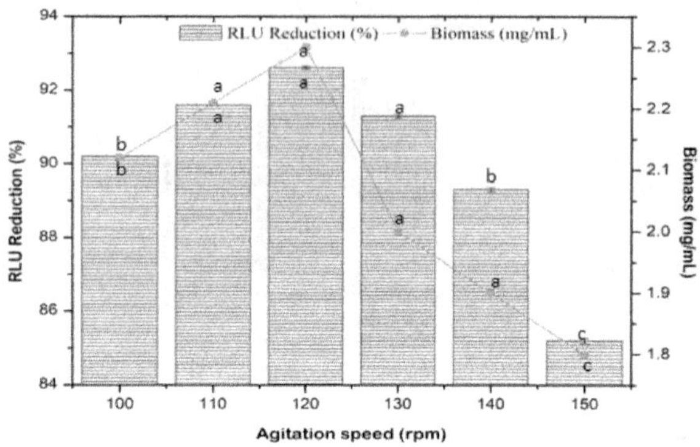

c

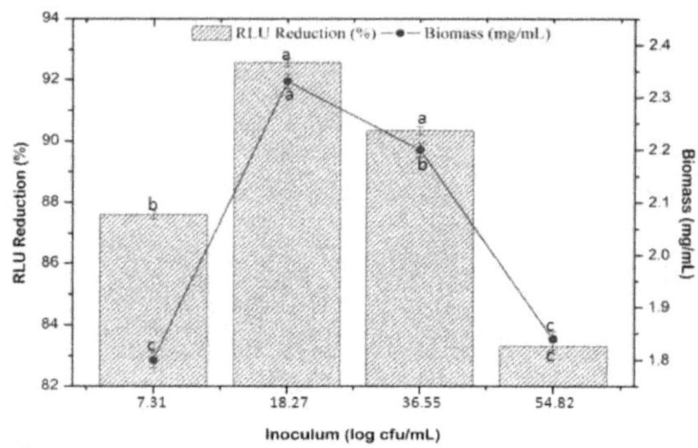

d

Continued……………

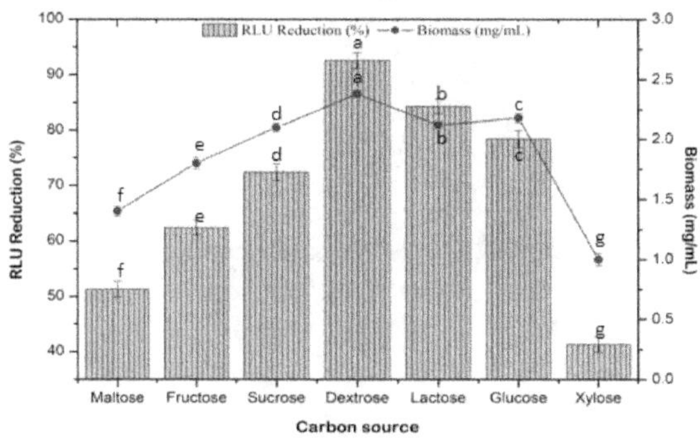

e

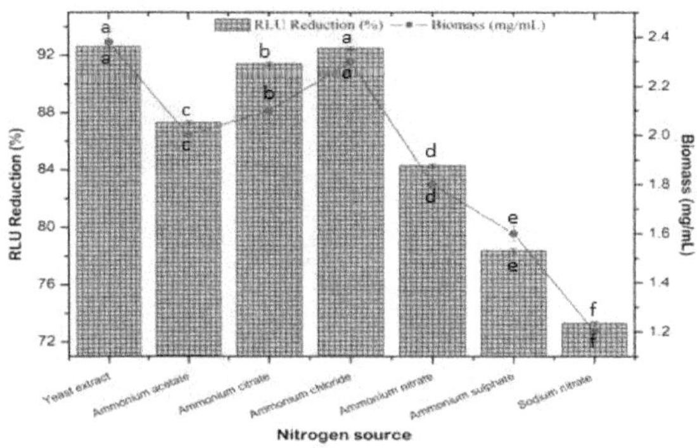

f

Continued…………

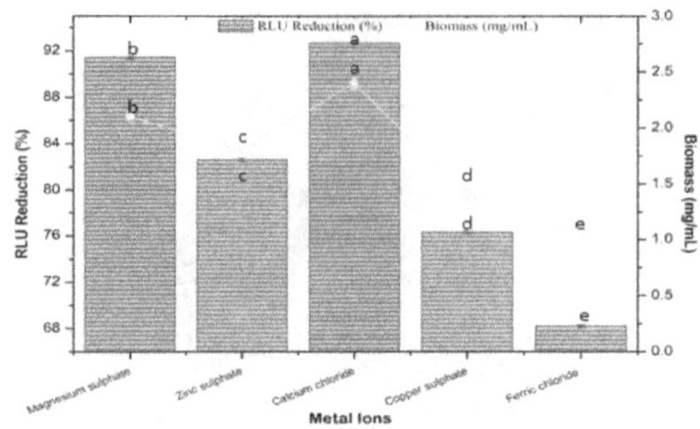

g

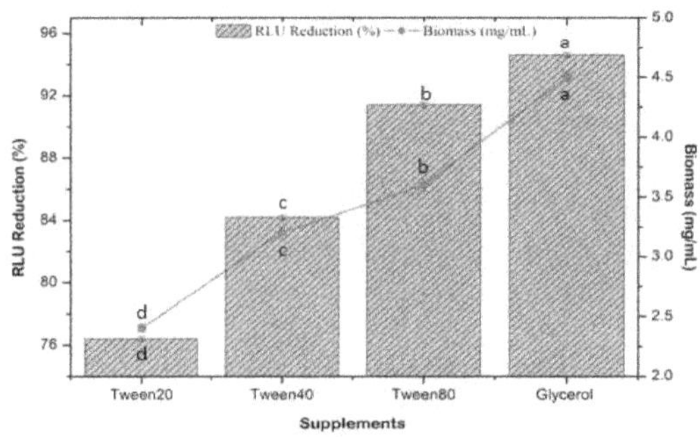

h

Figure 2: Effect of (a) pH, (b) temperature, (c) agitation speed, (d) inoculums, (e) carbon sources, (f) nitrogen sources, (g) metal ions, (h) supplements on anti-tubercular activities and biomass yield from strain MANF2 using OFAT method.

[Note: Values are represented as mean±SD of experiments carried out in triplicate (n = 3). [abcdefg]Values with different letters are significantly (P<0.05) different.]

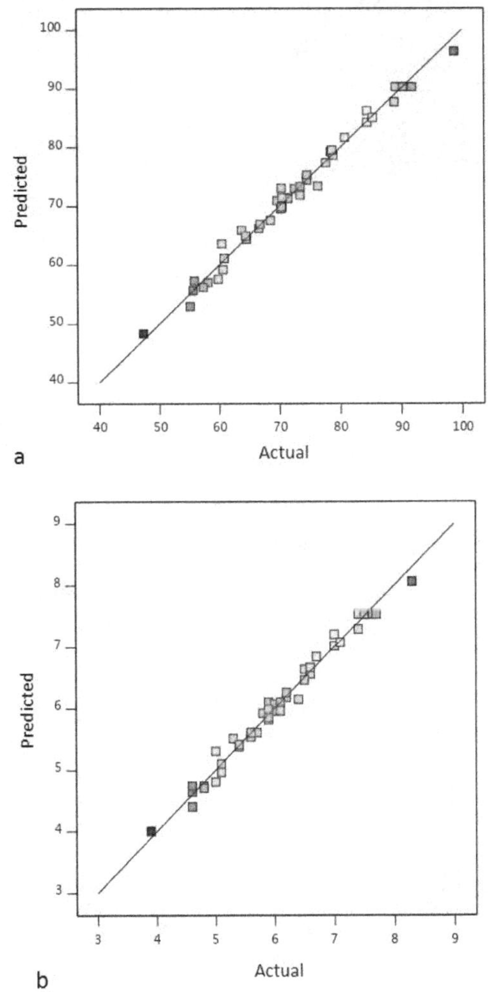

Figure 3: Observed and predicted values for (a) anti-tubercular activity and (b) biomass of strain MANF2. The response values were close to the diagonal line.

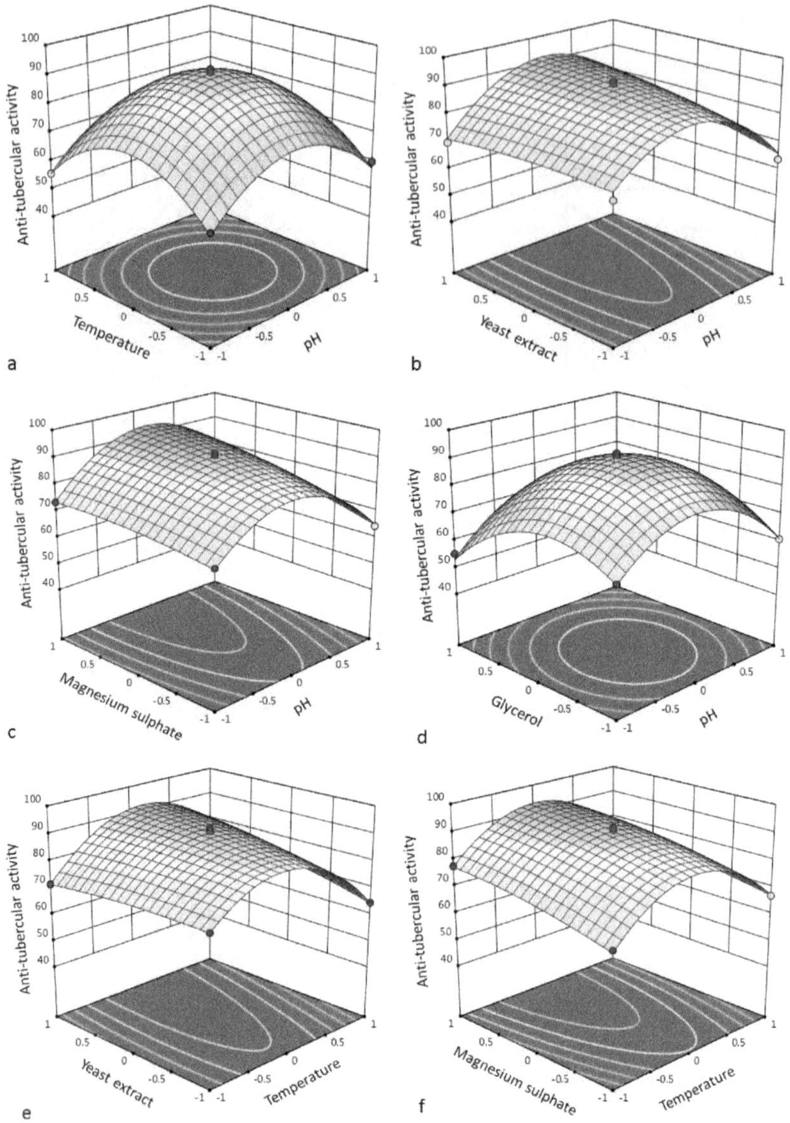

a
b
c
d
e
f
Anti-tubercular activity
Temperature
pH
Yeast extract
Magnesium sulphate
Glycerol

Continued………………

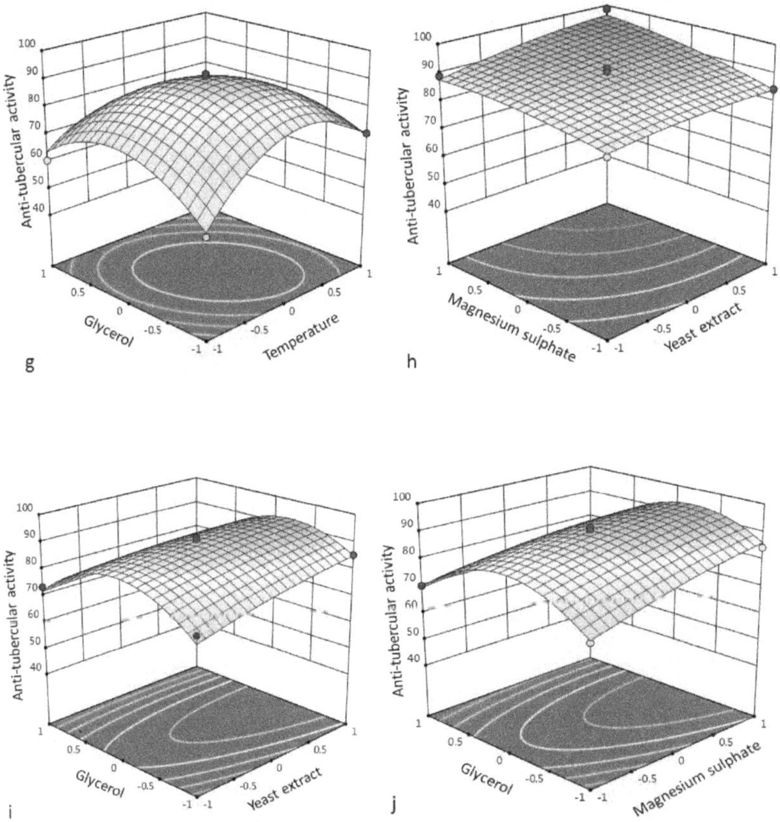

Figure 4: 3D response surface plots showing interdependent interaction between (a) pH and temperature, (b) pH and yeast extract, (c) pH and magnesium sulphate, (d) pH and glycerol, (e) temperature and yeast extract, (f) temperature and magnesium sulphate, (g) temperature and glycerol, (h) yeast extract and magnesium sulphate, (i) yeast extract and glycerol, and (j) magnesium sulphate and glycerol.

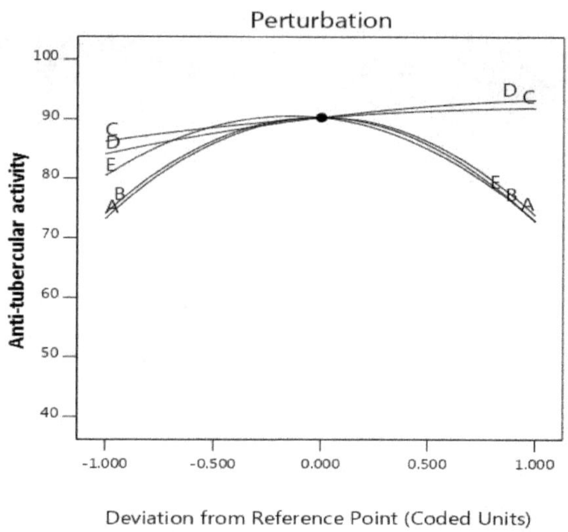

Figure 5: Perturbation graph showing effect of variables on anti-tubercular activity.

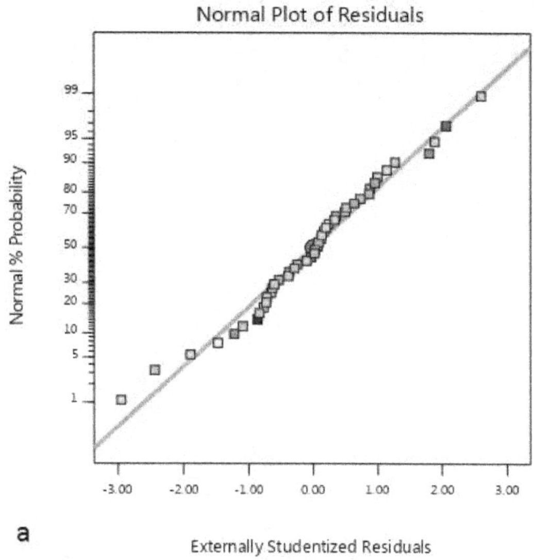

a

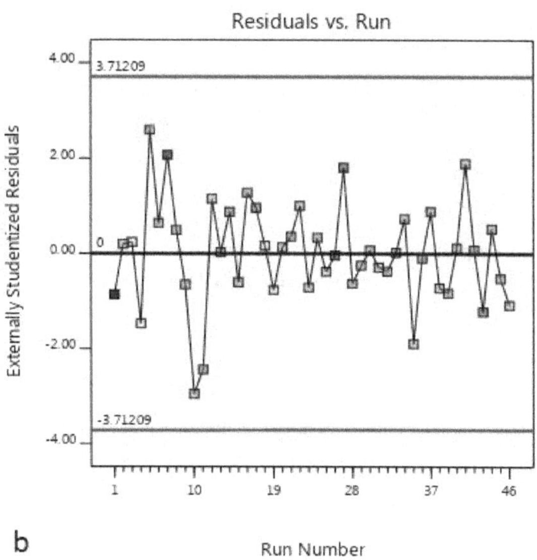

b

Figure 6: (a) Residuals vs. Factor or the probability plot of actual and predicted values of anti-tubercular activity and (b) Residuals vs. Run for anti-tubercular activities.

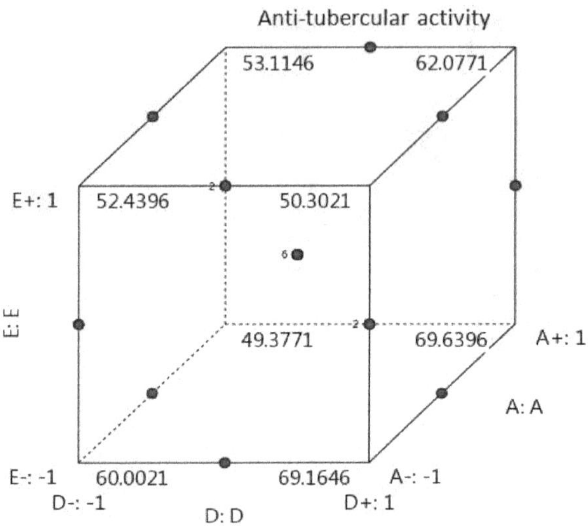

Figure 7: Cube plot showing varied predictions for distinct values of anti-tubercular activities.

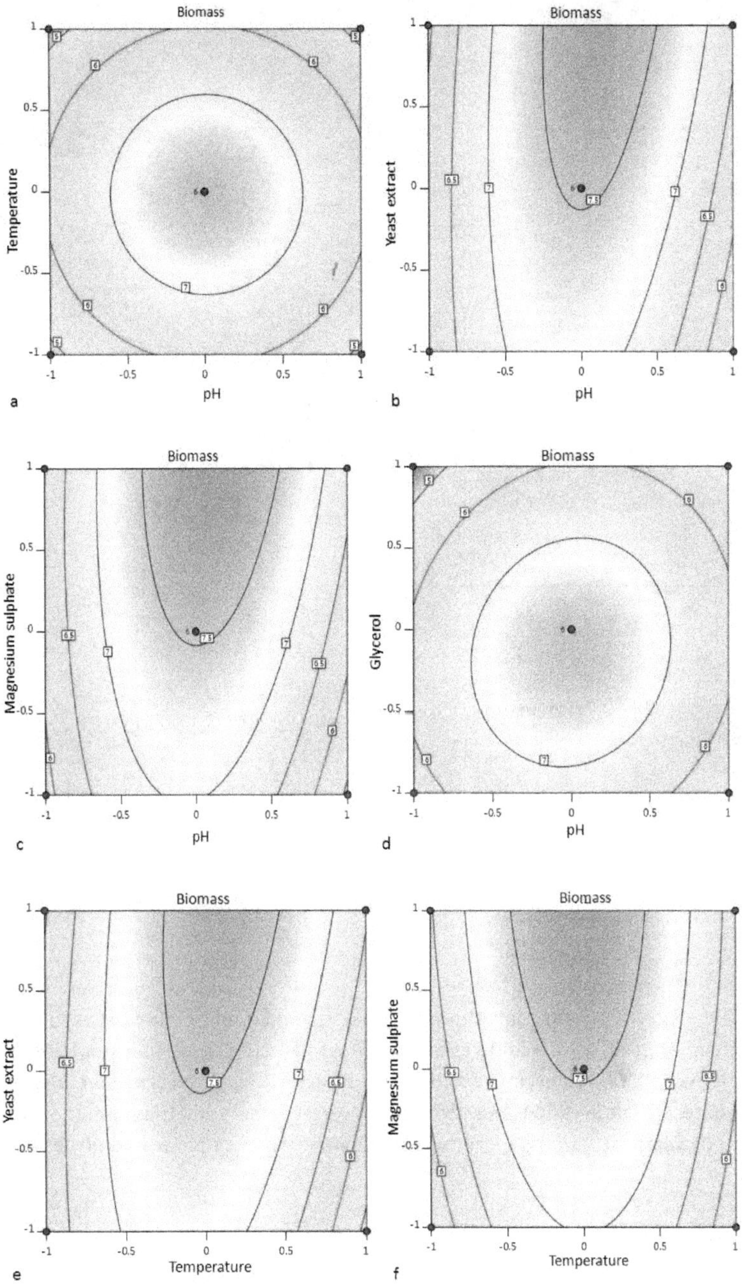
Biomass
Temperature
pH
Yeast extract
Magnesium sulphate
Glycerol
a
b
c
d
e
f

Continued…………

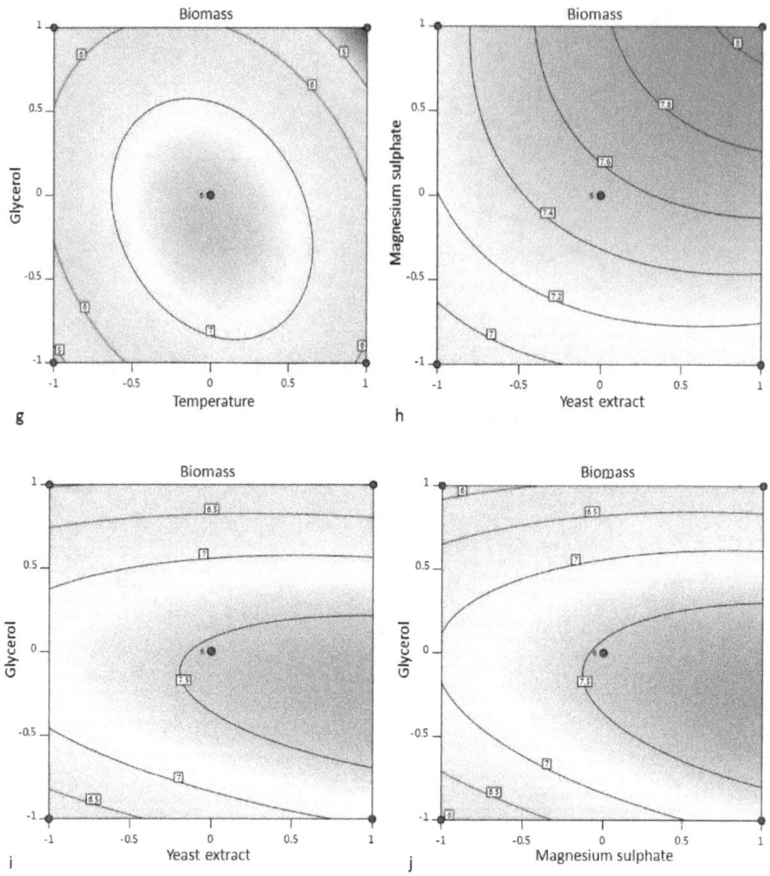

Figure 8: 2D Contour plots showing interdependent interaction between (a) pH and temperature, (b) pH and yeast extract, (c) pH and magnesium sulphate, (d) pH and glycerol, (e) temperature and yeast extract, (f) temperature and magnesium sulphate, (g) temperature and glycerol, (h) yeast extract and magnesium sulphate, (i) yeast extract and glycerol, and (j) magnesium sulphate and glycerol.

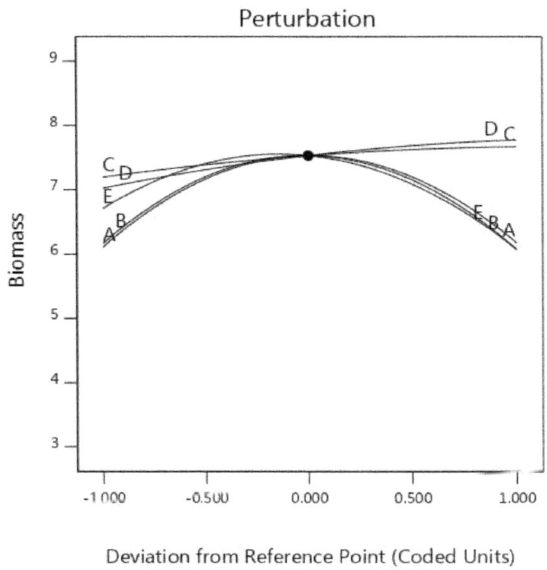

Figure 9: Perturbation graph showing effect of variables on biomass yield.

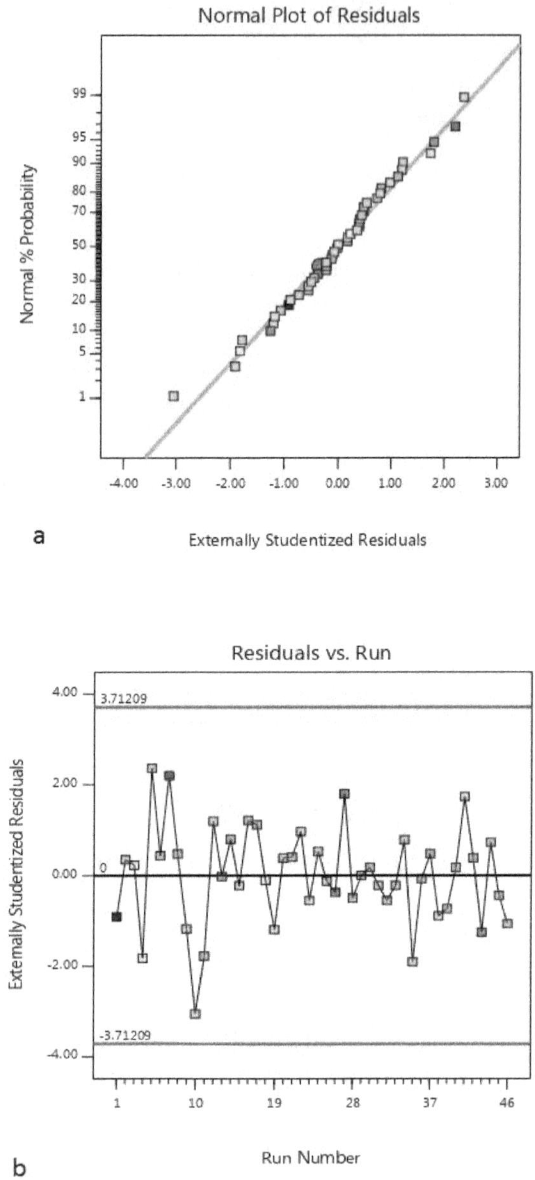

Figure 10: (a) Residuals vs. Factor or the probability plot of actual and predicted values of biomass yield and (b) Residuals vs. Run for biomass yield.

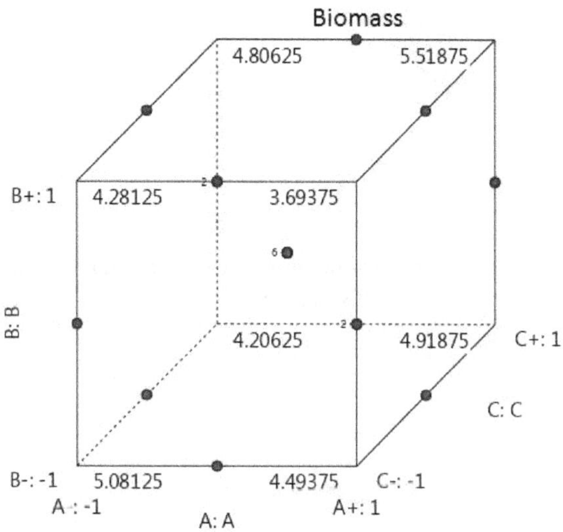

Figure 11: Cube plot showing varied predictions for distinct values of biomass yield.

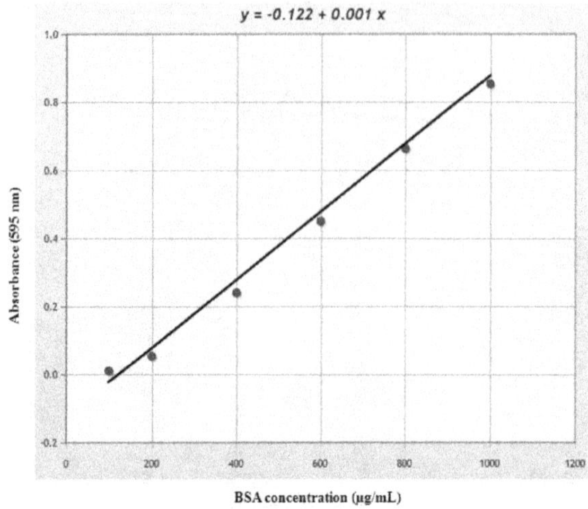

Figure 12: Regression curve equation for estimation of total protein content using BSA as standard.

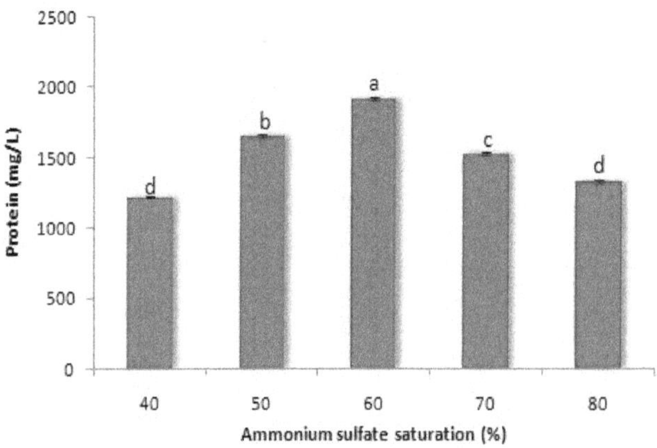

Figure 13: Total protein content determination at different saturation levels of ammonium sulphate.

[Note: Values are represented as mean±SD of experiments carried out in triplicate (n = 3). [abcd]Values with different letters are significantly ($P<0.05$) different.]

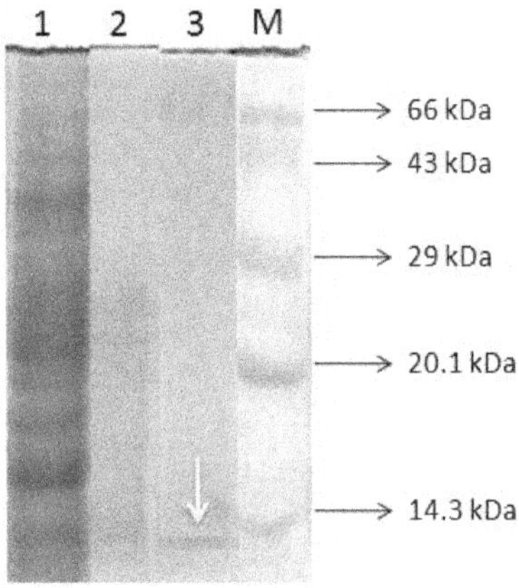

Lane 1: Ammonium sulphate precipitated sample
Lane 2: Dialysed sample
Lane 3: Purified sample
M: Protein marker

Figure 14: Molecular mass determination of purified protein using SDS-PAGE. Lane 3 showed a single homogeneous band corresponding to the molecular mass of approximately 8 kDa, indicated by yellow arrow.

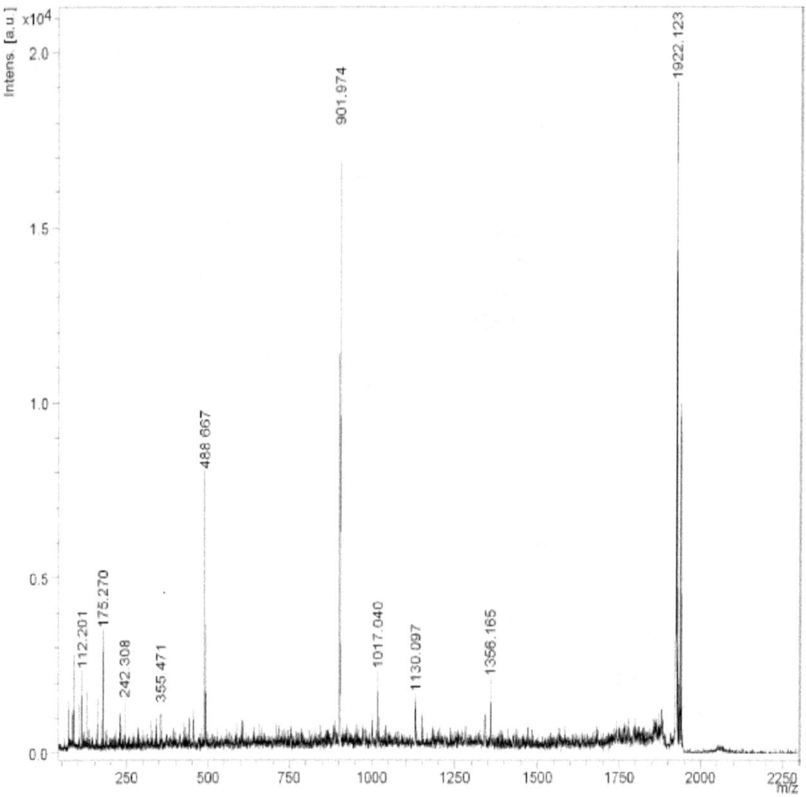

Figure 15: MALDI-TOF MS/MS spectrum of purified protein.

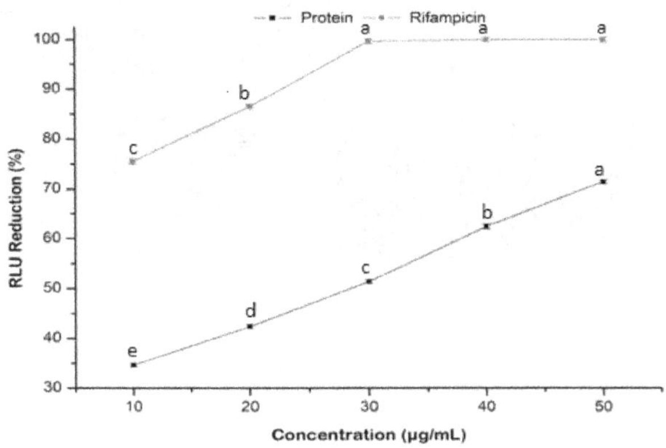

Figure 16: Anti-tubercular activities of purified protein and rifampicin at various concentrations.

[Note: Values are represented as mean±SD of experiments carried out in triplicate (n = 3). [abcde]Values with different letters are significantly ($P<0.05$) different.]

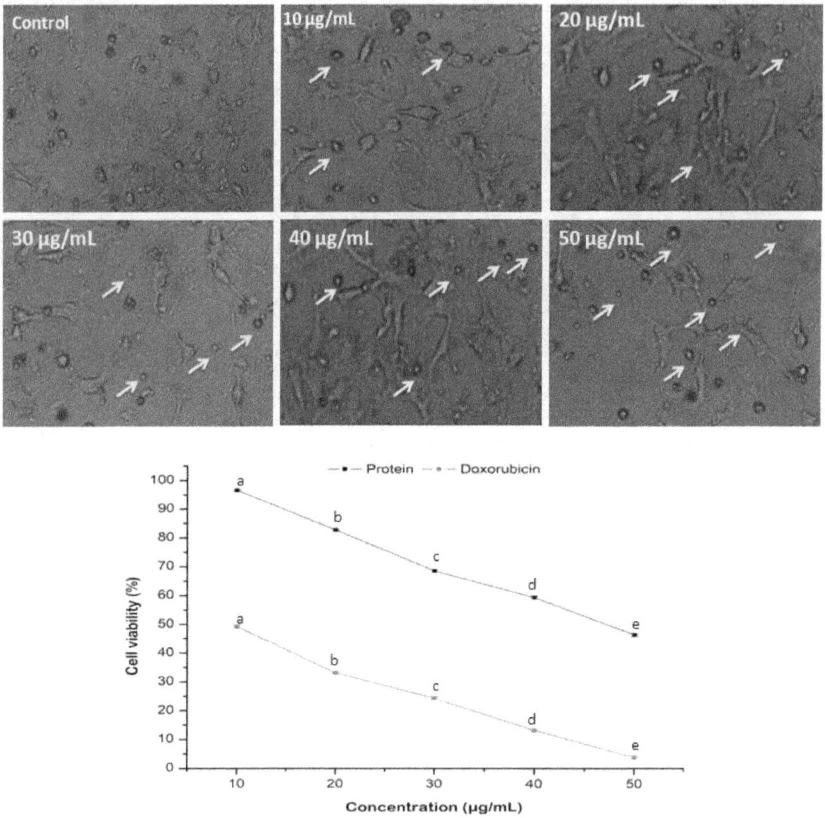

Figure 17: Morphological variations and reductions in the viabilities of A549 lung cancer cells in the presence of various concentrations of purified protein. Yellow arrows indicate morphological changes in the cancer cells.

[Note: Values are represented as mean±SD of experiments carried out in triplicate (n = 3). [abcde]Values with different letters are significantly (P<0.05) different.]

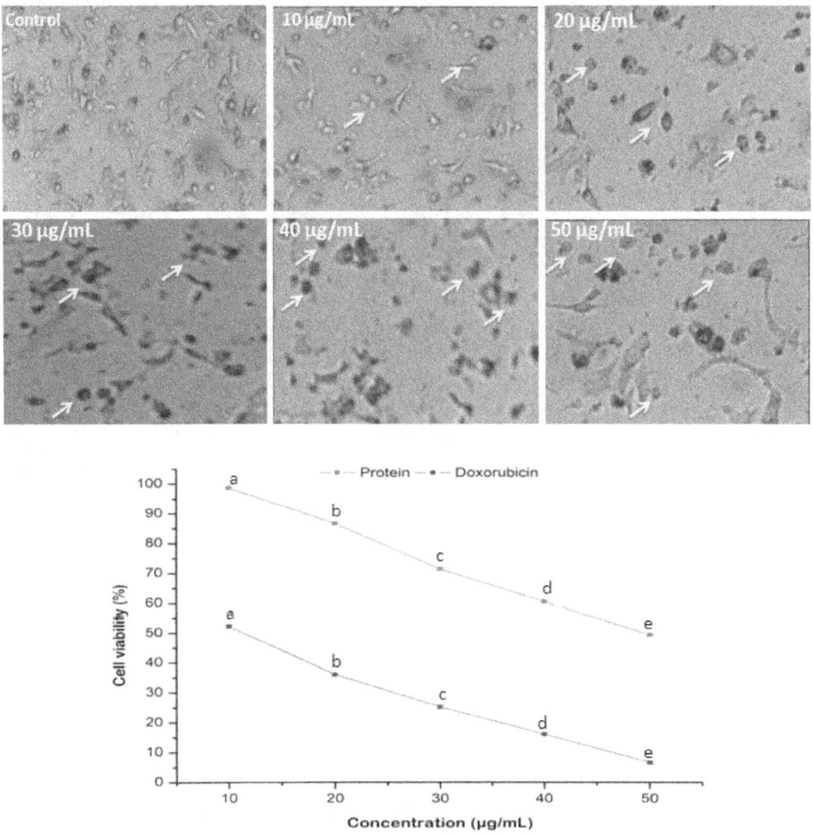

Figure 18: Morphological variations and reductions in the viabilities of HT-29 colon cancer cells in the presence of various concentrations of purified protein. Yellow arrows indicate morphological changes in the cancer cells.

[Note: Values are represented as mean±SD of experiments carried out in triplicate (n = 3). ^{abcde}Values with different letters are significantly (P<0.05) different.]

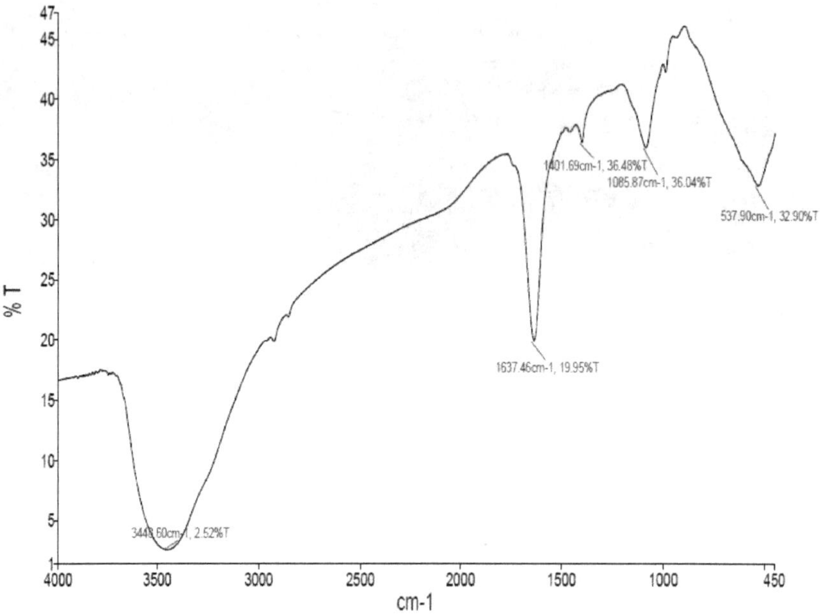

Figure 19: FT-IR spectrum of purified protein.

4. Discussion

Distinct groups of bacteria, indigenous to various fermented food products, play a critical role in the production of several bioactive metabolites (organic acids, alcohols, enzymes, proteins, antibiotics, and carbohydrates), which are known to contribute towards the safety and nutritional quality. Of them, CNS are often available as natural flora of fermented food products.

Abiotic factors and nutritional medium components are known to influence the production of antagonistic substances from probiotic bacteria. Several studies have been reported discussing the production of antibacterial substances from fermented food associated probiotic bacteria and its optimization by altering several physical factors as well as medium components (Parente *et al.*, 1994; Moortvedt-Abildgaard *et al.*, 1995; Aarti *et al.*, 2016). Probiotic bacteria and their bioactive constituents could be a promising alternative to existing antibiotics due to the pronounced activity against deadly pathogens. Considering this, there is a continuous effort by global researchers to optimize various nutritional and non-nutritional factors for the efficient production of antibacterial substances from probiotics in order to inhibit the growth of varied pathogens. In view of the continuous emergence of antibiotics resistant bacteria and the over demand of novel antagonistic agents as biotherapeutics, the present context was initially undertaken to screen the influence of physical factors and diverse nutritional constituents on the anti-tubercular activity and biomass yield of strain MANF2 using OFAT methods. This traditional method of optimization identified the significant ($P<0.05$) effect of pH, incubation temperature, carbon source (dextrose), nitrogen sources (yeast extract and ammonium chloride), metal ions (magnesium sulphate and calcium chloride), and supplement (glycerol) on the anti-tubercular activity and biomass production of strain MANF2. However, in spite of the wide applications of OFAT method in the optimization process, this time-consuming approach is being avoided at present due to large number of experiments to be carried out with probable misinterpretation of data, and certainly failure to determine the interactions between two factors (Khusro and Aarti, 2015). Hence, the statistical optimization tools were taken into further consideration for the enhancement of activity and biomass yield using the parameters selected through OFAT.

Statistical approaches have been employed constantly in recent years at varied phases of optimization strategy for targeted response(s). Taguchi OA is a fractional factorial experimental design that involves the implementation of predefined OA to study a maximal number of variables at selected levels with a minimal set of experiments. This tool determines the effect of individual factors and estimates the performance at the optimum levels obtained (Shehata and Abd El Aty, 2014). Currently, this methodology is employed for the optimization of various biotechnological processes to produce robust bioactive metabolites of interest. In the present study, we reported for the first time the statistical optimization strategy to improve anti-tubercular activity and biomass of *S. hominis* using Taguchi OA design. The ANOVA results showed the significant ($P \leq 0.05$) influence of pH, temperature, yeast extract, magnesium sulphate, and glycerol at particular assigned levels on the enhancement of anti-tubercular activity and biomass yield from strain MANF2.

The application of a good reliable statistical model is essential to develop better strategies for the optimization of valuable products (Shehata and Abd El Aty, 2014). In this regard, BBD was further implemented to enhance the anti-tubercular activity and biomass production from strain MANF2 using significant factors at different ranges. Experiments were performed considering the interaction between the control factors and operational conditions, thereby resulting in optimal performance. In our study, anti-tubercular activity and biomass yield were observed to be improved by optimizing pH, temperature, yeast extract, magnesium sulphate, and glycerol using BBD. However, yeast extract, magnesium sulphate, and glycerol revealed significant ($P \leq 0.05$) influence on both the responses. A good correlation between the experimental and predicted values verified the model and established the existence of the optimal points. The minor differences between experimental and predicted results were due to the determination coefficients (Khusro *et al.*, 2017).

The 3D response plots clearly depict that the model predicts the optimum region for responses at more or less central values of the variables. The elliptical nature of the two dimensional (2D) contour plots represents interdependent interaction between two predictor variables, whereas the circular contour plots illustrate insignificant interaction between two controlled variables. More or less similar to our findings, Arumugam and Kumar (2017) successfully investigated the enhancement of antimicrobial compounds and biomass yield from *Brevibacillus brevis* using statistical optimization tools. The present investigation and previous findings clearly suggest that these statistical optimization tools can undoubtedly be employed for modelling operational variables in order to maximize the antibacterial substances production and biomass yield from diversified potent isolates for remarkable therapeutic application.

Over the past few decades, antibacterial substances, particularly proteins or peptides of bacterial origin have gained immense interest as biotherapeutic agents. *Staphylococcus* spp. have been reported to produce a number of bioactive proteinaceous components (Bastos *et al.*, 2009). *S. hominis* MBBL 2-9, *S. pseudintermedius* strain 222, and *S. xylosus* produced novel antibacterial peptide with molecular mass of 6 kDa, 2038.4 Da, 5921.92 Da, respectively (Kim *et al.*, 2010; Wladyka *et al.*, 2015; Matikevičienė *et al.*, 2017). In this study, strain MANF2 produced anti-tubercular protein of molecular mass 7712.3 Da. Further, based on amino acid sequencing, the molecular mass of the most abundant peptide was determined as 1922.12 Da, which showed 95% homology with Glyceraldehyde-3-phosphate dehydrogenase, thereby categorizing it as new class of Glyceraldehyde-3-phosphate dehydrogenase-like protein in *S. hominis*. Also, the peptide was considered new due to the lack of homology of molecular mass with existing peptides previously reported from *Staphylococcus* spp., and thus this peptide was named as NMANF2. The purified protein exhibited promising mycobactericidal activity in a dose dependent manner, thereby indicating first report on the anti-tubercular potentiality of *S. hominis* associated protein.

Disparate pH treatment affected significantly the anti-tubercular activity of purified protein. The variation in the anti-tubercular property at lower or higher pH may be due to the denaturation of protein as electrostatic repulsion of intermolecular and breaking of hydrogen bonds (Yi *et al.*, 2016). Further, the protein lost its anti-tubercular activity at high temperature (>60^0C). It clearly suggests that heat resistance nature of protein depends on its stable structural characteristics (Kim *et al.*, 2010). The anti-tubercular trait of purified protein was lost completely after treatment with pepsin, trypsin, and protease K but its mycobactericidal attribute was retained by α-amylase treatment. Findings clearly represent that the purified product is proteinaceous in nature constituting amino acid residues, without carbohydrate moieties. Similar observations were reported by previous studies too (Kim *et al.*, 2010; Yi *et al.*, 2016).

In the present investigation, the cytotoxic activities of purified protein were determined against lung and colon cancer cells. The protein revealed comparatively higher anticancer activity against A549 cells with respect to HT-29 cells. Findings of the present study indicate the first report on the anticancer attribute of *S. hominis* associated protein. The purified protein can undeniably be used for designing new protein-based anticancer drug against lung and colon cancer.

The FT-IR spectroscopy is a powerful tool to provide information about the conformational and structural dynamics of a metabolite. In this study, the FT-IR spectrum of the purified protein indicates strong peaks, suggesting the presence of varied functional groups. The presence of different peaks in the protein was supposed to be obtained through stretching and bending vibrations in the region of infrared radiation.

5. Conclusions

In a nutshell, the anti-tubercular activity and biomass of strain MANF2 were successfully enhanced using Taguchi OA design and BBD of RSM. Among diversified controlled variables at assigned levels, the MRS medium of pH 6.5 constituting yeast extract (0.5% w/v), magnesium sulphate (0.1% w/v), and glycerol (1.5% v/v), being further incubated at 30^{0}C showed pronounced anti-tubercular activity (98.7%) and approximately 4 fold improvement in the biomass (8.3 mg/mL) of strain MANF2 with respect to the traditional OFAT method. The design and ANOVA of measured variables exhibited the significance of the model. Most importantly, the experimental values of response variables showed a close concordance with the predicted responding values, thereby confirming the validation of model. Further, the study represents the first report on the identification of anti-tubercular and anticancer protein from *S. hominis*. The nominal mass of the purified protein was obtained as 7712.3 Da, revealing sequence homology (95%) with Glyceraldehyde-3-phosphate dehydrogenase from *Staphylococcus* sp. It is a new Glyceraldehyde-3-phosphate dehydrogenase-like protein. The molecular mass of the most abundant peptide was observed as 1922.12 Da, and thus, the peptide was named as NMANF2. Protein purified from strain MANF2 can be used as an ideal therapeutic agent against TB and cancer (lung and colon).

Chapter 4

In silico modelling of anti-tubercular and anticancer peptide NMANF2: Stereo-chemical, physiochemical, functional, and docking insight

1. Introduction

Bacteria associated therapeutic peptides are ubiquitous in nature and have been investigated extensively in the past few decades for designing ideal antibiotics. Peptides are generally composed of short amino acids residues constituting small cationic and amphiphilic moieties. Based on the composition and structures, peptides have been grouped into distinct classes, possessing alpha (α)-helical structure (α family), beta (β)-strands (β family), both α-helical and β-strands (α β family), and neither α-helical structure nor β-strands (non-α β family) (Wang, 2013).

Plethora of studies has demonstrated that peptides could have many applications in medicine due to broad range of biological targets, thereby exhibiting remarkably high activity and potentially reduced toxicity than other small molecules (Craik *et al.*, 2013) Additionally, some peptides demonstrate multiple modes of action, which can be effective in improving biological potency and evading resistance process of pathogens (Schmitt *et al.*, 2011). Therefore, a number of research activities have focussed on the diverse applications of peptides towards the discovery of novel therapeutic drugs. Peptide properties viz. charge, hydrophobicity, primary and secondary structure, structure, and interaction with targets are leading parameters in the prediction of peptide to be pivotal therapeutic agents (Juretic *et al.*, 2009).

Peptide-protein interactions are important in several cellular functions. Hence, determination of the structure of peptide-protein complexes is crucial in order to understand the molecular mechanism of related biological processes and developing peptide-based drugs. The interaction between peptide and protein play a pivotal role in distinct biological processes such as signal transduction, immune responses, and cellular regulation (London *et al.*, 2013). About 40% of the protein-protein interactions are mediated by short peptides. Hence, determining the structure of peptide-protein complexes is important for understanding the molecular process and thus modulating the protein–protein interactions for therapeutic purposes (Fosgerau and Hoffmann, 2015). Now a days, very few peptide-protein complex structures are experimentally implied due to the high cost and technical difficulties. Therefore, molecular docking has been widely utilized towards the determination of peptide-protein complex structures. Peptide-protein docking predicts the complex structure by sampling plausible peptide binding conformations with an energy scoring function (London *et al.*, 2013).

Computational simulations or approaches are important for selecting therapeutic peptides as the hypothesis can be tested prior to the time-consuming and resource-demanding synthesis. In view of this, the present chapter was aimed not only to evaluate varied stereo-chemical and physiochemical properties of peptide NMANF2 (as discussed in previous chapter) but also design this very peptide-based drug against TB and cancer (lung and colon cancer cell lines) by means of *in silico* studies to aid efforts towards novel therapeutic strategy.

2. Materials and methods

2.1. Peptide of interest

Peptide NMANF2 was used in this investigation to predict its structure, stereo-chemical parameters, physiochemical properties, and molecular docking insight. The amino acid residues of NMANF2 were obtained as 'KAIGLVIPEIDGKLDGGAQRV', as mentioned in the previous chapter.

2.2. Structure prediction and model evaluation of peptide

The 3D conformations of peptide (21 amino acid residues) were predicted using online software PEP-FOLD (http://bioserv.rpbs.univ-paris-diderot.fr/services/PEP-FOLD3/) (Beaufays *et al.*, 2012) and iCn3D (https://www.ncbi.nlm.nih.gov/Structure/icn3d/full.html). The quality of peptide structure model was evaluated by determining different stereo chemical parameters such as Verify 3D, ERRAT, and WHATCHECK using PROCHECK (https://servicesn.mbi.ucla.edu/PROCHECK/) (Laskowski *et al.*, 1993). Verify 3D illustrates the compatibility of a model with its own amino acid residues by assigning a structural class based on its location as well as environment and comparing the outcome to valid structure. ERRAT determines the statistics of non-bonded interactions between different atom types and plots the value of the error function versus position of a 9-residue sliding window, calculated by a comparison with statistics from highly refined structures. WHATCHECK analyses stereo-chemical features of the residues in the valid model. The stereo-chemical parameters of peptide NMANF2 were checked by analyzing residue-by-residue and overall structure geometry.

2.3. Physiochemical properties of peptide

The physiochemical parameters viz. number of amino acids, theoretical pI (isoelectric point), instability index, aliphatic index, and Grand average of hydropathocity (GRAVY) were analyzed using ExPASy-ProtParam tool (http:// web.expasy.org/protparam) (Dunker *et al.*, 2001).

2.4. Primary structure analysis of peptide

The amino acid composition of peptide NMANF2 was determined using ExPASy-ProtParam tool (http:// web.expasy.org/protparam) (Dunker *et al.*, 2001).

2.5. Secondary structure analysis of peptide

Secondary structure of peptide was analysed using ExPASy SIB Bioinformatics SOPMA tool (http://npsa-prabi.ibcp.fr/cgi-bin/npsa_automat.pl?page=npsa_sopma.html) which determines number of α-helices, β-turn, extended strand, β-sheet, and coils. Sequences were submitted in FASTA format in order to utilize SOPMA. Ramachandran plot was constructed using PROCHECK (https://servicesn.mbi.ucla.edu/PROCHECK/) (Laskowski *et al.*, 1993). Ramachandran plot was used to visualize energetically allowed regions for backbone dihedral angles (Phi) ϕ against Ef (Φ) of amino acid residues of peptide NMANF2.

2.6. Functional analysis of peptide NMANF2

The membrane spanning or extracellular nature of peptide NMANF2 was analyzed using TMHMM tool (www.cbs.dtu.dk/services/TMHMM). A helical wheel diagram of the peptide was generated by Helical Wheel Projections (http://www.bioinformatics.nl/cgi-bin/emboss/pepwheel).

2.7. Molecular docking-

2.7.1. Ligands selection

The structure of peptide NMANF2 obtained using PEP-FOLD (http://bioserv.rpbs.univ-paris-diderot.fr/services/PEP-FOLD3/) was saved as Protein Data Bank (PDB) file and used for molecular docking. On the other hand, structure of rifampicin and doxorubicin were obtained from PubChem (https://pubchem.ncbi.nlm.nih.gov/) and were used for docking analysis too.

2.7.2. Targeted M. tuberculosis proteins

The 3D structures of receptors viz. alanine racemase, DNA gyrase, isocitrate lyase, LysA, and ribonucleotide reductase were retrieved from Research Collaboratory for Structural Bioinformatics (RCSB) PDB (http://www.rscb.org/pdb). The complexes bound to the receptor, such as non-essential water molecules and any inhibitors were removed while docking.

2.7.3. Targeted lung and colon cancer proteins

For targeting lung cancer (A540 cell line), the 3D structures of Bcl-2 (B cell lymphoma/leukemia type 2), H-Ras, and epidermal growth factor receptor (EGFR) tyrosine kinase were retrieved from RCSB PDB (http://www.rscb.org/pdb). The complexes bound to the receptor, such as non-essential water molecules and inhibitors were removed from the target receptors while docking.

Likewise, for targeting colon cancer (HT-29 cell line), Bcl-xL (B-cell lymphoma-extra large), CDK2 (cycline dependent kinase 2), and CDK4 (cycline dependent kinase 4) were retrieved from RCSB PDB (http://www.rscb.org/pdb). The complexes bound to the receptor, such as non-essential water molecules and inhibitors were removed from the target receptors while docking.

2.7.4. Peptide-protein docking and visualization

Molecular docking between ligands and targeted proteins of *M. tuberculosis* and cancer cell lines (A540 and HT-29) were analyzed and visualized using Hex 8.0.0 docking software (Macindoe *et al.*, 2010). Hex is an interactive molecular graphics program that reads in molecular coordinate files and displays *in silico* interaction in varied representations and colour schemes. The tool identifies the ligand with the best score and calculates the ligand-receptor interaction with the lowest free energy value.

The docking was performed by adjusting following parameters/features:

Correlation type - Shape + Electrostatics

FFT Mode - 3D

Post Processing - MM Energies

Grid Dimension - 0.6

Receptor range - 180

Ligand range - 180

Twist range - 360

Distance Range - 40

The binding energy (Kilo Joule per mole: KJ/mol) estimated after docking was tabulated.

3. Results

3.1. Structure prediction and model evaluation of peptide

Figure 1 shows modelled predicted structures such as 'Lines', 'Cartoon', 'Ribbon', 'Ball and Stick', 'Sphere', and 'Stick and Surface' of peptide NMANF2, as determined by PEP-FOLD and iCn3D online tool.

Verify 3D, ERRAT, and WHATCHECK were analyzed using PROCHECK server (Table 1). The quality of modelled peptide was analyzed by Verify 3D, and 100% residues of modelled peptide showed a score ≥0.2. Therefore, the average 3D-1D scores for all the residues of model were considered 'Pass'. The overall quality factor and compatibility of the model with amino acid residues was evaluated using ERRAT which was calculated as 91.66. In general, the modelled peptide is considered good if the quality factor is >50. Further, WHATCHECK evaluated the accuracy of modelled peptide structure, thereby indicated that the peptide NMANF2 structure was of reasonably good quality.

3.2. Physiochemical properties of peptide

Results for physiochemical parameters of peptide NMANF2 are shown in Table 1. The pI of the peptide NMANF2 (Total number of amino acids - 21) was calculated as 6.12. The instability index of the peptide was obtained as 19.3, thereby indicating its stability. Further, the aliphatic index and GRAVY of the peptide were calculated as 130.0 and 0.171, respectively.

3.3. Primary structure analysis of peptide

Figure 2 shows the amino acid composition of peptide NMANF2. The amino acids such as Glycine (19.0%) and Isoleucine (14.3%) were predominant in the peptide. On the other hand, 9.5% of Alanine, Aspartic acid, Leucine, Lysine, and Valine were present in the peptide. While, only 4.8% of Arginine, Glutamine, Glutamic acid, and Proline were available in the peptide.

3.4. Secondary structure analysis of peptide

Secondary structure of peptide NMANF2 was dominated by β-turn (42.86%), extended sheet region (33.33%), and random coil (23.81%) (Figure 3).

Figure 4 shows the percentage of residues in the most favourable regions, additionally allowed regions, generously allowed regions, and disallowed regions of Ramachandran plot. About 36% of residues were falling in favoured region, indicating slightly lower stability of this peptide.

3.5. *Functional analysis of peptide*

The membrane spanning or extracellular nature of peptide NMANF2 was analyzed using TMHMM tool which indicated lack of transmembrane domain in the peptide, thereby confirming the production of peptide NMANF2 extracellularly. Further, the helical wheel prediction of peptide NMANF2 is shown in Figure 5 which shows the presence of hydrophilic and positively charged residues.

3.6. *Molecular docking*

Structures of ligands used (peptide NMANF2, rifampicin, and doxorubicin) are shown in Figure 6. RCSB PDB IDs and metabolic pathways of *M. tuberculosis* receptors are illustrated in Table 2A. Likewise, the RCSB PDB IDs and metabolic pathways of cancer cells receptors are described in Table 2B.

Table 3A shows the binding affinity between peptide NMANF2 and targeted proteins of *M. tuberculosis* using Hex 8.0.0 docking software. The peptide exhibited highest negative energy value (E-value) of -635.15 KJ/mol with DNA gyrase, followed by -581.79, -551.88, -504.75, and -79.34 KJ/mol with ribonucleotide reductase, LysA, alanine racemase, and isocitrate lyase, respectively (Figure 7). Furthermore, rifampicin showed E-values with *M. tuberculosis* proteins in the order of alanine racemase (-332.23 KJ/mol) > ribonucleotide reductase (-324.09 KJ/mol) > LysA (-316.08 KJ/mol) > DNA gyrase (-300.01 KJ/mol) > isocitrate lyase (-248.83 KJ/mol) (Table 3B and Figure 8).

Among targeted proteins of A540 cell lines, peptide NMANF2 revealed highest docking score of -470.6 KJ/mol with Bcl-2 (Figure 9). On the other hand, the peptide showed highest negative E-value of -378.9 KJ/mol with CDK4 among targeted HT-29 cell lines (Table 4A and Figure 10). Molecular docking of doxorubicin with selected proteins of A540 and HT-29 cancer cells is shown in Figure 11 and Figure 12, respectively. Doxorubicin revealed highest docking score of -288.36 and -308.7 KJ/mol with Bcl-2 and CDK4, respectively (Table 4B).

Table 1: Stereo-chemical and physiochemical parameters of peptide.

Peptide	Stereo-chemical and physiochemical parameters							
NMANF2	Verify 3D	ERRAT	WHATCHECK	Number of amino acids	Theoretical pI	Instability index	Aliphatic index	GRAVY
	100%	91.66	Good	21	6.12	19.3	130.0	0.171

Table 2A: RCSB PDB IDs and metabolic pathways of *M. tuberculosis* targeted proteins.

S. No.	Proteins	RCSB PDB IDs	Metabolic pathways
1.	Alanine racemase	1XFC	Peptidoglycan biosynthesis
2.	DNA gyrase	3UC1	DNA synthesis
3.	Isocitrate lyase	1F8I	Replenishing of tricarboxylic acid cycle intermediates
4.	LysA	1HKV	Amino acid biosynthesis
5.	Ribonucleotide reductase	1UZR	DNA synthesis

Table 2B: RCSB PDB IDs and metabolic pathways of A540 and HT-29 proteins.

S. No.	Proteins	RCSB PDB IDs	Metabolic pathways
1.	Bcl-2	1G5M	Blocking apoptosis
2.	H-Ras	5P21	Signal transduction
3.	EGFR tyrosine kinase	1M17	Autophosphorylation and signal transduction
4.	Bcl-xL	1R2D	Anti-apoptosis
5.	CDK2	5IEY	Abnormal regulation of cell cycle
6.	CDK4	2W96	Phosphorylation of retinoblastoma gene product

Table 3A: Docking analysis of peptide NMANF2 with *M. tuberculosis* receptors.

S. No.	Proteins	RCSB PDB IDs	Docking E-value (KJ/mol)
1.	Alanine racemase	1XFC	-504.75
2.	DNA gyrase	3UC1	-635.15
3.	Isocitrate lyase	1F8I	-79.34
4.	LysA	1HKV	-551.88
5.	Ribonucleotide reductase	1UZR	-581.79

Table 3B: Docking analysis of rifampicin with *M. tuberculosis* receptors.

S. No.	Proteins	RCSB PDB IDs	Docking E-value (KJ/mol)
1.	Alanine racemase	1XFC	-332.23
2.	DNA gyrase	3UC1	-300.01
3.	Isocitrate lyase	1F8I	-248.83
4.	LysA	1HKV	-316.08
5.	Ribonucleotide reductase	1UZR	-324.09

Table 4A: Docking analysis of peptide NMANF2 with A540 and HT-29 cancer cells receptors.

S. No.	Proteins	RCSB PDB IDs	Docking E-value (KJ/mol)
1.	Bcl-2	1G5M	-470.6
2.	H-Ras	5P21	-416.78
3.	EGFR tyrosine kinase	1M17	-417.63
4.	Bcl-xL	1R2D	-374.83
5.	CDK2	5IEY	-353.62
6.	CDK4	2W96	-378.9

Table 4B: Docking analysis of doxorubicin with A540 and HT-29 cancer cells receptors

S. No.	Proteins	RCSB PDB IDs	Docking E-value (KJ/mol)
1.	Bcl-2	1G5M	-288.36
2.	H-Ras	5P21	-263.49
3.	EGFR tyrosine kinase	1M17	-32.45
4.	Bcl-xL	1R2D	-275.38
5.	CDK2	5IEY	-274.11
6.	CDK4	2W96	-308.7

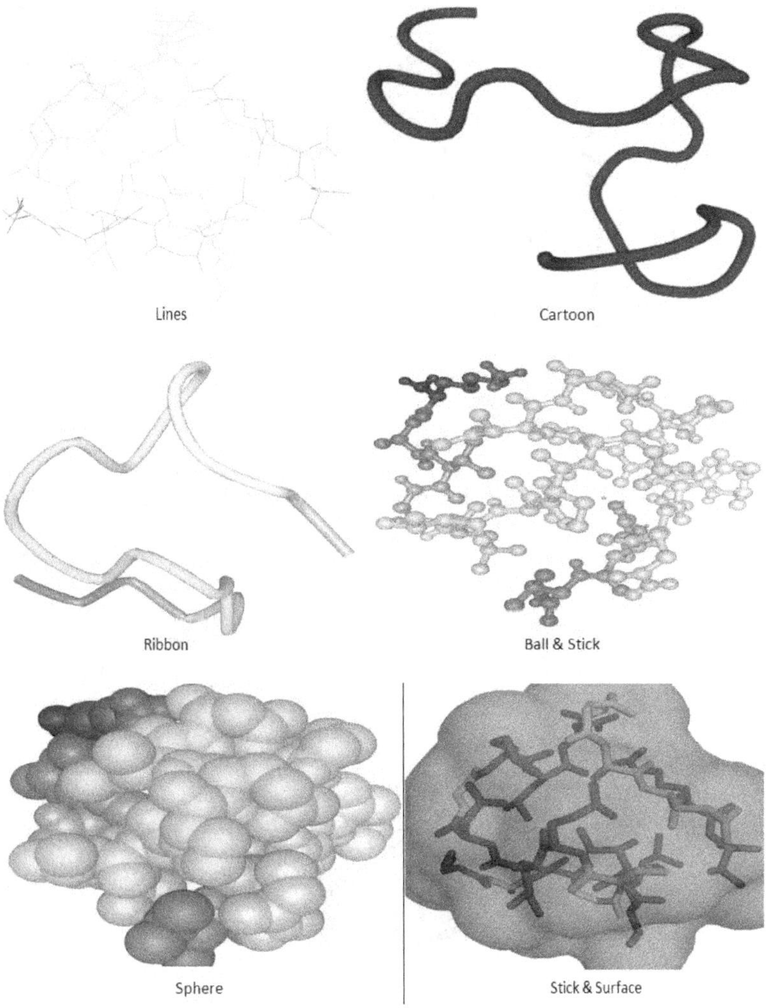

Figure 1: Structures of peptide NMANF2 obtained using PEP-FOLD and iCn3D.

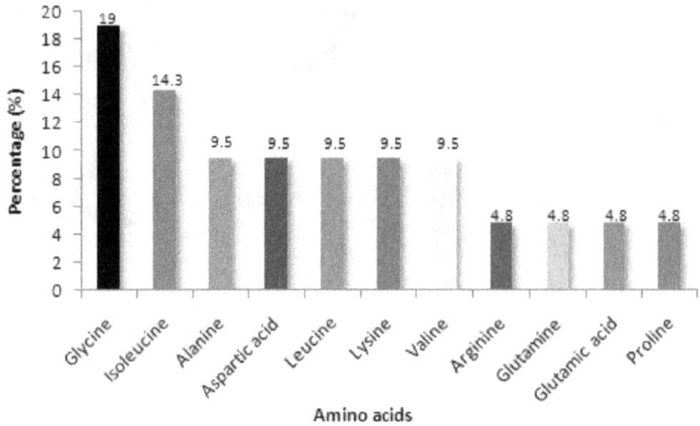

Figure 2: Amino acid composition (%) of peptide NMANF2.

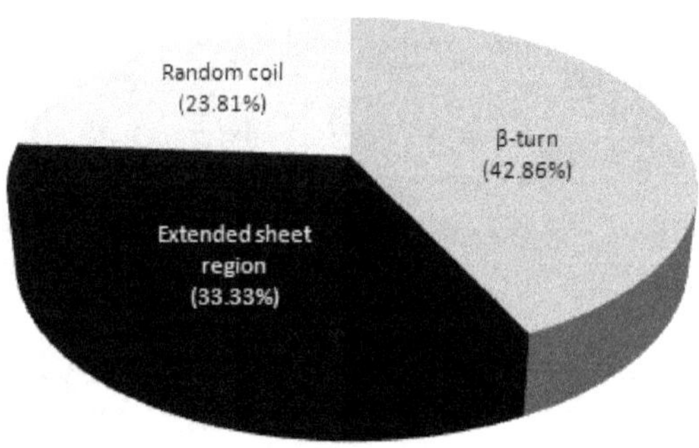

Figure 3: Secondary structure of peptide NMANF2 was dominated by β-turn, extended sheet region, and random coil.

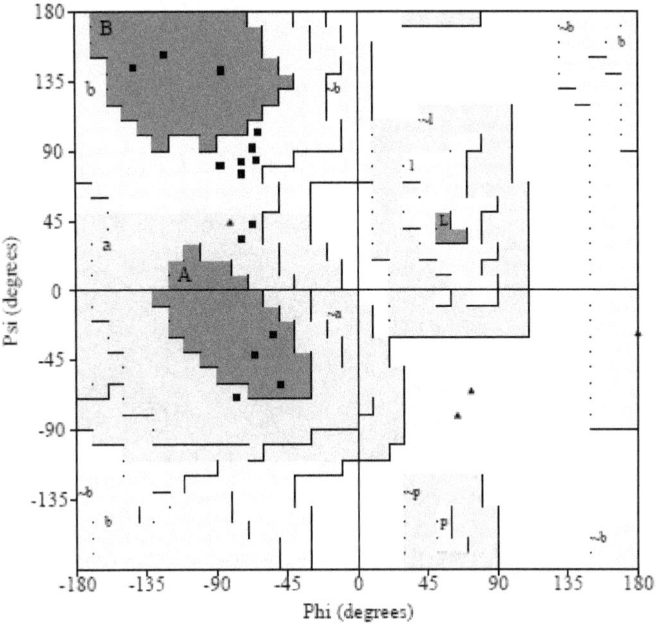

Plot statistics

Residues in most favoured regions [A,B,L]	5	35.7%
Residues in additional allowed regions [a,b,l,p]	9	64.3%
Residues in generously allowed regions [~a,~b,~l,~p]	0	0.0%
Residues in disallowed regions	0	0.0%
	----	------
Number of non-glycine and non-proline residues	14	100.0%
Number of end-residues (excl. Gly and Pro)	2	
Number of glycine residues (shown as triangles)	4	
Number of proline residues	1	

Total number of residues	21	

Figure 4: Ramachandran plot showing percentage of residues in the most favourable regions, additionally allowed regions, generously allowed regions, and disallowed regions.

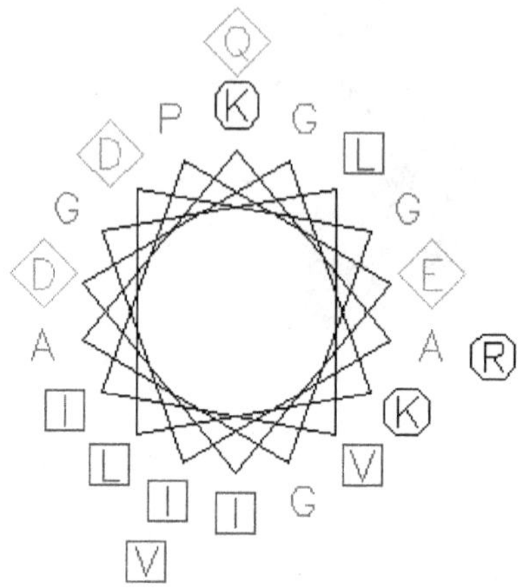

Figure 5: The helical wheel prediction of peptide NMANF2. Aliphatic residues are marked with squares, hydrophilic residues are marked with diamonds, and positively charged residues with octagons.

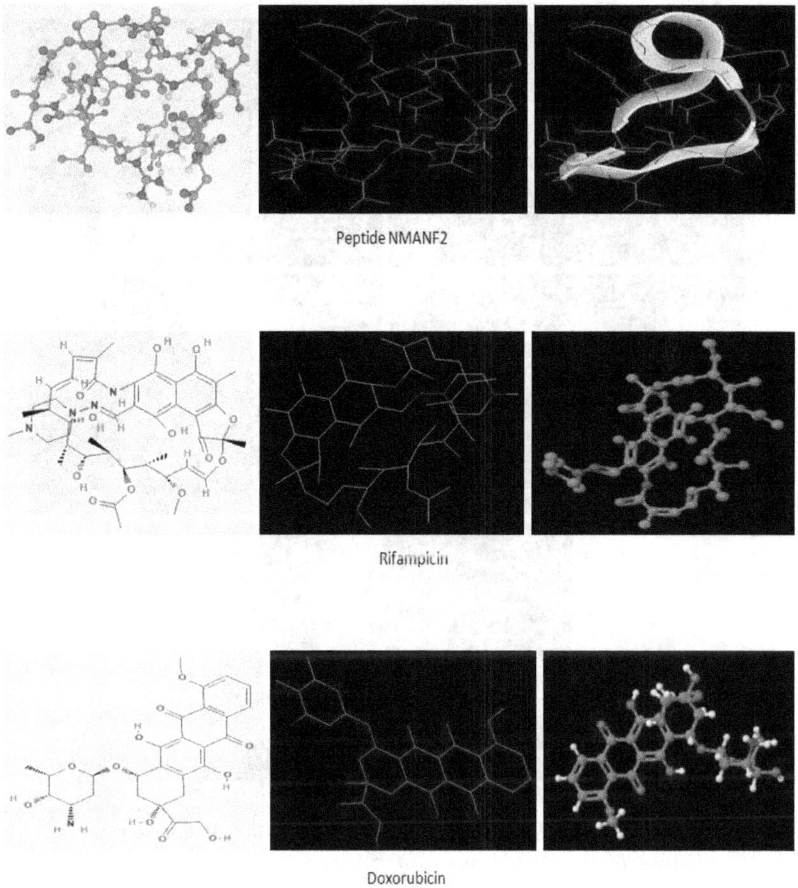

Figure 6: Different structures of ligands (peptide NMANF2, rifampicin, and doxorubicin).

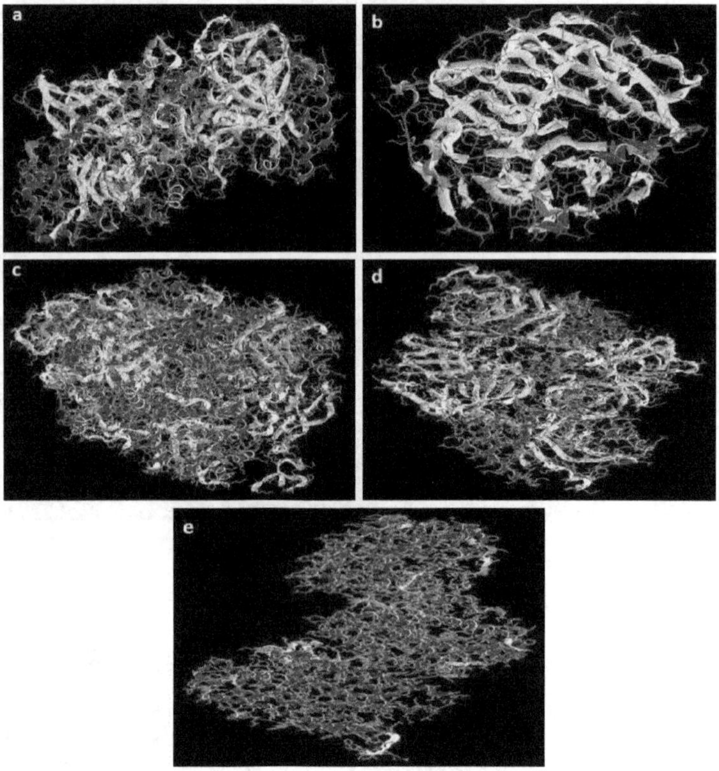

Figure 7: Molecular docking of peptide NMANF2 with (a) alanine racemase, (b) DNA gyrase, (c) isocitrate lyase, (d) LysA, and (e) ribonucleotide reductase.

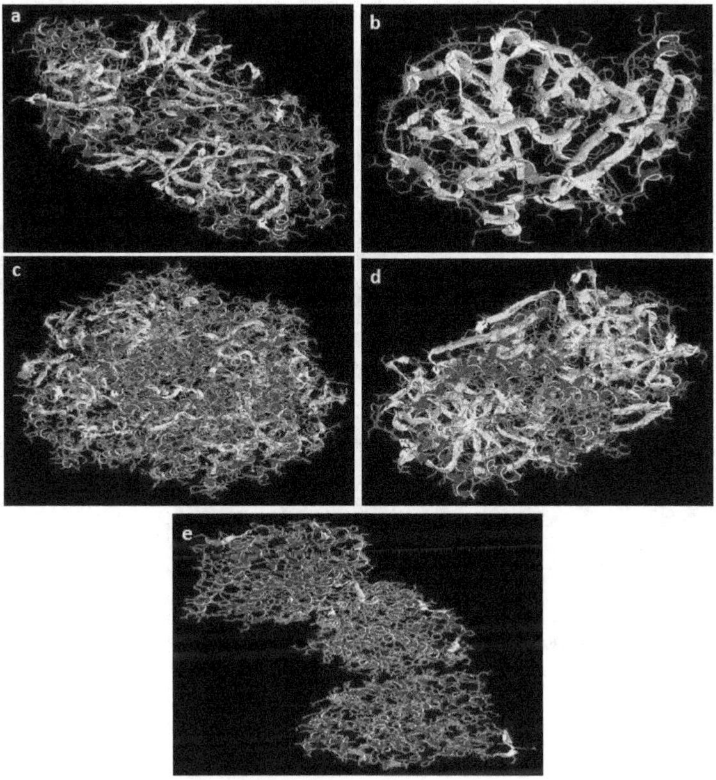

Figure 8: Molecular docking of rifampicin with (a) alanine racemase, (b) DNA gyrase, (c) isocitrate lyase, (d) LysA, and (e) ribonucleotide reductase.

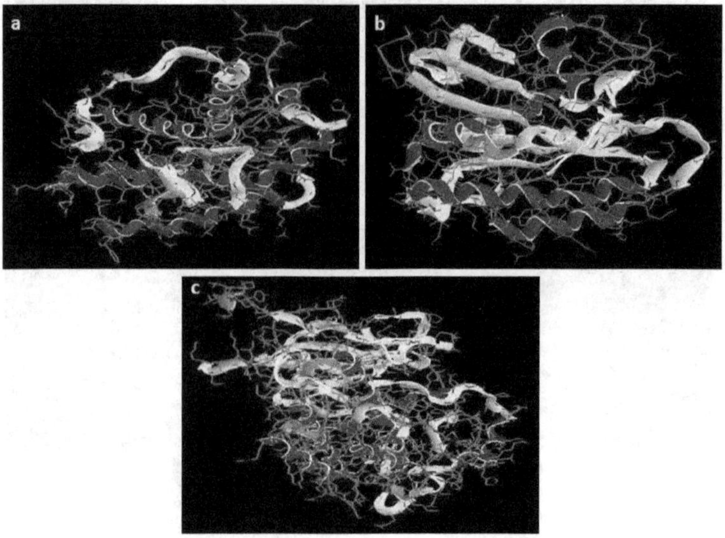

Figure 9: Molecular docking of peptide NMANF2 with (a) Bcl-2, (b) H-Ras, and (c) EGFR tyrosine kinase of A540 cell line.

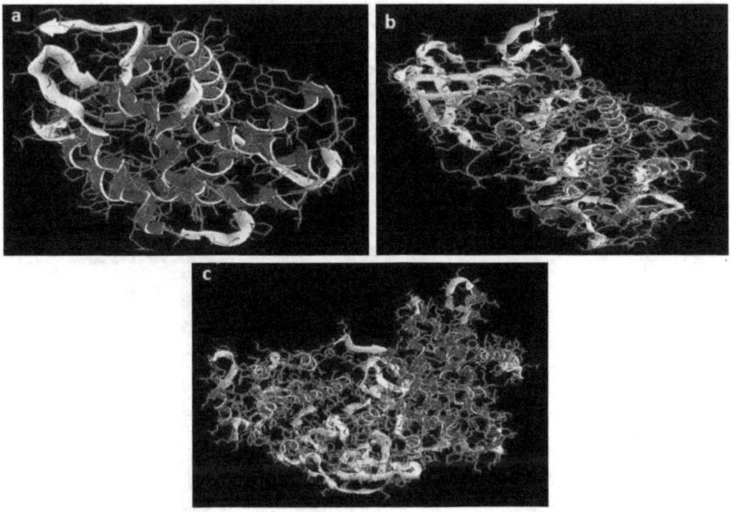

Figure 10: Molecular docking of peptide NMANF2 with (a) Bcl-xL, (b) CDK2, and (c) CDK4 of HT-29 cell line.

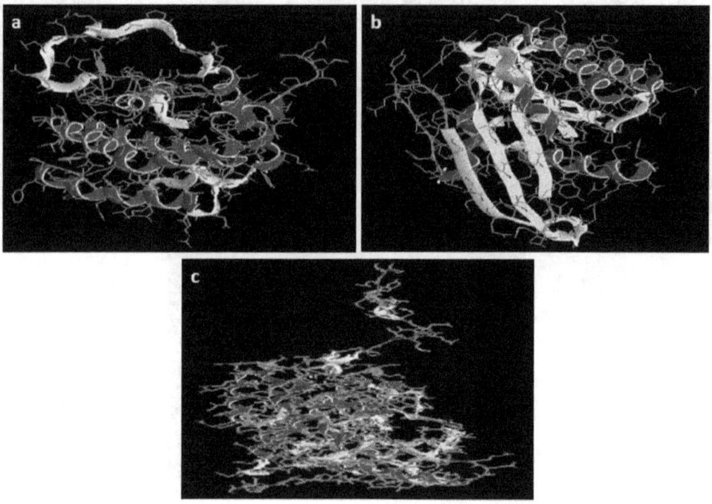

Figure 11: Molecular docking of Doxorubicin with (a) Bcl-2, (b) H-Ras, and (c) EGFR tyrosine kinase of A540 cell line.

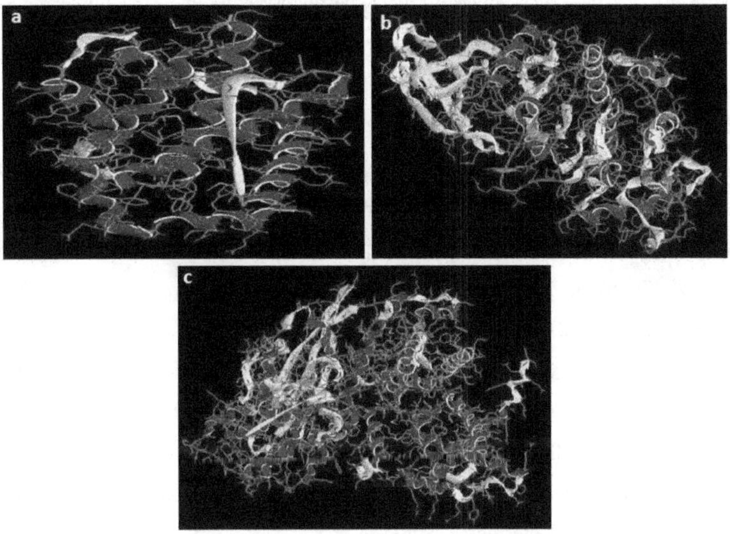

Figure 12: Molecular docking of Doxorubicin with (a) Bcl-xL, (b) CDK2, and (c) CDK4 of HT-29 cell line.

4. Discussion

Stereo-chemical parameters are used to assess the quality of protein or peptide structures generated through various tools. Verify 3D is one of the most important stereo-chemical parameters which is implemented to evaluate the residue profile of the 3D model of specific protein or peptide studied (Luthy *et al.*, 1992). In this study, Verify 3D showed 100% compatibility for the 3D model of peptide NMANF2. ERRAT is a structure evaluation server which predicts the quality assessment of stable models of proteins or peptides. In this study, ERRAT value of peptide NMANF2 is within the acceptable range. According to the report of Singh *et al.* (2016), any modelled structure exhibiting ERRAT score value of more than 50 is considered good. Likewise, WHATCHECK is another pivotal stereo-chemical parameter which is also used to assess the accuracy of modelled structure. WHATCHECK indicates that the structure of peptide NMANF2 is of reasonably good quality. Similar observation was reported by Singh *et al.* (2016) too.

Physiochemical parameters are the preliminary properties of proteins or peptides which depicts their uniqueness. The pI is the pH at which the surface of protein is charged but net charge of protein is zero (Dutta *et al.*, 2018). The nature of the macromolecule is alkaline if the theoretical pI value is more than 7. The theoretical pI below 7 indicates the acidic nature of the molecule. In this study, theoretical pI of peptide NMANF2 was determined acidic in nature. Instability index is another crucial parameter which evaluates the uniqueness of the protein or peptide. Instability index value of any protein below 40 is considered stable (Dutta *et al.*, 2018). In our study, the instability index value of peptide NMANF2 was calculated as 19.3, thereby indicating stability of this peptide. The relative volume of protein or peptide occupied by aliphatic amino acids in the side chain is determined by its aliphatic index value. A high aliphatic index value more than 50 represents that the particular protein is temperature stable. In general, higher the aliphatic index, greater the thermo-stability of the protein or peptide (Dutta *et al.*, 2018). In this study, peptide NMANF2 exhibited the aliphatic index value of 130.0, which indicates its stability towards high temperature. Hydropathicity is the relative hydrophobicity or hydrophilicity of amino acids that are present in the protein or peptide sequence (Kusumaningtyas *et al.*, 2016). In this study, the GRAVY value of peptide NMANF2 represents its potential interaction with water.

Primary structure analysis depicts the amino acid composition of peptides. In this context, Glycine (19.0%) and Isoleucine (14.3%) were predominant in the peptide NMANF2. On the other hand, Alanine, Aspartic acid, Leucine, Lysine, Valine, Arginine, Glutamine, Glutamic acid, and Proline were present in comparatively lower amount. Hydrophilic amino acids are known to seek contact with aqueous phase. In general, the predominance of Glycine provides high flexibility to the protein or peptide (Dutta *et al.*, 2018).

Secondary structure of peptide NMANF2 was dominated by β-turn (42.86%), extended sheet region (33.33%), and random coil (23.81%). Thus, the finding illustrates that the peptide is slightly lower stable in structure as it is predominantly composed of β-turn. Ramachandran angles determine the rotation of the polypeptide backbone around the bonds between N-C_α (Φ) and C_α-C (ϕ). The torsion angles (Φ and ϕ) provide the variable flexibility required for a polypeptide backbone to take up certain fold and steric effects from their side-chains (Singh *et al.*, 2016). Ramachandran plot shows the percentage of residues in the most favourable regions, additionally allowed regions, generously allowed regions, and disallowed regions. The higher residues in favoured region indicate more stability of the protein or peptide. In this study, about 36% of residues were falling in favoured region, indicating slightly lower stability of this peptide. The membrane spanning or extracellular nature of the peptide was analyzed using TMHMM tool which indicated extracellular production of peptide NMANF2. Further, the helical wheel prediction of peptide NMANF2 showed the presence of hydrophilic and positively charged residues, thus, supporting the findings of Xin *et al.* (2017).

Target proteins of *M. tuberculosis* were docked with the peptide NMANF2 and rifampicin using Hex 8.0.0 software in order to demonstrate their molecular interactions and binding energy. In the present investigation, peptide NMANF2 and rifampicin were reported as the most potent inhibitors against DNA gyrase and alanine racemase of *M. tuberculosis*, respectively, thereby showing higher E-values and strong interaction with receptors. Peptide NMANF2 exhibited higher docking score than rifampicin. This might be due to the fact that rifampicin had comparatively lower interaction with these selected targeted receptors. Likewise, peptide NMANF2 showed higher docking score with Bcl-2 and CDK4 of A540 and HT-29 cancer cells. Doxorubicin also revealed higher docking score with Bcl-2 and CDK4 of A540 and HT-29 cancer cells. However, the E-values obtained due to the interaction with doxorubicin were reported to be lower than that of peptide NMANF2. This might also be due to the fact that doxorubicin had comparatively lower interaction with these targeted receptors. Recent *in silico* studies had successfully used Hex 8.0.0 software for evaluating the molecular interaction between ligand of interest and various receptors of diverse diseases (Suryawanshi and Chouhan, 2017; Ashwini *et al.*, 2017; Menakha *et al.*, 2018). Our findings provided further promising role of Hex 8.0.0 tool in understanding peptide-protein based interaction towards designing ideal drugs against TB and cancer (lung and colon) in future.

5. Conclusions

In silico investigations clearly indicated the promising stereo-chemical, physiochemical, and functional characteristics of peptide NMANF2. Further, the peptide showed affinity with DNA gyrase, ribonucleotide reductase, LysA, alanine racemase, and isocitrate lyase of *M. tuberculosis*. Similarly, among targeted proteins of A540 cell line, peptide NMANF2 revealed potential docking with Bcl-2. On the other hand, the peptide was reported to be potential inhibitor of CDK4 among targeted HT-29 cell line.

Chapter 5

Anti-tubercular and anticancer protein synthesis in *S. hominis* strain MANF2 under mild stress condition

1. Introduction

Bacteria are exposed to stress in diversified challenging environmental conditions. They are often adapted to the stress environment by inducing various defence systems. As a matter of fact, the desideratum purpose of the defence mechanisms towards the unfavourable conditions is to protect bacteria by repairing the damages, altering the metabolism of cells, activating the signal transduction cascade, and synthesizing specific group of proteins, thereby maintaining the function of bacteria in the stress environment (Swiecilo and Zych-Wezyk, 2013). Most importantly, bacteria "switch on/off" a catalogue of genes or up-regulate and down-regulate many transcripts under stress conditions which lead to affect protein promoters (Goh *et al*., 2002).

Antimicrobial agents or antimicrobials are pronounced lethal substances exhibiting broad spectrum inhibition of bacterial growth by modulating transcription mechanism in cells. Among ideal antimicrobials, medicinal plants at low concentrations provide stress to bacteria, thereby causing variations in the physiology and metabolism of the cell (Subramanian *et al*., 2012). Antibiotics are another promising bactericidal agents which cause the inhibition of bacterial growth by degrading cell wall and blocking transcriptional machinery (Greenwood and Eley, 1982). In like manner, the exposure of toxic heavy metals is known to affect the microbiota by influencing their growth, morphology, and other biochemical activities. In fact, bacterial metabolism is induced due to the sub-lethal concentration exposure of certain toxic heavy metals (Roane and Pepper, 1999).

The physiological activities and functionalities of the probiotics are being affected by the stresses (Kheadr *et al*., 2007). Probiotic bacteria exhibit varied molecular processes to evade the detrimental environmental stresses. In fact, external signals can elicit dramatic alteration in the expression of various stress-related genes encoding proteins which is in fact thought to enhance adaptation towards the changing environment (Sawatari and Yokota, 2007). Since, antimicrobials at sub-lethal concentrations can stimulate the production of bioactive proteins from bacteria, hence, stress responses of probiotic bacteria can be exploited for the production of therapeutic proteins.

In spite of the exposure of diverse unfavourable conditions such as high temperature, salt concentration, acidity, alkalinity, and oxidative stress to bacteria, there are very few studies assessing the potentiality of new categories of antimicrobials as signalling agents to trigger biological characteristics in bacteria, probably unavailable in fermented food associated coagulase-negative *Staphylococcus* sp. Considering this, in this chapter, a significant attempt was undertaken to optimize statistically and synthesize bioactive protein in strain MANF2 under mild stress of certain antimicrobials (medicinal plant, antibiotic, and heavy metal) and to evaluate its anti-tubercular and anticancer properties.

2. Materials and methods

2.1. Antimicrobials of interest

Three different categories of antimicrobials viz. medicinal plants [*Allium sativum* (garlic), *Allium cepa* (onion), *Mentha piperita* (peppermint), *Curcuma longa* (turmeric), and *Zingiber officinale* (ginger)], antibiotics [streptomycin, penicillin G ($C_{16}H_{18}N_2O_4S$), chloramphenicol ($C_{11}H_{12}Cl_2N_2O_5$), kanamycin ($C_{18}H_{38}N_4O_{15}S$), gentamicin ($C_{21}H_{43}N_5O_7$), nalidixic acid ($C_{12}H_{12}N_2O_3$), and rifampicin), and heavy metals [mercuric chloride ($HgCl_2$), silver nitrate ($AgNO_3$), zinc chloride ($ZnCl_2$), copper sulphate, and lead nitrate ($Pb(NO_3)_2$] were selected for this study (Figure 1).

2.2. Preparation of antimicrobials

All the medicinal plants were purchased freshly from the local market of Nungambakkam, Chennai and stored at 4^{0}C. The outer layers of *A. sativum*, *A. cepa*, *C. longa*, and *Z. officinale* were peeled, surface sterilized using 95% (v/v) ethanol, and washed with autoclaved distilled water. Likewise, fresh leaves of *M. piperita* were collected, surface sterilized using 95% (v/v) ethanol, and washed with autoclaved distilled water too. All the medicinal plants were homogenized separately using grinder (Prestige Iris), filtered through six layers of muslin cloth, and then centrifuged at 6000 *g* for 15 min. The supernatant of each sample was collected, filter sterilized using 0.2 µm syringe filter, and considered as 100%. All the samples were stored at 4^{0}C for further studies. Antibiotics were prepared at standard concentrations using sterilized distilled water or DMSO and considered 100%. Similarly, each heavy metal was dissolved in sterilized distilled water at the concentration of 25 mg/L (25 ppm) and considered

100%. Antibiotics and heavy metals were stored at 4^{0}C too for further experimental analyses.

2.3. *Antibacterial activities of antimicrobial agents*

The antibacterial activities of antimicrobial agents were determined against strain MANF2 using disc diffusion assay method (Bauer *et al*., 1966). Strain MANF2 was inoculated into sterilized MRS broth aseptically and incubated at 30^{0}C for 24 h. After required period of incubation, the culture was swabbed into freshly prepared MRS agar medium using sterile cotton swab. On the other hand, commercially available sterile discs (6 mm diameter) were soaked with 25 μL of all the antimicrobial agents prepared and allowed to dry for 30 min. Discs were placed aseptically over previously prepared MRS agar plates (seeded with the test bacteria) using ethanol dipped and flamed forceps. Plates were incubated at 30^{0}C and observed for the zone of inhibition after 48 h of incubation period. The diameter of zone of inhibition was measured in millimetres (mm) and results were recorded.

2.4. *Determination of minimum inhibitory concentration (MIC) and sub-MIC*

Based on antibacterial tests, *M. piperita*, penicillin G, and mercuric chloride showed maximum activities against strain MANF2. Hence, these very potent antibacterial agents were selected to determine MIC and sub-MIC values against the indicator bacteria. The MIC values of *M. piperita*, penicillin G, and mercuric chloride were determined by microdilution assay as per the methodology of Eloff (1998) with slight modifications. Fifty microlitres of overnight grown bacterial inoculum were added into each well of the microtitre plate containing 50 μL of *M. piperita*, penicillin G, and mercuric chloride as per the dilutions (100-1% concentrations) mentioned in Table 1A, 1B, and 1C, respectively. Dilutions of antimicrobials were made using MRS broth. The well containing only bacterial inoculums was considered control. The microtitre plate was incubated at 30^{0}C for 48 h. After required incubation period, the viability of bacteria was observed by adding 40 μL of MTT solution as an indicator into each well of the microtitre plate. The microtiter plate was further incubated at 30^{0}C for 30 min and observed for colour change. The colour change of the suspension from yellow to dark purple indicates the bacterial growth, while yellow colour in remaining wells indicates lack of bacterial growth. The lowest concentration of antimicrobials inhibiting the growth of strain MANF2 was considered as MIC value. Half of the value of the MIC was calculated as sub-MIC of antimicrobials.

2.5. Growth curve analysis of strain MANF2

Growth curve was analyzed to determine the lag phase and log phase of strain MANF2. One millilitre of bacterium was inoculated aseptically into freshly prepared MRS broth and incubated at 30^{0}C under shaking condition. The absorbance was read at 600 nm using UV-Vis spectrophotometer every 1 h interval.

2.6. Optimization of total protein content under antimicrobials stress-

2.6.1. Statistical optimization

Central composite design (CCD) of RSM was employed to optimize three parameters (yeast extract, glycerol, and antimicrobial agent) in order to enhance extracellular protein production from strain MANF2 under stress. Parameters such as yeast extract and glycerol were selected in this study based on their significant impact on biomass yield from strain MANF2 (identified previously in chapter 3). Each variable in the design matrix was tested at 5 different levels (-α, -1, 0, +1, +α). The design involved 6 central points with an α value being ±2. The total number of experimental combinations is $2^k + 2k + n$, where 'k' is the number of variables and 'n' is the number of repetition of experiments at the central point. The experimental design consisted of 20 runs of three variables for enhancing the protein production under mild stress of *M. piperita*, penicillin G, and mercuric chloride. All variables were set at a central coded value of zero. The efficacy of selected variables to the response was calculated by a second-order polynomial equation as given below:

$$Y \text{ (mg/mL)} = \beta_0 + \beta_1 A + \beta_2 B + \beta_3 C + \beta_{11} A^2 + \beta_{22} B^2 + \beta_{33} C^2 + \beta_{12} AB + \beta_{13} AC + \beta_{23} BC$$

[Equation 1]

where, Y is dependent variable (protein production)

β_0 is intercept

β_1, β_2, and β_3 are linear coefficients

β_{11}, β_{22}, and β_{33} are squared coefficients

β_{12}, β_{13}, and β_{23} are interaction coefficients

A, B, C, A^2, B^2, C^2, AB, AC, and BC are variables levels.

The accuracy of polynomial model was inferred by R^2. The parameters affecting significantly the production of protein from strain MANF2 was analyzed by ANOVA.

2.6.2. *M. piperita stress*

M. piperita at sub-MIC concentration was used to provide stress during lag and log phase of strain MANF2, as determined through growth curve. Fifty millilitres of MRS broth medium (pH 6.5) containing varied concentrations of yeast extract and glycerol was autoclaved into 250 mL of conical flasks and allowed to cool. Overnight grown culture of strain MANF2 was added into each production medium aseptically. Different concentrations (0.2-2.0% v/v) of *M. piperita* at sub-MIC values were added into the culture broth during lag and log phase of bacteria. Flasks were incubated at 30^{0}C under shaking condition and total protein content was estimated after 48 h of incubation period.

2.6.3. *Penicillin G stress*

Penicillin G at sub-MIC concentration was used to provide stress during lag and log phase of strain MANF2, as determined through growth curve. Fifty millilitres of MRS broth medium containing varied concentrations of yeast extract and glycerol was autoclaved into 250 mL of conical flasks and allowed to cool. Overnight grown culture of strain MANF2 was added into each production medium aseptically. Different concentrations (0.2-2.0% v/v) of penicillin G at sub-MIC values were added into the culture broth during lag and log phase of bacteria. Flasks were incubated at 30^{0}C under shaking condition and total protein content was estimated after 48 h of incubation period.

2.6.4. *Mercuric chloride stress*

Mercuric chloride at sub-MIC concentration was used to provide stress during lag and log phase of strain MANF2, as determined through growth curve. Fifty millilitres of MRS broth medium containing varied concentrations of yeast extract and glycerol was autoclaved into 250 mL of conical flasks and allowed to cool. Overnight grown culture of strain MANF2 was added into each production medium aseptically. Different concentrations (0.2-2.0% v/v) of mercuric chloride at sub-MIC values were added into the culture broth during lag and log phase of bacteria. Flasks were incubated at 30^{0}C under shaking condition and total protein content was estimated after 48 h of incubation period.

2.6.5. *Estimation of protein*

Protein content of each run was estimated according to the methodology of Bradford (1976) using BSA as standard. After required period of incubation period, culture grown under antimicrobials stress was centrifuged at 8000 *g* for 10 min and supernatant of each sample was collected. Hundred microlitres of supernatant from each sample were taken out in clean tubes and volumes were made up to 1 mL using autoclaved distilled water. Five millilitres of Bradford reagent were added into each tube and mixed thoroughly. One millilitre of autoclaved distilled water + 5 mL of Bradford reagent were used as blank. Absorbance of samples was read at 595 nm using UV-Vis spectrophotometer. Protein content of each sample was estimated against the standard curve of BSA. The BSA standard and Bradford reagent were prepared according to methodologies mentioned in chapter 3.

2.6.7. Experiment validation

The statistical optimization was validated by carrying out the experiments using optimized parameters of selected variables under submerged fermentation. The maximum production of protein from strain MANF2 under mild stress of antimicrobials was compared with the non-optimized conditions (without antimicrobials stress). The production of protein was estimated based on the methodology as described above.

2.7. Purification of protein-

In this study, strain MANF2 exhibited maximum production of protein due to the supplementation of mild concentration of *M. piperita* at log phase of bacterial growth. Hence the protein was purified from strain MANF2 after inoculation of *M. piperita* (1.5% v/v) during log phase of bacterial growth only.

2.7.1. Medium preparation

One litre of MRS medium was prepared using statistically optimized parameters and autoclaved. The overnight grown culture of strain MANF2 was inoculated into cooled MRS medium aseptically and incubated at 30^{0}C under shaking conditions. *M. piperita* (1.5% v/v) was added into the bacterial culture during its log phase and incubated up to 48 h.

2.7.2. Ammonium sulphate precipitation

The bacterial culture was centrifuged at 8000 *g* for 15 min at 4^{0}C. The supernatant was collected, neutralized, and precipitated with varied saturation levels (40, 50, 60, 70, and 80%) of ammonium sulphate. As per the saturation level, ammonium sulphate was weighed and powdered using mortar and pestle. The powdered ammonium sulphate was added in small amount into the supernatant and stirred for 4 h at 4^{0}C using magnetic stirrer. Further, samples were incubated at 4^{0}C in refrigerator for the complete precipitation of protein. The precipitated protein samples were collected after centrifugation at 10000 *g* for 15 min at 4^0C. The resulting pellets were re-suspended in sodium phosphate buffer (1M, pH 7.0) for the determination of total protein content using Bradford assay (Bradford, 1976).

2.7.3. Dialysis-

2.7.3.1. Pre-treatment of dialysis membrane

Dialysis membrane (1.0 kDa cut-off) was pre-treated using freshly prepared 10mM EDTA, 2% (w/v) sodium bicarbonate, distilled water (65^0C), and distilled water (room temperature). The dialysis membrane was dipped into the solutions in the sequential order of distilled water (65^0C) for 5 min, 10mM EDTA for 5 min, 2% (w/v) sodium bicarbonate for 5 min, and distilled water (room temperature) for 5-10 min. The pre-treated dialysis membrane was used for dialysis process.

2.7.3.2. Dialysis of sample

One end of the pre-treated dialysis membrane was tied with thread and filled with the ammonium sulphate precipitated sample. About 1 mL of sodium phosphate buffer (1M, pH 7.0) was added again into the sample and tied another end of the membrane with thread. The sample was mixed by gentle hand press. The sample containing membrane was dipped into approximately 1 L of sodium phosphate buffer (1M, pH 7.0) and kept under slow stirring at cold condition for 2-3 h. The buffer was changed every 2-3 h and continued the process for 4 cycles under cold condition. Total protein content of dialysed sample was estimated according to Bradford assay (Bradford, 1976) as discussed earlier and used for further process.

2.7.4. DEAE-Cellulose column chromatography

DEAE-Cellulose (1.5 g) was soaked in 0.1M (pH 7.0) phosphate buffer. The column was washed using distilled water and then with the buffer. The column was packed with pre-soaked DEAE cellulose and excess buffer was eluted. The dialyzed sample was loaded into the column. After 30 min, sample was eluted using the same buffer at the flow rate of 0.5 mL/min. The gradient elution was carried out using 0.2, 0.3, 0.4, 0.5M sodium chloride in the same buffer. Fractions were collected and tested for anti-tubercular activities according to the methodology mentioned in chapter 1. Fractions showing maximum anti-tubercular activities were pooled together for determining total protein content (Bradford, 1976) and electrophoresed using SDS-PAGE for the determination of molecular mass.

2.7.5. Molecular mass determination

The purity and molecular mass of the most active fractions were determined using SDS-PAGE with 4% stacking gel and 12% separating gel.

Preparation of separating gel (10 mL)-

Acrylamide:	3.3 mL
Separating buffer (pH 8.8):	2.5 mL
Distilled water:	4 mL
SDS (10%):	100 μL
APS (10%):	100 μL
TEMED:	5 μL

Preparation of stacking gel (10 mL)-

Acrylamide:	670 μL
Stacking buffer (pH 8.8):	500 μL
Distilled water:	2.7 mL
SDS (10%):	40 μL
APS (10%):	40 μL
TEMED:	4 μL

Clean notched and rectangular glass plates were assembled and kept in vertical position by placing them in a gel casting stand. The separating gel mixture was prepared and poured into the glass plates uniformly without any leakage. After polymerization of the separating gel, the stacking gel so prepared was poured over it and the comb was inserted gently. This setup was kept for few minutes to allow the gel to polymerize completely. The comb was then carefully removed and wells formed in the gel were rinsed with distilled water completely. Protein samples (50 μL) were mixed with 50 μL of sample solubilising buffer (1:1) and the mixture was heated at 95^{0}C in water bath for 10 min.

Preparation of solubilising buffer-

Sucrose:	20 g
SDS:	10 g
Stacking buffer:	22.5 mL
Distilled water:	60 mL
Mercaptoethanol:	10 mL
Bromophenol blue:	20 mg

Protein samples along with standard protein marker were then loaded into the respective wells. The gel was electrophoresed at 50-100V for 3-4 h in order to allow the samples run completely into the gel. After electrophoresis, the gel was placed in CBB staining solution for 1 h and washed thoroughly with distilled water.

Preparation of CBB staining solution-

Methanol:	125 mL
Acetic acid:	25 mL
Distilled water:	100 mL
CBB G250:	0.05 g

The stained gel was then placed in destaining solution. Destaining solution was prepared as mentioned below:

Preparation of destaining solution-

Methanol:	125 mL
Acetic acid:	25 mL
Distilled water:	100 mL

Destaining solution was changed every 30 min and the destaining was continued till the bands are clearly observed. Protein band was observed and its molecular mass was calculated based on the relative mobility of the standard marker (14.3-66 kDa).

2.8. Mass spectrometry and N- terminal amino acid sequencing

After SDS-PAGE, the protein band of interest was excised from the gel and kept in 50% (v/v) methanol. MALDI-TOF MS/MS was used to determine the molecular mass of the purified protein. The protein was digested using trypsin at 37^0C for 12 h. An equal volume of CHCA solution (10 mg/mL CHCA in 70% acetonitrile, 0.03% trifluoro acetic acid) was added to the trypsinized protein. MALDI-TOF spectrum depicts the fragmentation of protein into various peptides. The PMF was carried out to examine the sequence of the peptide fragments of protein. Mass spectra were recorded in the range of 100-2250 m/z. The *N*- amino acid sequence was compared with the sequence available in BLAST, NCBI algorithm (http://www.ncbi.nlm.nih.gov/) with the MASCOT search program (http://matrixscience.com).

2.9. Fourier-transform infrared spectroscopy

Three milligrams of purified protein were mixed with 300 mg of KBr (FT-IR grade) and pressed into a pellet in a hydraulic press by applying 500 kg/m^3 pressure.

The pellet was put into the sample holder and FT-IR spectra were recorded ranging 4000-400 cm^{-1} using FT-IR spectrometer.

2.10. Anti-tubercular activity of purified protein

M. tuberculosis H37Rv was grown in the presence of various concentrations (10-50 μg/mL) of purified protein and the anti-tubercular activities were estimated according to the methodology as mentioned in chapter 1. Rifampicin was used as positive control.

2.11. Characterization of protein-

2.11.1. Effect of pH

pH of the purified protein (1 mg/mL) was adjusted from 3.0 to 8.0 using 1N HCl and 1N NaOH. Samples were incubated at 37^0C for 3 h and residual anti-tubercular activities were calculated against the control (pH 6.5).

2.11. 2. Effect of temperature

To investigate the thermal effect on residual anti-tubercular activities, purified protein (1 mg/mL) at optimum pH level was incubated at 40^0C for 2 h, 60^0C for 1 h, 80^0C 30 min, 100^0C for 20 min, and 121^0C for 15 min. The protein sample without heat treatment was considered as control.

2.11.3. Effect of enzymes

Enzymes (1 mg/mL; pepsin - pH 3.0, trypsin - pH 7.5, protease K - pH 7.5, and α-amylase - pH 7.5) were mixed with purified protein at optimal pH and temperature. The mixture was incubated for 1 h and then subsequently heated at 100^0C for 5 min in order to inactivate the enzymes. Residual anti-tubercular activities were calculated according to the methodology mentioned earlier. The purified protein without the addition of enzymes was used as control.

2.12. Anticancer activity of purified protein-

2.12.1. Cell culture

Human lung cancer cells (A549) and human colon cancer cells (HT-29) were purchased from the National Centre for Cell Sciences, Pune, India. Cells were maintained in DMEM supplemented with 2mM L-glutamine and BSS adjusted to contain 1.5 g/L Na_2CO_3, 0.1mM non-essential amino acids, 1mM sodium pyruvate, 2mM L-glutamine, 1.5 g/L glucose, 10mM HEPES and 10% fetal bovine serum (GIBCO, USA). Penicillin and streptomycin (100 IU/100μg) were adjusted to 1 mL/L. Cells were maintained at 37^0C with 5% CO_2 in a humidified CO_2 incubator.

2.12.2. *In vitro cytotoxicity*

Anticancer activity of purified protein (10-50 μg/mL) was evaluated using MTT assay (Mosmann, 1983). Cancer cells were grown (1×10^4 cells/well) in a 96-well plate for 48 h into 75% confluence. The medium was replaced with fresh medium containing protein sample, and cells were further incubated for 48 h. The culture medium was removed, MTT solution (100 μL) was added to each well, and incubated at 37°C for 4 h. After removal of the supernatant, 50 μL of DMSO was added to each of the wells and incubated for 10 min to solubilise the formazan crystals. The absorbance was measured at 620 nm using an ELISA multi-well plate reader. Doxorubicin was used as positive control. The absorbance value was used to calculate the percentage of viability using the following formula:

$$\%\ \text{viability} = \frac{\text{Absorbance of sample}}{\text{Absorbance of control}} \times 100 \qquad \text{[Equation 2]}$$

The minimum concentration of protein required for 50% inhibition of cell viability (IC_{50}) was calculated using linear regression curve statistics (https://www.graphpad.com/quickcalcs/linear1/).

2.13. *Statistical analyses and softwares used*

Experiments were demonstrated in triplicate and values were expressed in terms of mean±SD. The statistical optimization process was interpreted using Design Expert Version 11.0.0 (Stat-Ease Inc., Minneapolis, Minnesota, USA) software. Data were validated using ANOVA and values $P\leq0.05$ were considered statistically significant.

3. Results

3.1. *Antibacterial activities of antimicrobial agents*

Among all the medicinal plants tested, *M. piperita* exhibited promising antibacterial activity against strain MANF2 with maximum zone of inhibition of 20.3±0.03 mm. *A. sativum* showed comparatively lower activity with moderate zone of inhibition of 18.3±0.03 mm. On the other hand, *A. cepa*, *C. longa*, and *Z. officinale* revealed no activity against the indicator bacterium (Figure 2a).

Figure 2b illustrates the susceptibility patterns of strain MANF2 to conventional antibiotics. All the strains showed varied degree of sensitivity towards the tested antibiotics in the order of penicillin G (32.3±0.3 mm) > gentamicin (31.3±0.4 mm) > rifampicin (30.3±0.5 mm) > kanamycin (22.3±0.6 mm) > chloramphenicol (21.3±0.5 mm) > streptomycin (13.3±0.4 mm). The strain was resistant to nalidixic acid.

Results for antibacterial activities of heavy metals are shown in Figure 2c. Mercuric chloride and silver nitrate revealed antibacterial activities against strain MANF2 with zones of inhibition of 21.3±0.6 and 11.3±0.6 mm, respectively. On the other hand, zinc chloride, copper sulphate, and lead nitrate showed complete lack of activity against the isolate.

3.2. Determination of MIC and sub-MIC

The MIC values of *M. piperita*, penicillin G, and mercuric chloride against strain MANF2 were observed as 25.0, 10.0, and 16.67%, respectively (Figure 3). Likewise, the sub-MIC values of *M. piperita*, penicillin G, and mercuric chloride against strain MANF2 were calculated as 12.5, 5.0, and 8.3%, respectively (Table 2A-C).

3.3. Growth curve analysis of strain MANF2

Figure 4 represents the growth curve of strain MANF2. The lag and log phase of the bacterium were achieved at 2 and 9 h. Antimicrobials stresses were provided to bacterium at lag and log phase and total protein content was estimated further.

3.4. Statistical optimization of total protein content under antimicrobials stress

Shake flask fermentation was carried out to provide antimicrobials stresses to strain MANF2 during lag (Figure 5) and log phase (Figure 6) of its growth. Protein production from strain MANF2 under mild stress of antimicrobials was optimized using CCD of RSM. Table 3A-C shows selected variables with their respective ranges employed in CCD tool. Table 4A represents the CCD matrix of selected variables in coded units along with observed as well as predicted values of protein production under mild stress of *M. piperita*, provided at lag phase of strain MANF2.

The response (*Y*) optimized through CCD was estimated by the following model equation:

$$Y\text{ (mg/mL)} = 3.04 + 1.02A - 0.5009B + 1.08C - 0.6307AB + 0.5211AC + 0.1693BC + 0.2324A^2 - 0.0935B^2 + 0.3738C^2 \quad \text{[Equation 3]}$$

A total of 20 experiments were conducted at diverse combinations of selected variables and the maximum protein production of 6.4 mg/mL was achieved from Run No. 14, consisting of medium with yeast extract (0.5% w/v), glycerol (1.5% v/v) and *M. piperita* (1.5% v/v). The experimental protein production from strain MANF2 was estimated to be close to the predicted value (6.2 mg/mL).

Table 4B represents ANOVA for protein production quadric model. The model F-value of 48.47 implies the model is significant. There is only 0.01% chance that a large "Model F-value" could occur due to noise. Values of "Prob > F" < 0.05 indicate model terms are significant. In this study, A, B, C, AB, AC, A^2, and C^2 are significant model terms. The "Lack of Fit F-value" of 1.02 implies the Lack of Fit is non-significant relative to the pure error. Non-significant lack of fit is good for the model to fit. The R^2 (0.9776) indicates appropriate correlation between experimental and predicted response values, and thus reveals the accuracy of the model. In this study, a low C.V. (8.62%) represents the reliability of the experiments. The "Predicted R^2" of 0.8834 is in reasonable agreement with the "Adj R^2" of 0.9574. "Adeq Precision" ratio of 22.52 indicates an adequate signal, and thereby suggests the navigation of design space.

Table 5A represents the CCD matrix of selected variables in coded units along with observed as well as predicted values of protein production under mild stress of *M. piperita*, provided at log phase of strain MANF2.

The response (Y) optimized through CCD was estimated by the following model equation:

$$Y\,(\text{mg/mL}) = 6.03 + 1.22A - 0.6139B + 1.33C - 0.6974AB + 0.4253AC + 0.1776BC + 0.1172A^2 - 0.1317B^2 + 0.2586C^2 \quad \text{[Equation 4]}$$

A total of 20 experiments were conducted at diverse combinations of selected variables and the maximum protein production of 9.4 mg/mL was achieved from Run No. 14, consisting of medium with yeast extract (0.5% w/v), glycerol (1.5% v/v) and *M. piperita* (1.5% v/v). The experimental protein production from strain MANF2 was estimated to be close to the predicted value (9.3 mg/mL).

Table 5B represents ANOVA for protein production quadric model. The model F-value of 66.73 implies the model is significant. There is only 0.01% chance that a large "Model F-value" could occur due to noise. Values of "Prob > F" < 0.05 indicate model terms are significant. In this study, A, B, C, AB, AC, and C^2 are significant model terms. The "Lack of Fit F-value" of 0.981 implies the Lack of Fit is non-significant relative to the pure error. Non-significant lack of fit is good for the model to fit. The R^2 (0.9836) indicates appropriate correlation between experimental and predicted response values, and thus reveals the accuracy of the model. In this study, a low C.V. (4.66%) represents the reliability of the experiments. The "Predicted R^2" of

0.9208 is in reasonable agreement with the "Adj R^2" of 0.9689. "Adeq Precision" ratio of 26.29 indicates an adequate signal, and thereby suggests the navigation of design space.

Table 6A represents the CCD matrix of selected variables in coded units along with observed as well as predicted values of protein production under mild stress of penicillin G, provided at lag phase of strain MANF2.

The response (Y) optimized through CCD was estimated by the following model equation:

Y (mg/mL) = 2.05 + 0.9337A - 0.3388B + 0.8558C - 0.4011AB + 0.5843AC + 0.1239BC + 0.3045A^2 - 0.0581B^2 + 0.4106C^2 [Equation 5]

A total of 20 experiments were conducted at diverse combinations of selected variables and the maximum protein production of 5.4 mg/mL was achieved from Run No. 14, consisting of medium with yeast extract (0.5% w/v), glycerol (1.5% v/v) and penicillin G (1.5% v/v). The experimental protein production from strain MANF2 was estimated to be close to the predicted value (5.1 mg/mL).

Table 6B represents ANOVA for protein production quadric model. The model F-value of 43.14 implies the model is significant. There is only 0.01% chance that a large "Model F-value" could occur due to noise. Values of "Prob > F" < 0.05 indicate model terms are significant. In this study, A, B, C, AB, AB, AC, A^2, and C^2 are significant model terms. The "Lack of Fit F-value" of 0.69 implies the Lack of Fit is non-significant relative to the pure error. Non-significant lack of fit is good for the model to fit. The R^2 (0.9749) indicates appropriate correlation between experimental and predicted response values, and thus reveals the accuracy of the model. In this study, a low C.V. (10.41%) represents the reliability of the experiments. The "Predicted R^2" of 0.9039 is in reasonable agreement with the "Adj R^2" of 0.9523. "Adeq Precision" ratio of 20.31 indicates an adequate signal, and thereby suggests the navigation of design space.

Table 7A represents the CCD matrix of selected variables in coded units along with observed as well as predicted values of protein production under mild stress of penicillin G, provided at log phase of strain MANF2.

The response (Y) optimized through CCD was estimated by the following model equation:

Y (mg/mL) = 5.03 + 1.22A - 0.6139B + 1.33C - 0.6974AB + 0.4253AC + 0.1776BC + 0.1172A^2 - 0.1317B^2 + 0.2586C^2 [Equation 6]

A total of 20 experiments were conducted at diverse combinations of selected variables and the maximum protein production of 8.4 mg/mL was achieved from Run No. 14, consisting of medium with yeast extract (0.5% w/v), glycerol (1.5% v/v) and penicillin G (1.5% v/v). The experimental protein production from strain MANF2 was estimated to be close to the predicted value (8.3 mg/mL).

Table 7B represents ANOVA for protein production quadric model. The model F-value of 66.73 implies the model is significant. There is only 0.01% chance that a large "Model F-value" could occur due to noise. Values of "Prob > F" < 0.05 indicate model terms are significant. In this study, A, B, C, AB, AC, and C^2 are significant model terms. The "Lack of Fit F-value" of 0.98 implies the Lack of Fit is non-significant relative to the pure error. Non-significant lack of fit is good for the model to fit. The R^2 (0.9836) indicates appropriate correlation between experimental and predicted response values, and thus reveals the accuracy of the model. In this study, a low C.V. (5.56%) represents the reliability of the experiments. The "Predicted R^2" of 0.9208 is in reasonable agreement with the "Adj R^2" of 0.9689. "Adeq Precision" ratio of 26.29 indicates an adequate signal, and thereby suggests the navigation of design space.

Table 8A represents the CCD matrix of selected variables in coded units along with observed as well as predicted values of protein production under mild stress of mercuric chloride, provided at lag phase of strain MANF2.

The response (Y) optimized through CCD was estimated by the following model equation:

Y (mg/mL) = 1.71 + 0.6281A - 0.2453B + 0.6704C - 0.2386AB + 0.5938AC - 0.1136BC + 0.2689A^2 - 0.0468B^2 + 0.2865C^2 [Equation 7]

A total of 20 experiments were conducted at diverse combinations of selected variables and the maximum protein production of 4.4 mg/mL was achieved from Run No. 5, consisting of medium with yeast extract (0.5% w/v), glycerol (1.5% v/v) and mercuric chloride (1% v/v). The experimental protein production from strain MANF2 was estimated to be close to the predicted value (4.1 mg/mL).

Table 8B represents ANOVA for protein production quadric model. The model F-value of 28.02 implies the model is significant. There is only 0.01% chance that a large "Model F-value" could occur due to noise. Values of "Prob > F" < 0.05 indicate model terms are significant. In this study, A, B, C, AB, AC, A^2, and C^2 are significant model terms. The "Lack of Fit F-value" of 1.16 implies the Lack of Fit is non-significant relative to the pure error. Non-significant lack of fit is good for the model to fit. The R^2 (0.9619) indicates appropriate correlation between experimental and predicted response values, and thus reveals the accuracy of the model. In this study, a low C.V. (12.12%) represents the reliability of the experiments. The "Predicted R^2" of 0.8201 is in reasonable agreement with the "Adj R^2" of 0.9275. "Adeq Precision" ratio of 17.20 indicates an adequate signal, and thereby suggests the navigation of design space.

Table 9A represents the CCD matrix of selected variables in coded units along with observed as well as predicted values of protein production under mild stress of mercuric chloride, provided at log phase of strain MANF2.

The response (Y) optimized through CCD was estimated by the following model equation:

$$Y \text{ (mg/mL)} = 4.03 + 1.13A - 0.6181B + 1.27C - 0.7045AB + 0.5291AC + 0.1705BC + 0.1812A^2 - 0.1192B^2 + 0.2695C^2 \quad \text{[Equation 8]}$$

A total of 20 experiments were conducted at diverse combinations of selected variables and the maximum protein production of 7.4 mg/mL was achieved from Run No. 5, consisting of medium with yeast extract (0.5% w/v), glycerol (1.5% v/v) and mercuric chloride (1% v/v). The experimental protein production from strain MANF2 was estimated to be close to the predicted value (7.4 mg/mL).

Table 9B represents ANOVA for protein production quadric model. The model F-value of 63.07 implies the model is significant. There is only 0.01% chance that a large "Model F-value" could occur due to noise. Values of "Prob > F" < 0.05 indicate model terms are significant. In this study, A, B, C, AB, AC, A^2, and C^2 are significant model terms. The "Lack of Fit F-value" of 0.93 implies the Lack of Fit is non-significant relative to the pure error. Non-significant lack of fit is good for the model to fit. The R^2 (0.9827) indicates appropriate correlation between experimental and predicted response values, and thus reveals the accuracy of the model. In this study, a low C.V. (6.72%) represents the reliability of the experiments. The "Predicted R^2" of 0.9133 is in reasonable agreement with the "Adj R^2" of 0.9671. "Adeq Precision" ratio of 26.10 indicates an adequate signal, and thereby suggests the navigation of design space.

The optimized conditions obtained using CCD were used for the authentication experiment. The observed protein production of strain MANF2 was estimated to be very much close to the predicted value, thereby indicating the authentication of model towards the improvement of protein production. Further, Figure 7 shows that the protein production from strain MANF2 under mild stress of antimicrobials was enhanced extensively with respect to the non-optimized conditions (1.8±0.3 mg/mL). The protein production was estimated to be increased due to the antimicrobials stress provided during log phase of strain MANF2. *M. piperita*, penicillin G, and mercuric chloride stresses provided at lag phase of strain MANF2 estimated comparatively lower protein production. In brief, medium containing yeast extract (0.5% w/v) and glycerol (1.5% v/v), and supplementation of *M. piperita* (1.5% v/v) at log phase of strain MANF2 revealed enhanced protein content (9.4±0.4 mg/mL).

3.5. Purification of protein

The anti-tubercular protein was purified using standard protein purification techniques including ammonium sulphate precipitation, dialysis, and DEAE-Cellulose column chromatography. Initially, ammonium sulphate at varied saturation levels (40–80%) was implied to precipitate the protein. Total protein content was estimated based on regression curve equation [Y = -0.122+0.001X (discussed in chapter 3)] obtained. Proteins precipitated at 60% saturation showed relatively higher total protein content (9546.3±69.3 mg/L) than that of other saturations (Figure 8). The protein precipitated with 60% saturation was used for dialysis which revealed total protein content of 340.3 mg with 79.1% recovery and purification fold of 29.1 (Table 10). The dialysed product was further purified using DEAE-Cellulose column chromatography. After column chromatography, the yield and purification fold of protein were estimated to be 72.3% and 1372.1, respectively (Table 10). A total of 16 fractions (2 mL) were collected from the elution process and tested for anti-tubercular activities as well as total protein content determination. Among all the fractions tested, fraction 6 showed maximum protein content and activity. This fraction was lyophilized for molecular mass determination.

3.6. *Molecular mass determination*

The molecular mass of the purified protein was observed using SDS-PAGE which showed a single homogeneous band corresponding to the molecular mass of approximately 52 kDa based on relative mobility (Figure 9).

3.7. *Mass spectrometry and N- terminal amino acid sequencing*

Figure 10 shows MALDI-TOF MS/MS spectrum of purified protein. The nominal mass of the purified protein was found to be 51293 Da as obtained from PMF analysis. Each peak in the spectrum represents peptides present in the tryptic digest of purified protein. The size of the peptide ion varies from *m/z* 1689.63 to 3555.06. The most abundant peptide ion is *m/z* 2110.87. Identification of protein using database which contains theoretical tryptic digests of all known proteins revealed the sequence homology (100%) with 1-1321 amino acids of proline dehydrogenase (ProDH). The amino acid sequence of the most abundant peptide (*m/z* = 2110.87) in the purified protein was identified as 'Leu-Val-Ser-Thr-His-Asn-Glu-Ala-Gly-Leu-Thr-Ser-Ser-Leu-Asn-Arg-Leu-Ile-Gly-Lys' (LVSTHNEAGLTSSLNRLIGK).

3.8. *Fourier transform infra-red spectroscopy*

The FT-IR spectrum of the purified protein is shown in Figure 11. The high absorption bands at 3422.2, 2966.9, 2344.72, 1641.32, 1451.9, and 1105.75 cm^{-1} indicate the presence of strong N-H stretch, C-H bond of Amide I, C-N bond, C=O stretch, and C-H bending.

3.9. *Anti-tubercular activity of protein*

The anti-tubercular activities of purified protein were estimated to be increased in a concentration dependent manner (10-50 μg/mL) ranging from RLU reduction of 36.8±0.3 to 78.5±0.4% with respect to the standard (75.5±0.5 to 99.9±0.5%) (Figure 12).

3.10. *Characterization of protein*

The impact of pH, temperature, and enzymes on the residual anti-tubercular activities of purified protein is shown in Table 11. The anti-tubercular activities of protein varied significantly ($P<0.05$) at various pHs. The protein retained its activity at pH 6.0 and 7.0 with residual activities of 93.5±0.5 and 96.6±0.4%. The residual anti-tubercular activities of protein were reduced at acidic and alkaline pHs.

The heat treatment on purified protein revealed significant ($P<0.05$) variations in residual anti-tubercular activities. The protein retained maximum residual activity of

97.2±0.4% at 40°C for 2 h. The residual anti-tubercular activities were drastically reduced (10.8±0.4%) at high temperature (121°C for 15 min).

The anti-tubercular activity of purified protein was lost completely after treatment with pepsin, trypsin, and protease K. On the other hand, the protein was found resistant to α-amylase, showing residual activity of 98.2±0.5%.

3.11. Anticancer activity of purified protein

The anticancer activity of protein against A549 cell line is shown in Figure 13. After treatment with purified protein at various doses, cell shrinkage followed by rounding of cells and reduction in cell counts occur. The viabilities of A549 cells were estimated (92.6±0.3-41.3±0.4%) to be reduced significantly ($P<0.05$) with increase in the protein concentrations. A similar morphological alteration was observed in HT-29 cells after treatment with purified protein (Figure 14). The viabilities of HT-29 cell lines were also estimated (94.6±0.3-48.5±0.4%) to be reduced significantly ($P<0.05$) with increase in the protein concentrations. The purified protein revealed comparatively higher anticancer activity against A549 cells with respect to HT-29 cells. The IC_{50} values of purified protein against A549 and HT-29 cells were calculated as 42.2 and 48.4 µg/mL, respectively. In contrary to this, doxorubicin exhibited pronounced anticancer activities with IC_{50} values of 7.4 and 9.6 µg/mL against A549 and HT-29 cells, respectively.

Table 1A: Dilutions of *M. piperita*.

Sample	Concentration (%)	Volume of *M. piperita* (μL)	Volume of MRS broth (μL)
1	100.0 (Pure)	100	0
2	50.0	50	50
3	33.33	50	100
4	25.0	50	150
5	20.0	50	200
6	16.67	50	250
7	14.29	50	300
8	12.5	50	350
9	11.11	50	400
10	10.0	50	450
11	9.09	50	500
12	8.3	50	550
13	7.6	50	600
14	7.1	50	650
15	6.6	50	700
16	6.25	50	750
17	5.8	50	800
18	5.5	50	850
19	5.2	50	900
20	5.0	50	950
21	4.7	50	1000
22	4.5	50	1050
23	4.0	50	1200
24	3.5	50	1350
25	3.03	50	1600
26	2.5	50	1950
27	2.12	50	2300
28	2.0	50	2450
29	1.81	50	2700
30	1.75	50	2800
31	1.72	50	2850
32	1.0	50	4950

Table 1B: Dilutions of penicillin G.

Sample	Concentration (%)	Volume of penicillin G (μL)	Volume of MRS broth (μL)
1	100.0 (Pure)	100	0
2	50.0	50	50
3	33.33	50	100
4	25.0	50	150
5	20.0	50	200
6	16.67	50	250
7	14.29	50	300
8	12.5	50	350
9	11.11	50	400
10	10.0	50	450
11	9.09	50	500
12	8.3	50	550
13	7.6	50	600
14	7.1	50	650
15	6.6	50	700
16	6.25	50	750
17	5.8	50	800
18	5.5	50	850
19	5.2	50	900
20	5.0	50	950
21	4.7	50	1000
22	4.5	50	1050
23	4.0	50	1200
24	3.5	50	1350
25	3.03	50	1600
26	2.5	50	1950
27	2.12	50	2300
28	2.0	50	2450
29	1.81	50	2700
30	1.75	50	2800
31	1.72	50	2850
32	1.0	50	4950

Table 1C: Dilutions of mercuric chloride.

Sample	Concentration (%)	Volume of mercuric chloride (µL)	Volume of MRS broth (µL)
1	100.0 (Pure)	100	0
2	50.0	50	50
3	33.33	50	100
4	25.0	50	150
5	20.0	50	200
6	16.67	50	250
7	14.29	50	300
8	12.5	50	350
9	11.11	50	400
10	10.0	50	450
11	9.09	50	500
12	8.3	50	550
13	7.6	50	600
14	7.1	50	650
15	6.6	50	700
16	6.25	50	750
17	5.8	50	800
18	5.5	50	850
19	5.2	50	900
20	5.0	50	950
21	4.7	50	1000
22	4.5	50	1050
23	4.0	50	1200
24	3.5	50	1350
25	3.03	50	1600
26	2.5	50	1950
27	2.12	50	2300
28	2.0	50	2450
29	1.81	50	2700
30	1.75	50	2800
31	1.72	50	2850
32	1.0	50	4950

Table 2A: MIC value of *M. piperita* against strain MANF2.

M. piperita concentration (%)	Strain MANF2
100.0	-
50.0	-
33.33	-
25.0	-*
20.0	+
16.67	+
14.29	+
12.5	+**
11.11	+
10.0	+
9.09	+
8.3	+
5.0	+
4.7	+
2.5	+
1.0	+

[Note: - = No growth, + = Growth, -* = MIC, +** = Sub-MIC]

Table 2B: MIC value of penicillin G against strain MANF2.

Penicillin G concentration (%)	Strain MANF2
100.0	-
50.0	-
33.33	-
25.0	-
20.0	-
16.67	-
14.29	-
12.5	-
11.11	-
10.0	*-
9.09	+
8.3	+
5.0	+**
4.7	+
2.5	+
1.0	+

[Note: - = No growth, + = Growth, -* = MIC, +** = Sub-MIC]

Table 2C: MIC value of mercuric chloride against strain MANF2.

Mercuric chloride concentration (%)	Strain MANF2
100.0	-
50.0	-
33.33	-
25.0	-
20.0	-
16.67	**-***
14.29	+
12.5	+
11.11	+
10.0	+
9.09	+
8.3	**+****
5.0	+
4.7	+
2.5	+
1.0	+

[Note: - = No growth, + = Growth, -* = MIC, +** = Sub-MIC]

Table 3A: Variables with their ranges and levels for CCD.

Variables	Code	Unit	Range and levels				
			-α	-1	0	+1	+α
Yeast extract	A	% w/v	0.02	0.05	0.1	0.5	1.0
Glycerol	B	% v/v	0.5	1.0	1.5	2.0	2.5
M. piperita	C	% v/v	0.2	0.5	1.0	1.5	2.0

Table 3B: Variables with their ranges and levels for CCD.

Variables	Code	Unit	Range and levels				
			-α	-1	0	+1	+α
Yeast extract	A	% w/v	0.02	0.05	0.1	0.5	1.0
Glycerol	B	% v/v	0.5	1.0	1.5	2.0	2.5
Penicillin G	C	% v/v	0.2	0.5	1.0	1.5	2.0

Table 3C: Variables with their ranges and levels for CCD.

Variables	Code	Unit	Range and levels				
			-α	-1	0	+1	+α
Yeast extract	A	% w/v	0.02	0.05	0.1	0.5	1.0
Glycerol	B	% v/v	0.5	1.0	1.5	2.0	2.5
Mercuric chloride	C	% v/v	0.2	0.5	1.0	1.5	2.0

Table 4A: Experimental and predicted values of protein production from strain MANF2 under mild stress of *M. piperita* provided at lag phase.

Run order	Yeast extract (A)	Glycerol (B)	*M. piperita* (C)	Protein content (mg/mL)	
				Experimental	Predicted
1	0	-α	0	3.8	3.6
2	0	0	0	3.4	3.04
3	0	0	0	3.4	3.04
4	0	0	-α	2.6	2.2
5	+1	0	0	5.4	5.2
6	0	0	0	2.9	3.04
7	0	0	0	2.8	3.04
8	-α	0	0	2.2	1.9
9	0	+α	0	1.9	1.9
10	0	0	0	2.8	3.04
11	-1	-1	+1	2.8	2.7
12	+1	-1	-1	4.2	4.2
13	-1	+1	+1	3.4	3.3
14	**+1**	**0**	**+1**	**6.4**	**6.2**
15	-1	-1	-1	1.7	2.01
16	+1	+1	-1	1.6	1.6
17	0	0	0	2.9	3.04
18	0	0	+α	5.7	5.9
19	+α	0	0	5.3	5.4
20	-1	+1	-1	1.8	1.9

Table 4B: Analysis of variance for protein production from strain MANF2 under mild stress of *M. piperita* provided at lag phase.

Source	Sum of Squares	df	Mean Square	*F*-value	*P*-value	
Model	36.42	9	4.05	48.47	<0.0001	significant
A-A	13.61	1	13.61	163.01	<0.0001	
B-B	2.90	1	2.90	34.77	0.0002	
C-C	15.21	1	15.21	182.20	<0.0001	
AB	2.43	1	2.43	29.14	0.0003	
AC	2.0	1	2.0	23.90	0.0006	
BC	0.1752	1	0.1752	2.10	0.1780	
A^2	0.7682	1	0.7682	9.20	0.0126	
B^2	0.1227	1	0.1227	1.47	0.2533	
C^2	1.99	1	1.99	23.81	0.0006	
Residual	0.8348	10	0.0835			
Lack of Fit	0.4214	5	0.0843	1.02	0.4917	not significant
Pure Error	0.4133	5	0.0827			
Cor Total	37.25	19				

R^2 - 0.9776, Adj R^2 - 0.9574, Predicted R^2 - 0.8834, CV – 8.62%, Adeq precision – 22.52, df - degree of freedom, Significant – $P < 0.05$, Non-significant – $P > 0.05$.

Table 5A: Experimental and predicted values of protein production from strain MANF2 under mild stress of *M. piperita* provided at log phase.

Run order	Yeast extract (A)	Glycerol (B)	*M. piperita* (C)	Protein content (mg/mL)	
				Experimental	Predicted
1	0	-α	0	6.8	6.6
2	0	0	0	6.4	6.1
3	0	0	0	6.4	6.1
4	0	0	-α	4.6	4.5
5	+1	0	0	8.4	8.1
6	0	0	0	5.9	6.1
7	0	0	0	5.8	6.1
8	-α	0	0	4.2	4.3
9	0	+α	0	4.3	4.6
10	0	0	0	5.8	6.1
11	-1	-1	+1	5.8	5.6
12	+1	-1	-1	7.2	7.2
13	-1	+1	+1	6.4	6.2
14	**+1**	**0**	**+1**	**9.4**	**9.3**
15	-1	-1	-1	4.1	4.2
16	+1	+1	-1	4.3	4.2
17	0	0	0	5.9	6.1
18	0	0	+α	8.7	8.9
19	+α	0	0	8.3	8.4
20	-1	+1	-1	4.2	4.1

Table 5B: Analysis of variance for protein production from strain MANF2 under mild stress of *M. piperita* provided at log phase.

Source	Sum of Squares	df	Mean Square	*F*-value	*P*-value	
Model	49.9	9	5.47	66.73	<0.0001	significant
A-A	19.41	1	19.41	236.92	<0.0001	
B-B	4.36	1	4.36	53.22	<0.0001	
C-C	22.80	1	22.80	278.31	<0.0001	
AB	2.97	1	2.97	36.31	0.0001	
AC	1.33	1	1.33	16.22	0.0024	
BC	0.1928	1	0.1928	2.35	0.1559	
A^2	0.1955	1	0.1955	2.39	0.1534	
B^2	0.2432	1	0.2432	2.97	0.1156	
C^2	0.9517	1	0.9517	11.62	0.0067	
Residual	0.8191	10	0.0819			
Lack of Fit	0.4057	5	0.0811	0.9816	0.5079	not significant
Pure Error	0.4133	5	0.0827			
Cor Total	50.01	19				

R^2 - 0.9836, Adj R^2 - 0.9689, Predicted R^2 - 0.9208, CV – 4.66%, Adeq precision – 26.29, df - degree of freedom, Significant – $P < 0.05$, Non-significant – $P > 0.05$.

Table 6A: Experimental and predicted values of protein production from strain MANF2 under mild stress of penicillin G provided at lag phase.

Run order	Yeast extract (A)	Glycerol (B)	*M. piperita* (C)	Protein content (mg/mL)	
				Experimental	Predicted
1	0	-α	0	2.8	2.7
2	0	0	0	2.4	2.05
3	0	0	0	2.4	2.05
4	0	0	-α	1.6	1.7
5	+1	0	0	4.4	4.5
6	0	0	0	1.9	2.05
7	0	0	0	1.8	2.05
8	-α	0	0	1.4	1.3
9	0	+α	0	1.6	1.6
10	0	0	0	1.8	2.05
11	-1	-1	+1	1.8	1.9
12	+1	-1	-1	3.2	3.1
13	-1	+1	+1	2.4	2.3
14	**+1**	**0**	**+1**	**5.4**	**5.1**
15	-1	-1	-1	1.8	1.6
16	+1	+1	-1	1.7	1.4
17	0	0	0	1.9	2.05
18	0	0	+α	4.7	4.6
19	+α	0	0	4.3	4.4
20	-1	+1	-1	1.5	1.5

Table 6B: ANOVA for protein production from strain MANF2 under mild stress of penicillin G provided at lag phase.

Source	Sum of Squares	df	Mean Square	*F*-value	*P*-value	
Model	27.13	9	3.01	43.14	< 0.0001	significant
A-A	11.32	1	11.32	161.97	< 0.0001	
B-B	1.33	1	1.33	19.00	0.0014	
C-C	9.51	1	9.51	136.08	< 0.0001	
AB	0.9836	1	0.9836	14.08	0.0038	
AC	2.51	1	2.51	35.90	0.0001	
BC	0.0939	1	0.0939	1.34	0.2733	
A^2	1.32	1	1.32	18.88	0.0015	
B^2	0.0474	1	0.0474	0.6779	0.4295	
C^2	2.40	1	2.40	34.33	0.0002	
Residual	0.6987	10	0.0699			
Lack of Fit	0.2854	5	0.0571	0.6904	0.6529	not significant
Pure Error	0.4133	5	0.0827			
Cor Total	27.83	19				

R^2 - 0.9749, Adj R^2 - 0.9523, Predicted R^2 - 0.9039, CV – 10.41%, Adeq precision – 20.31, df - degree of freedom, Significant – $P < 0.05$, Non-significant – $P > 0.05$.

Table 7A: Experimental and predicted values of protein production from strain MANF2 under mild stress of penicillin G provided at log phase.

Run order	Yeast extract (A)	Glycerol (B)	*M. piperita* (C)	Protein content (mg/mL)	
				Experimental	Predicted
1	0	-α	0	5.8	5.6
2	0	0	0	5.4	5.03
3	0	0	0	5.4	5.03
4	0	0	-α	3.6	3.5
5	+1	0	0	7.4	7.1
6	0	0	0	4.9	5.03
7	0	0	0	4.8	5.03
8	-α	0	0	3.2	3.3
9	0	+α	0	3.3	3.6
10	0	0	0	4.8	5.03
11	-1	-1	+1	4.8	4.6
12	+1	-1	-1	6.2	6.2
13	-1	+1	+1	5.4	5.2
14	**+1**	**0**	**+1**	**8.4**	**8.3**
15	-1	-1	-1	3.1	3.2
16	+1	+1	-1	3.3	3.2
17	0	0	0	4.9	5.03
18	0	0	+α	7.7	7.9
19	+α	0	0	7.3	7.4
20	-1	+1	-1	3.2	3.06

Table 7B: ANOVA for protein production from strain MANF2 under mild stress of penicillin G provided at log phase.

Source	Sum of Squares	df	Mean Square	*F*-value	*P*-value	
Model	49.19	9	5.47	66.73	< 0.0001	Significant
A-A	19.41	1	19.41	236.92	< 0.0001	
B-B	4.36	1	4.36	53.22	< 0.0001	
C-C	22.80	1	22.80	278.31	< 0.0001	
AB	2.97	1	2.97	36.31	0.0001	
AC	1.33	1	1.33	16.22	0.0024	
BC	0.1928	1	0.1928	2.35	0.1559	
A^2	0.1955	1	0.1955	2.39	0.1534	
B^2	0.2432	1	0.2432	2.97	0.1156	
C^2	0.9517	1	0.9517	11.62	0.0067	
Residual	0.8191	10	0.0819			
Lack of Fit	0.4057	5	0.0811	0.9816	0.5079	not significant
Pure Error	0.4133	5	0.0827			
Cor Total	50.01	19				

R^2 - 0.9836, Adj R^2 - 0.9689, Predicted R^2 - 0.9208, CV – 5.56%, Adeq precision – 26.29, df - degree of freedom, Significant – $P < 0.05$, Non-significant – $P > 0.05$.

Table 8A: Experimental and predicted values of protein production from strain MANF2 under mild stress of mercuric chloride provided at lag phase.

Run order	Yeast extract (A)	Glycerol (B)	*M. piperita* (C)	Protein content (mg/mL)	
				Experimental	Predicted
1	0	-α	0	1.8	1.9
2	0	0	0	1.4	1.7
3	0	0	0	1.4	1.7
4	0	0	-α	1.3	1.3
5	**+1**	**0**	**0**	**4.4**	**4.1**
6	0	0	0	1.9	1.7
7	0	0	0	1.8	1.7
8	-α	0	0	1.5	1.4
9	0	+α	0	1.3	1.1
10	0	0	0	1.8	1.7
11	-1	-1	+1	1.8	1.7
12	+1	-1	-1	2.2	1.9
13	-1	+1	+1	1.4	1.5
14	+1	0	+1	3.4	3.5
15	-1	-1	-1	1.5	1.4
16	+1	+1	-1	1.3	1.2
17	0	0	0	1.9	1.7
18	0	0	+α	3.7	3.6
19	+α	0	0	3.3	3.5
20	-1	+1	-1	1.6	1.6

Table 8B: ANOVA for protein production from strain MANF2 under mild stress of mercuric chloride provided at lag phase.

Source	Sum of Squares	df	Mean Square	*F*-value	*P*-value	
Model	15.26	9	1.70	28.02	< 0.0001	Significant
A-A	5.12	1	5.12	84.66	< 0.0001	
B-B	0.6958	1	0.6958	11.50	0.0069	
C-C	5.83	1	5.83	96.44	< 0.0001	
AB	0.3480	1	0.3480	5.75	0.0374	
AC	2.59	1	2.59	42.83	< 0.0001	
BC	0.0789	1	0.0789	1.30	0.2801	
A^2	1.03	1	1.03	17.00	0.0021	
B^2	0.0307	1	0.0307	0.5074	0.4925	
C^2	1.17	1	1.17	19.31	0.0013	
Residual	0.6049	10	0.0605			
Lack of Fit	0.3249	5	0.0650	1.16	0.4372	not significant
Pure Error	0.2800	5	0.0560			
Cor Total	15.86	19				

R^2 - 0.9619, Adj R^2 - 0.9275, Predicted R^2 - 0.8201, CV – 12.12%, Adeq precision – 17.20, df - degree of freedom, Significant – $P < 0.05$, Non-significant – $P > 0.05$.

Table 9A: Experimental and predicted values of protein production from strain MANF2 under mild stress of mercuric chloride provided at log phase.

Run order	Yeast extract (A)	Glycerol (B)	*M. piperita* (C)	Protein content (mg/mL)	
				Experimental	Predicted
1	0	-α	0	4.8	4.7
2	0	0	0	4.4	4.03
3	0	0	0	4.4	4.03
4	0	0	-α	2.6	2.6
5	**+1**	**0**	**0**	**7.4**	**7.4**
6	0	0	0	3.9	4.03
7	0	0	0	3.8	4.03
8	-α	0	0	2.5	2.6
9	0	+α	0	2.3	2.6
10	0	0	0	3.8	4.03
11	-1	-1	+1	3.8	3.7
12	+1	-1	-1	5.2	5.2
13	-1	+1	+1	4.4	4.2
14	+1	0	+1	6.4	6.1
15	-1	-1	-1	2.5	2.5
16	+1	+1	-1	2.3	2.2
17	0	0	0	3.9	4.03
18	0	0	+α	6.7	6.9
19	+α	0	0	6.3	6.4
20	-1	+1	-1	2.6	2.4

Table 9B: ANOVA for protein production from strain MANF2 under mild stress of mercuric chloride provided at log phase.

Source	Sum of Squares	df	Mean Square	F-value	P-value	
Model	45.20	9	5.02	63.07	< 0.0001	Significant
A-A	16.56	1	16.56	207.93	< 0.0001	
B-B	4.42	1	4.42	55.49	< 0.0001	
C-C	20.90	1	20.90	262.45	< 0.0001	
AB	3.04	1	3.04	38.11	0.0001	
AC	2.06	1	2.06	25.83	0.0005	
BC	0.1777	1	0.1777	2.23	0.1661	
A^2	0.4669	1	0.4669	5.86	0.0360	
B^2	0.1991	1	0.1991	2.50	0.1449	
C^2	1.03	1	1.03	12.98	0.0048	
Residual	0.7963	10	0.0796			
Lack of Fit	0.3830	5	0.0766	0.9266	0.5323	not significant
Pure Error	0.4133	5	0.0827			
Cor Total	46.00	19				

R^2 - 0.9827, Adj R^2 - 0.9671, Predicted R^2 - 0.9133, CV – 6.72%, Adeq precision – 26.10, df - degree of freedom, Significant – $P < 0.05$, Non-significant – $P > 0.05$.

Table 10: Purification of protein from strain MANF2.

Purification step	**Volume (mL)**	**RLU (%)**	**Total protein (mg)**	**Specific activity**	**Purification fold**	**Yield (%)**
CFNS	1000	98.8	12535.3	0.0079	1	100
Ammonium sulphate precipitation	1000	84.3	9546.3	0.009	1.14	85.3
Dialysis	10	78.1	340.3	0.23	29.1	79.1
DEAE - Cellulose column chromatography	2	71.5	6.6	10.84	1372.1	72.3

Table 11: Effect of pH, temperature, and enzymes on residual anti-tubercular activity of protein.

Treatment	Residual activity (%)
pH	
Control	100±0.5^{a}
3	40.4±0.4^{f}
4	44.8±0.4^{e}
5	54.6±0.5^{d}
6	93.5±0.5^{c}
7	96.6±0.4^{b}
8	54.5±0.4^{d}
Temperature	
Control	100±0.5^{a}
40°C, 2 h	97.2±0.4^{b}
60°C, 1 h	54.5±0.4^{c}
80°C, 30 min	26.8±0.5^{d}
100°C, 20 min	14.4±0.5^{e}
121°C, 15 min	10.8±0.4^{f}
Enzymes	
Control	100±0.5^{a}
Pepsin	0.00±0.00
Trypsin	0.00±0.00
Protease K	0.00±0.00
α-amylase	97.8±0.5^{b}

Values represent mean±SD of experiments carried out in triplicate (n = 3).

^{a,b,c,d,e,f}Means followed by different superscripts are significantly different (*P*<0.05).

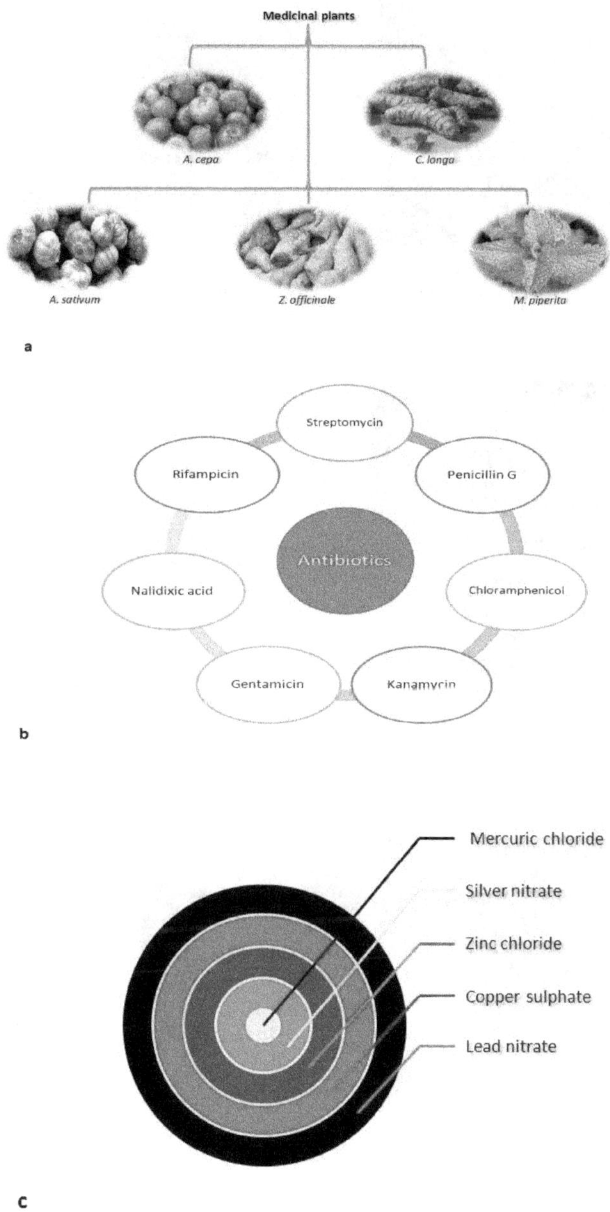

Figure 1: Three different categories of antimicrobials viz. (a) medicinal plants, (b) antibiotics, and (c) heavy metals used.

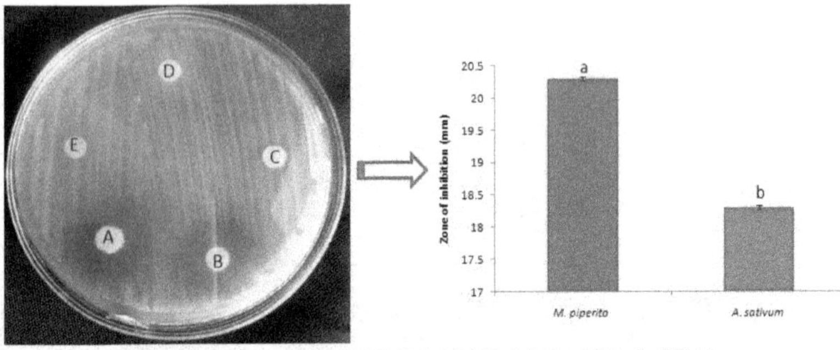

[Note: A – *M. piperita*, B – *A. sativum*, C – *A. cepa*, D – *C. longa*, and E – *Z. officinale*
[ab]Values with different letters are significantly ($P<0.05$) different]

a

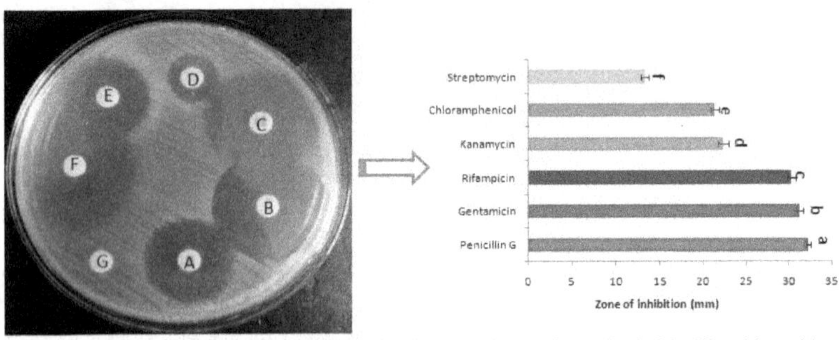

[Note: A – Kanamycin, B – Penicillin G, C – Gentamicin, D – Streptomycin, E – Chloramphenicol, F – Rifampicin, and G – Nalidixic acid
[abcdef]Values with different letters are significantly ($P<0.05$) different]

b

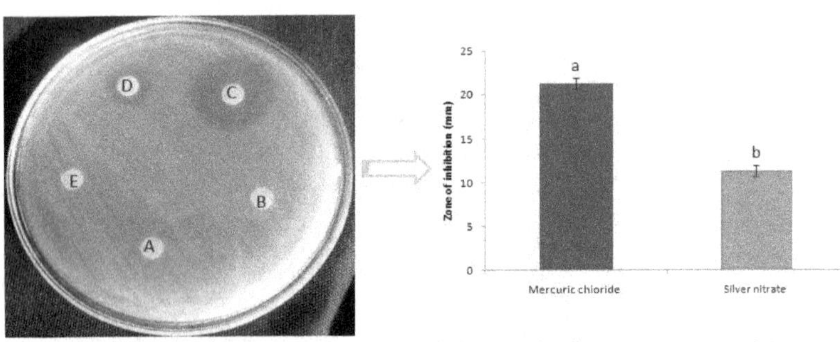

[Note: A – Zinc chloride, B – Copper sulphate, C – Mercuric chloride , D – Silver nitrate , and E – Lead nitrate
[ab]Values with different letters are significantly ($P<0.05$) different]

c

Figure 2: Antibacterial activities of (a) medicinal plants, (b) antibiotics, and (c) heavy metals against strain MANF2.

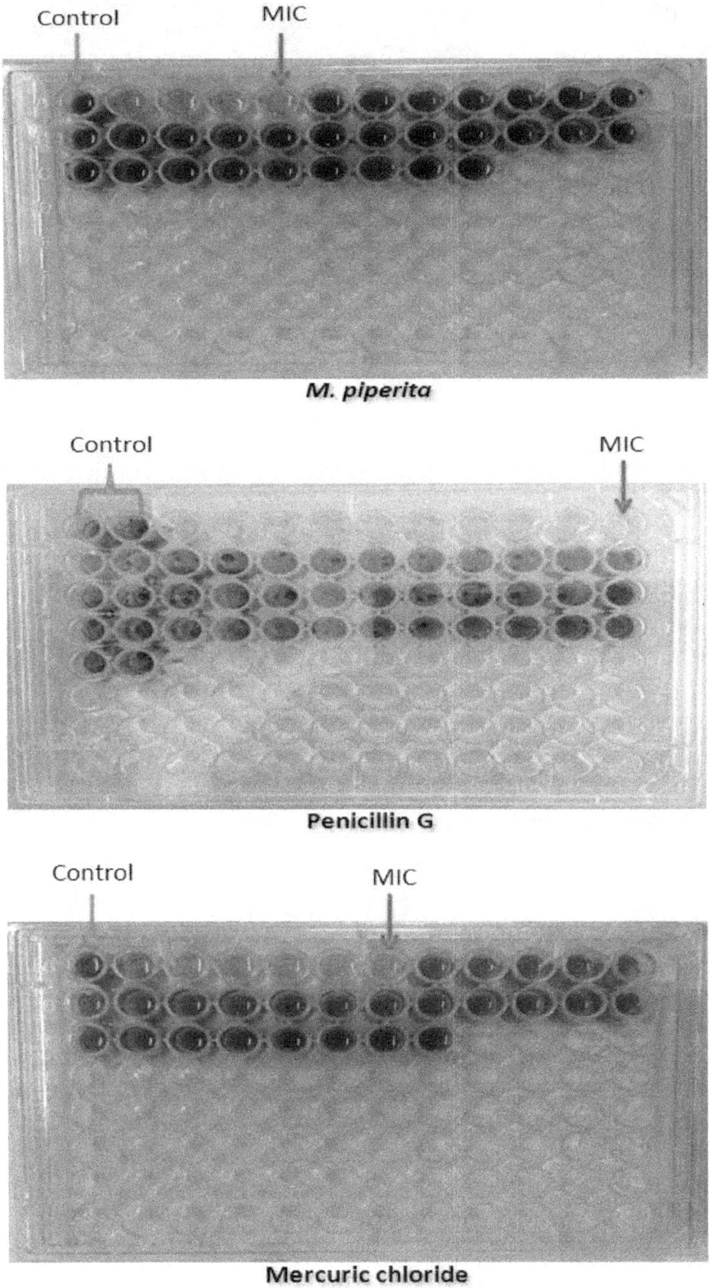

Figure 3: MIC determination of potent antimicrobial agents.

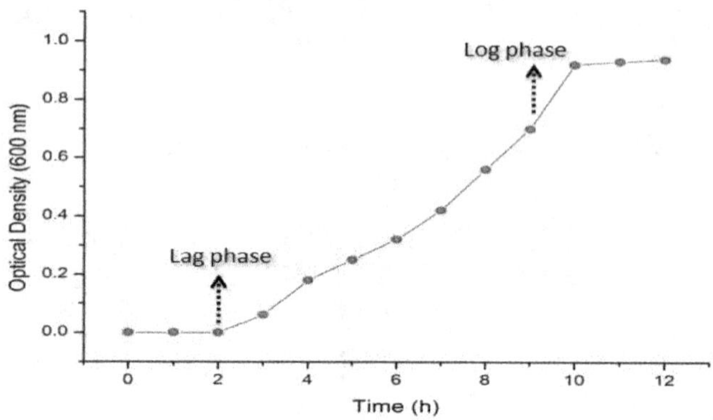

Figure 4: Growth curve analysis of strain MANF2.

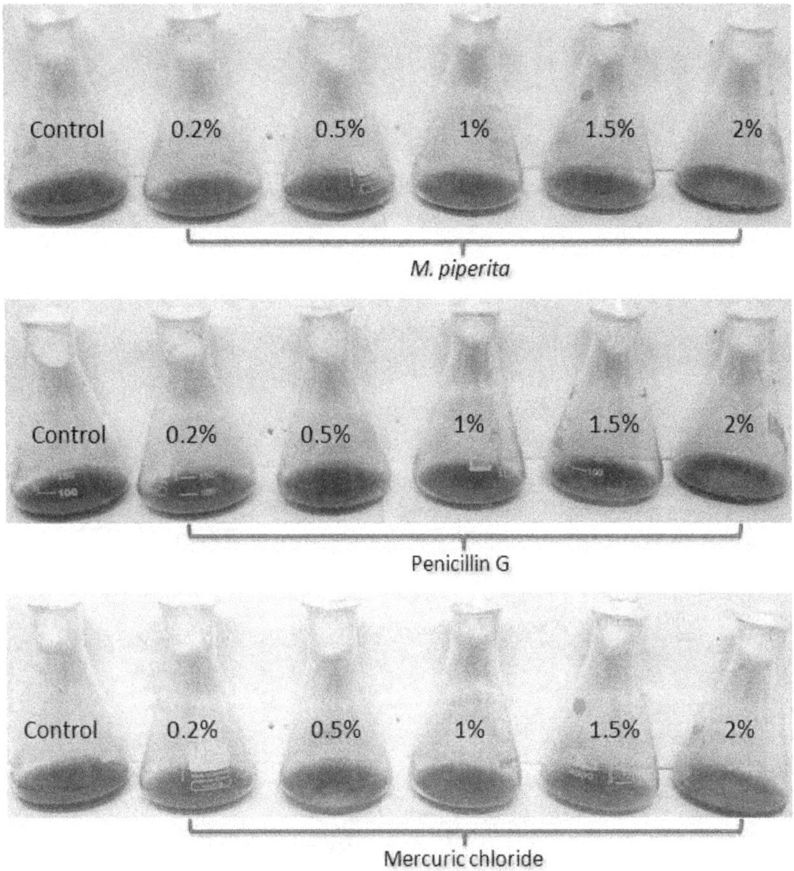

Figure 5: Shake flask fermentation in the presence of potent antimicrobials of varied concentration (0.2-2%). Stress was provided at lag phase of strain MANF2.

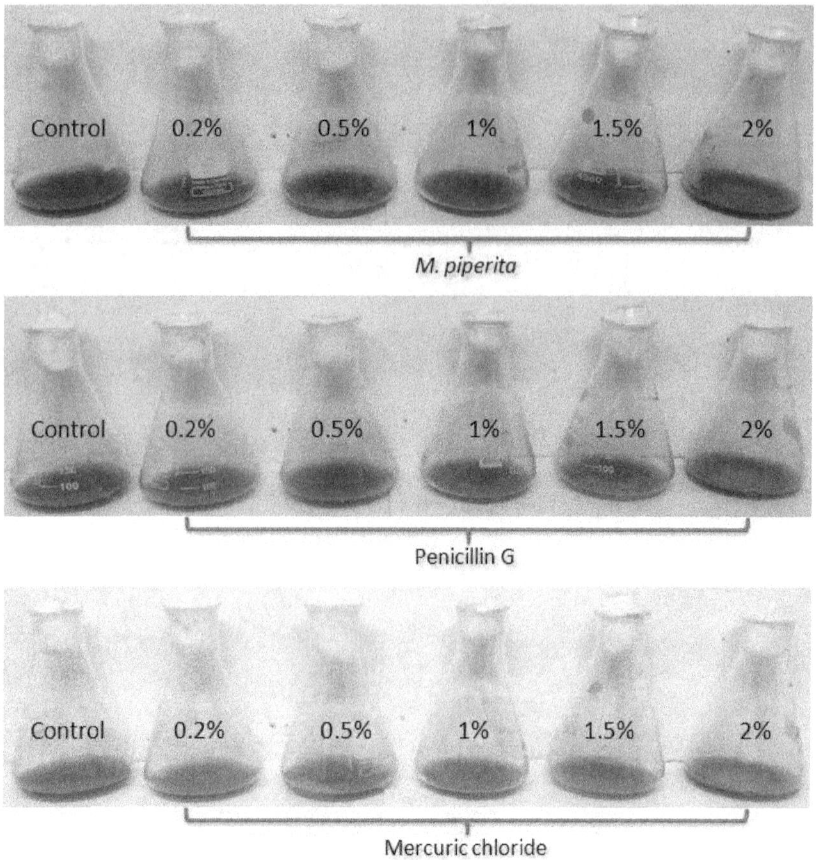

Figure 6: Shake flask fermentation in the presence of potent antimicrobials of varied concentration (0.2-2%). Stress was provided at log phase of strain MANF2.

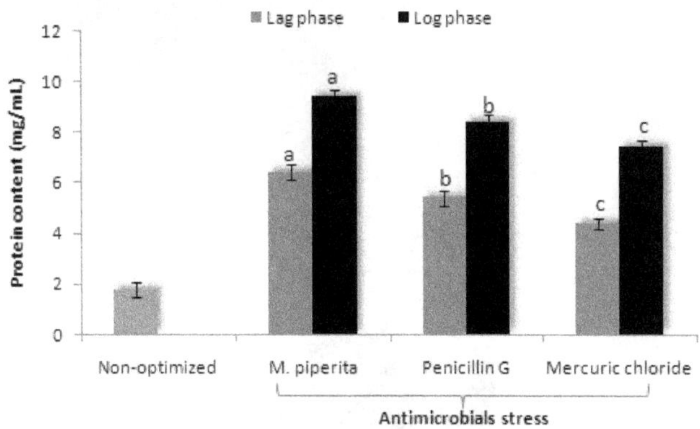

Figure 7: Protein production from strain MANF2 under mild stress of antimicrobials with respect to the non-optimized conditions.

[Note: Values are represented as mean±SD of experiments carried out in triplicate (n = 3). [abc]Values with different letters are significantly (P<0.05) different.]

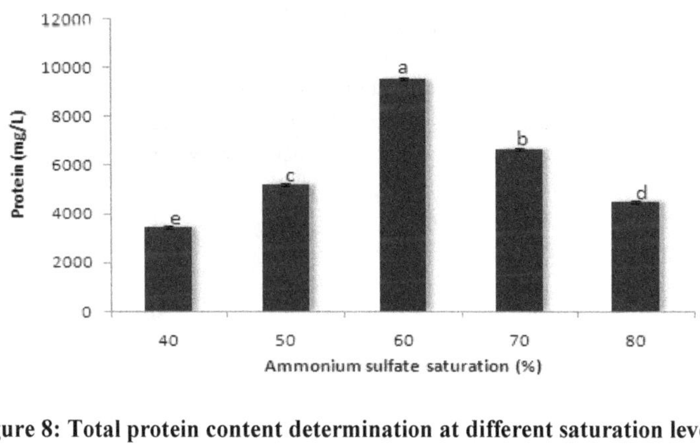

Figure 8: Total protein content determination at different saturation levels of ammonium sulphate.

[Note: Values are represented as mean±SD of experiments carried out in triplicate (n = 3). [abcde]Values with different letters are significantly (P<0.05) different.]

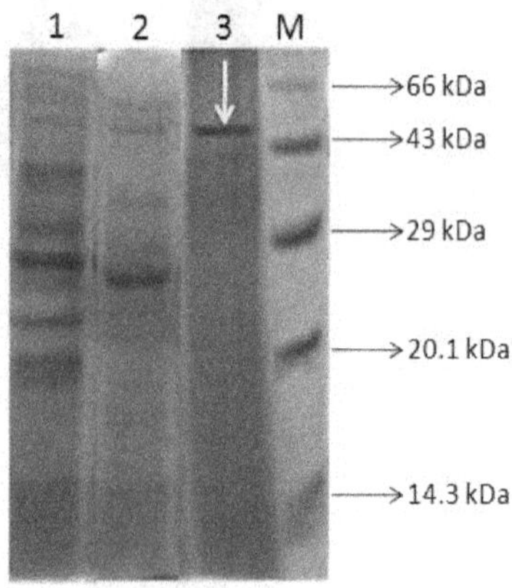

Lane 1: Ammonium sulphate precipitated sample
Lane 2: Dialysed sample
Lane 3: Purified sample
M: Protein marker

Figure 9: Molecular mass determination of purified protein using SDS-PAGE. Lane 3 showed a single homogeneous band corresponding to the molecular mass of approximately 52 kDa, indicated by yellow arrow.

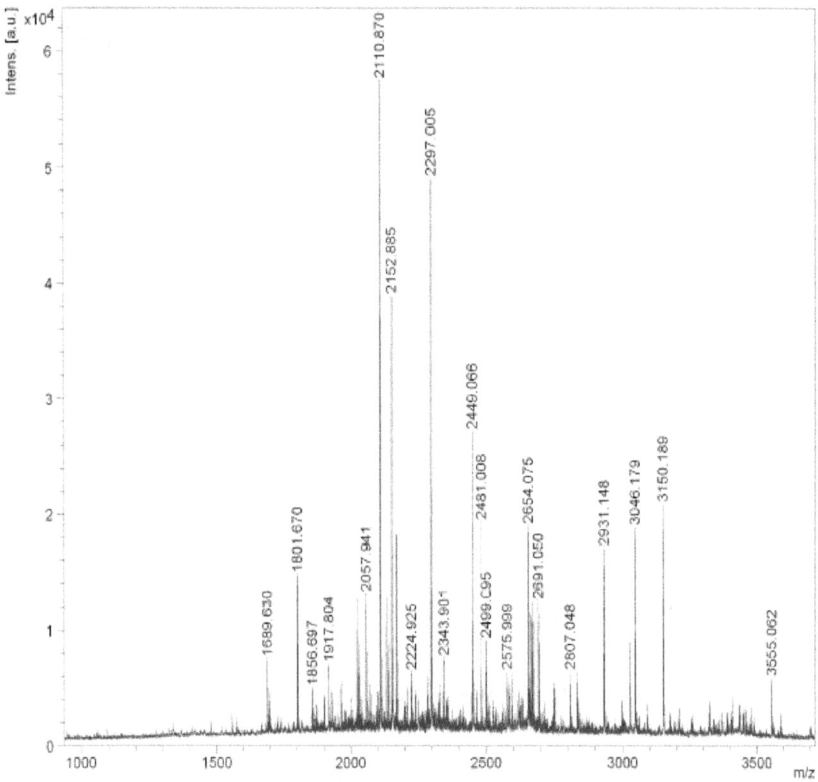

Figure 10: MALDI-TOF MS/MS spectrum of purified protein.

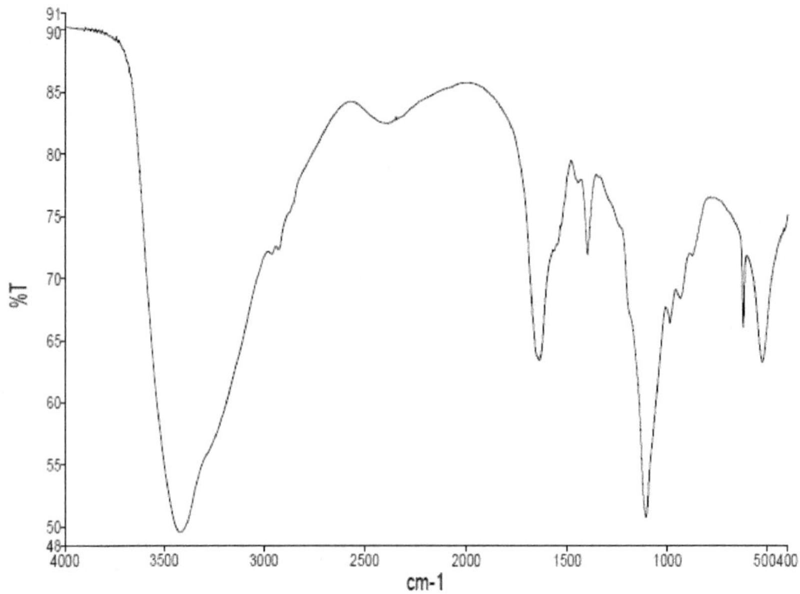

Figure 11: FT-IR spectrum of purified protein.

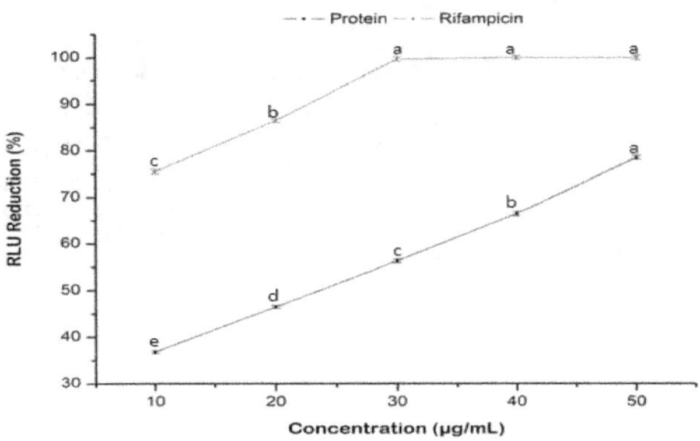

Figure 12: Anti-tubercular activities of purified protein and rifampicin at various concentrations.

[Note: Values are represented as mean±SD of experiments carried out in triplicate (n = 3). [abcde]Values with different letters are significantly (P<0.05) different.]

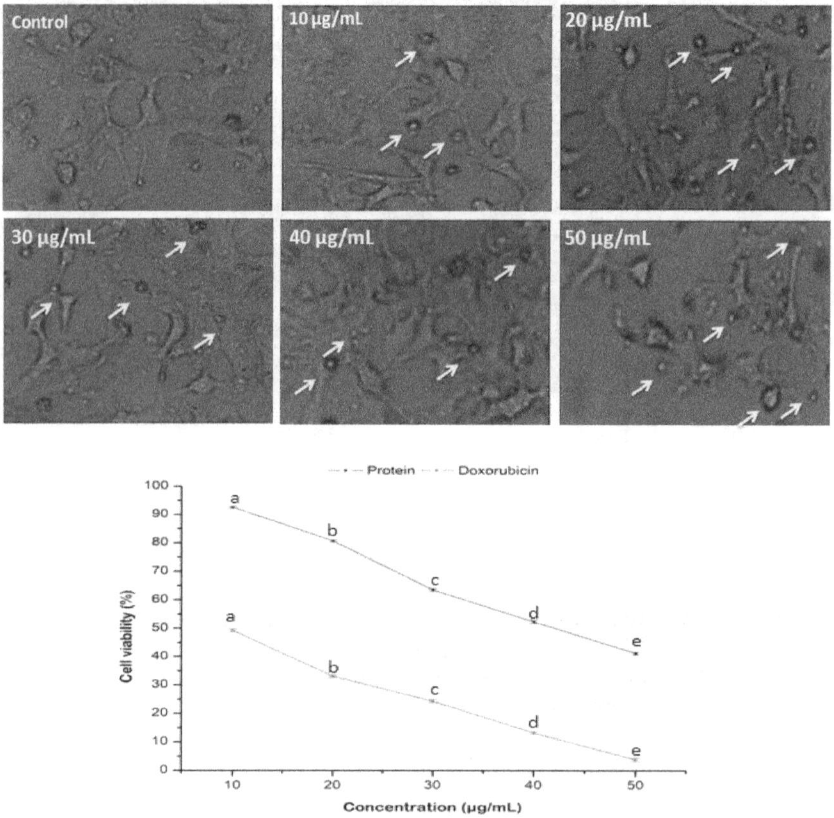

Figure 13: Morphological variations and reductions in the viabilities of A549 cancer cells in the presence of various concentrations of purified protein. Yellow arrows indicate morphological changes in the cancer cells.

[Note: Values are represented as mean±SD of experiments carried out in triplicate (n = 3). [abcde]Values with different letters are significantly (*P*<0.05) different.]

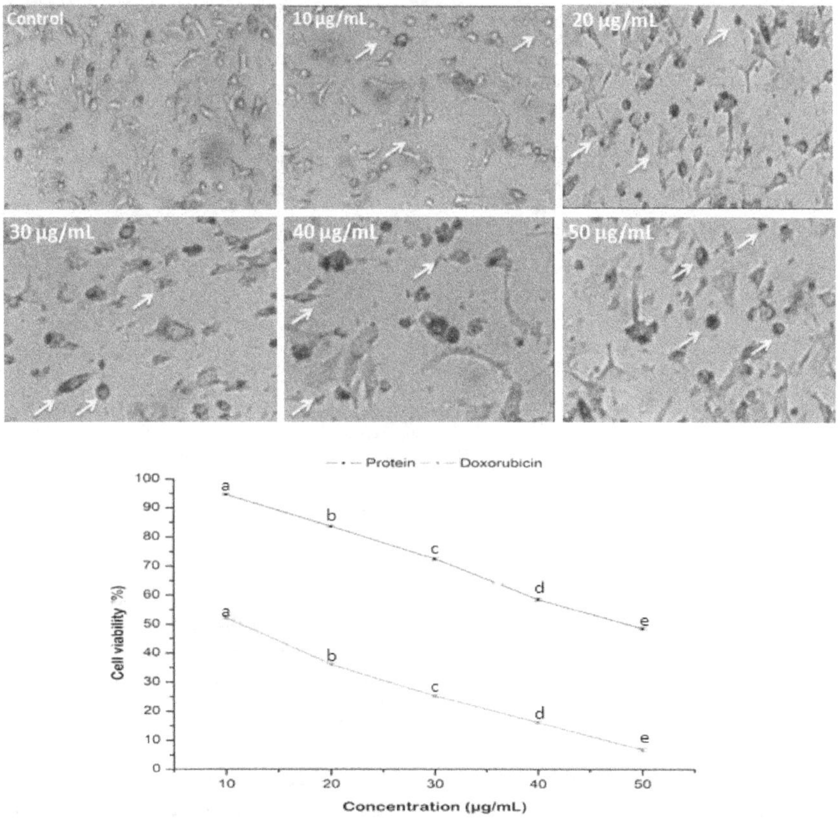

Figure 14: Morphological variations and reductions in the viabilities of HT-29 cancer cells in the presence of various concentrations of purified protein. Yellow arrows indicate morphological changes in the cancer cells.

[Note: Values are represented as mean±SD of experiments carried out in triplicate (n = 3). [abcde]Values with different letters are significantly (*P*<0.05) different.]

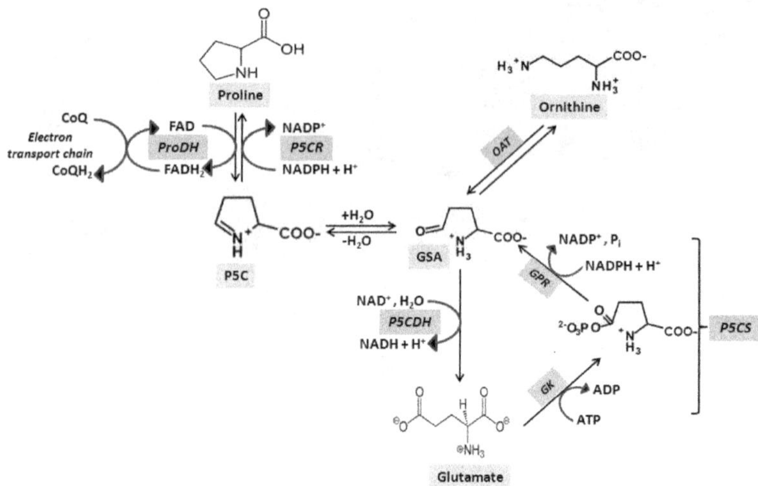

Figure 15: Pathway of proline metabolism. Proline is synthesized from glutamate starting with the enzymes glutamate kinase (GK) and γ-glutamyl phosphate reductase (GPR), which in plants and animals are fused together in the bifunctional enzyme Δ^1-pyrroline-5-carboxylate synthetase (P5CS). The intermediate, γ-glutamate-semialdehyde (GSA) spontaneously cyclises to Δ^1-pyrroline-5-carboxylate (P5C), which is then reduced to proline by P5C reductase (P5CR). Alternatively, proline can be formed from ornithine, which is converted into P5C/GSA via ornithine-δ-aminotransferase (OAT). P5C is then reduced to proline by P5C reductase (P5CR).

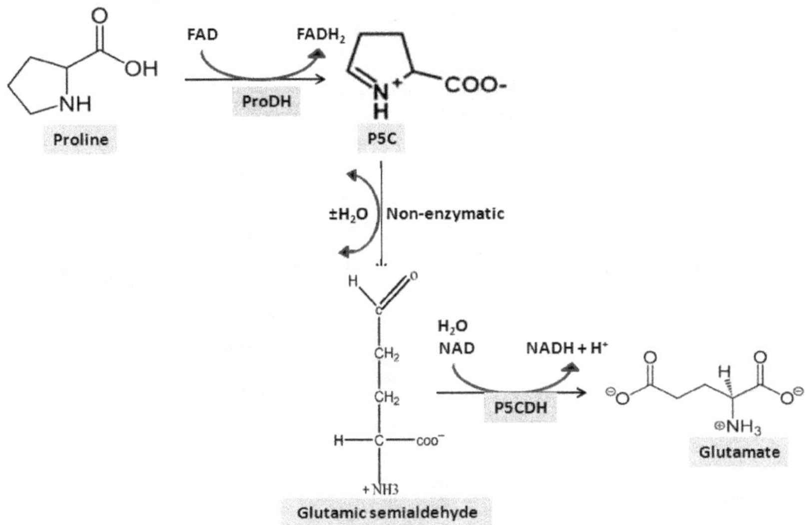

Figure 16: Metabolism of proline to glutamate through the catalytic reaction of ProDH. The first enzymatic step transforms proline to Δ^1-pyrroline-5-carboxylate (P5C), which is non-enzymatically hydrolyzed to glutamic semialdehyde. The semialdehyde is oxidized in the second enzymatic step to glutamate by the catalytic action of Δ^1-pyrroline-5-carboxylate dehydrogenase.

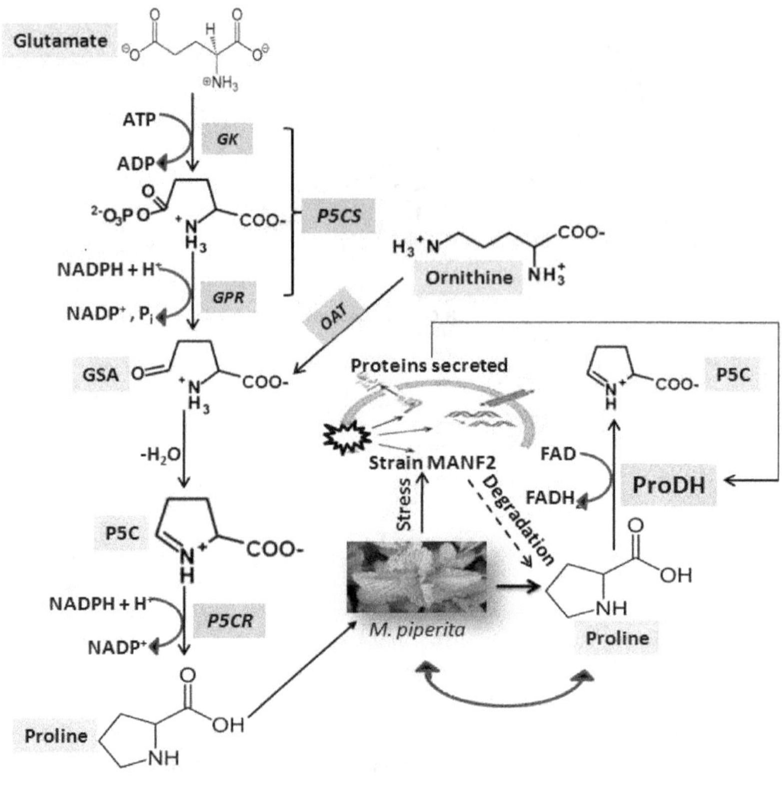

Figure 17: Proposed pathway for ProDH production from strain MANF2 under mild stress of *M. piperita.* Proline was synthesized in *M. piperita* from glutamate through proline metabolism pathway. *M. piperita* at mild concentration exposed strain MANF2 to proline which caused the secretion of bioactive proteins from bacterium into the medium for its degradation. Proline was degraded by ProDH which was purified further through chromatographic techniques.

4. Discussion

Bacteria are exposed to diversified kinds of stresses in the environment which impair their metabolism. The potentiality to adapt rapidly the changing environmental conditions is one of the most important hallmarks of bacterial survival ability. Mild or drastic variations in the environment can cause alteration in the transcriptome of bacterial cells. As a matter of fact, stress can elicit dramatic variations in the expression pattern of stress-related genes encoding proteins which improve adaptation toward the changing environment. The sensing of any kind of stress sends alarming signals to bacteria, and thus, the mechanisms within them start working overtime to neutralize or pump out the undesired environment as well as to repair damaged constituents of the cell. This situation triggers transcriptional variations in the bacteria and produces or secretes new proteins (Ismail *et al.*, 2013).

In this study, antimicrobials agents such as *M. piperita*, penicillin G, and mercuric chloride at sub-MIC concentrations were used to provide stress to strain MANF2 during its lag and log phase. Mild concentrations of antimicrobials supplemented at log phase of strain MANF2 showed significant ($P<0.05$) enhancement in total protein production using statistical optimization tool. The finding suggested that the protein content from bacteria can be enhanced by supplementing the particular doses of antimicrobials at specific growth period of bacteria. It is supported by the previous study of Khusro and Sankari (2015) who evaluated exemplary role of *A. sativum* in improving total protein production from *Bacillus* sp. using non-statistical tool. Our findings revealed first report on the promising role of *M. piperita*, penicillin G, and mercuric chloride in enhancement of total protein content from fermented food associated coagulase-negative *Staphylococcus* sp.

Extracellular stimulations cause alterations in the metabolic activities of bacteria. In the present investigation, strain MANF2 showed rapid variations in their cellular responses after exposure of *M. piperita* at mild concentrations. The mild stress of antimicrobial agents might induce the production of metabolism associated distinct proteins. It should be noteworthy that bacteria obtain energy for growth through metabolic processes. A stimulus can over express a variety of genes which produce metabolism related new proteins inside the bacterial cells. An immediate defensive response is required for the survival of bacteria in the presence of external stimuli. In this regard, translational regulation of pre-existing mRNAs provides a fast and efficient strategy for controlling the expression of various genes (Ismail *et al.*, 2013). Notably, the stress-induced attenuation of global translation is often accompanied by a switch to the selective translation of proteins that are essential for the survival of bacteria under stress (Harding *et al.*, 2000). In the current study, protein involved in the translation process were differentially expressed by strain MANF2 following exposure to *M. piperita* stress at log phase of bacterial growth.

Strain MANF2 under *M. piperita* stress produced anti-tubercular protein of molecular mass 51293 Da. Further, based on amino acid sequencing, the molecular mass of the most abundant peptide was determined as 2110.87 Da, which showed 100% homology with ProDH, thereby categorizing it as new class of ProDH- like protein in *S. hominis*. Also, the peptide was considered new due to the lack of homology of molecular mass with existing peptides previously reported from *Staphylococcus* spp., and thus this peptide was named as SMANF2. The findings established the fact that because of stress, translation is regulated to mitigate energy consumption and to selectively synthesize new proteins for the proper establishment of tolerance. Further, the FT-IR spectrum of the purified protein indicates strong peaks, suggesting the presence of varied functional groups. The presence of different peaks in the protein was supposed to be obtained through stretching and bending vibrations in the region of infrared radiation. Reports on the purification of ProDH from bacterial sources are scarce. Previous studies have revealed the purification of ProDH from *P. aeruginosa* (Meile and Leisinger, 1982), *E. coli* (Baban *et al.*, 2004), *P. entomophila* (Shahbaz-Mohammadi and Omidinia, 2011), and *P. putida* (Shahbaz-Mohammadi and Omidinia, 2012). Interestingly, our findings represent the first report on the purification of ProDH from *S. hominis*.

Oxidation of amino acids is a central part of energy metabolism. Proline ($C_5H_9NO_2$) is a proteinogenic secondary amino acid, which plays essential roles not only in primary metabolism but also in redox homeostasis, osmotic adjustment, protection against stress, and signalling in all organisms and plants. The chemical reactions of the proline metabolic pathway are shown in Figure 15. Proline is synthesized from glutamate starting with the enzymes glutamate kinase and γ-glutamyl phosphate reductase, which in plants and animals are fused together in the bifunctional enzyme Δ^1-pyrroline-5-carboxylate synthetase. The intermediate, γ-glutamate-semialdehyde (GSA) spontaneously cyclises to Δ^1-pyrroline-5-carboxylate (P5C), which is then reduced to proline by P5C reductase (P5CR). Alternatively, proline can be formed from ornithine, which is converted into P5C/GSA via ornithine-δ-aminotransferase (Liang *et al.*, 2013).

Proline acts as energy supplier and may stabilize DNA, protein, and membrane structure and function of plants (Kavir-Kishor *et al.*, 2005). *M. piperita* contains promising amount of proline, as investigated by Askary *et al.* (2017) and Samandari-Gikloo *et al.* (2018). Despite the presence of proline originally into the plant, proline accumulation in plants also occurs due to various stresses, including salt, drought, UV radiation, and heavy metal ions (Liang *et al.*, 2013). Besides, proline accumulation is a common phenomenon observed in response to environmental stress in bacteria too (Csonka, 1981). In this study, *M. piperita* was used as antimicrobial agent to provide mild stress to strain MANF2, which clearly indicates growth of bacteria in the presence of proline. The oxidative pathway for proline degradation consists of two enzymatic steps and an intervening non-enzymatic equilibrium. ProDH and Δ^1-pyrroline-5-carboxylate dehydrogenase (P5CDH) catalyze L-proline into glutamate (Menzel and Roth, 1981). The first enzymatic step transforms proline to P5C, which is non-enzymatically hydrolyzed to glutamic semialdehyde. The semialdehyde is oxidized in the second enzymatic step to glutamate (Figure 16) (adapted from Shahbaz-Mohammadi and Omidinia, 2012).

ProDH catalyzes the oxidation of L-proline to P5C leading to the release of electrons, which can be transferred to either electron transfer systems or to molecular oxygen. ProDH is essential not only for proline catabolism but also provides energy. In most bacteria, ProDH and P5CDH activities are combined in a single bifunctional enzyme known as Proline utilization A. Studies of the bacterial enzymes have shown that ProDH is an flavin adenine dinucleotide -dependent enzyme.

The proposed hypothesis for the ProDH production pathway from strain MANF2 under mild stress of *M. piperita* is shown in Figure 17. The supplementation of mild concentration of *M. piperita* exposed the bacterium to proline present in this plant, as synthesized through proline metabolism pathway. The ProDH encoding gene might have been ‘switched on’ through the signalling mechanism due to the presence of external stimulus. ProDH was secreted into the medium to catalyze the proline oxidation mechanisms; thereby the production of extracellular ProDH from strain MANF2 was obtained.

Proteins synthesized in bacteria under mild stress of antimicrobial agents such as *A. sativum* and streptomycin sulphate have shown pronounced activities against human pathogens (Ismail *et al.*, 2013; Hanina *et al.*, 2014). In this context, we have taken further significant attempt to synthesize new protein in coagulase-negative *Staphylococcus* sp. under mild stress of *M. piperita* for its anti-tubercular and anticancer properties. The purified protein exhibited promising anti-tubercular activities in a dose dependent manner. Different pH treatments affected significantly the anti-tubercular activities of purified protein. Variations in the anti-tubercular properties at lower or higher pH may be due to the denaturation of the purified protein as electrostatic repulsion of intermolecular and breaking of hydrogen bonds (Yi *et al.*, 2016). Further, the protein lost its anti-tubercular activity at high temperature (>60^{0}C). It clearly suggests that heat resistance nature of protein depends on its stable structural characteristics (Kim *et al.*, 2010). The anti-tubercular trait of purified protein was lost completely after treatment with pepsin, trypsin, and protease K but its attribute was retained by α-amylase treatment. Findings clearly represent that the purified product is proteinaceous in nature constituting amino acid residues, without carbohydrate moieties. Similar observations were reported by Yi *et al.* (2016) too.

In the present investigation, the cytotoxic activity of purified protein was determined against lung and colon cancer cells. The protein revealed comparatively higher anticancer activity against A549 cells with respect to HT-29 cells. Findings of the present study indicated the first report on the anticancer attribute of *S. hominis* associated protein synthesized under mild stress of *M. piperita*. The protein synthesized in bacteria under mild stress conditions of certain antimicrobials may be used for designing new protein/peptide-based anti-tubercular and anticancer drugs in future.

5. Conclusions

Total protein content from strain MANF2 was enhanced in the presence of *M. piperita*, penicillin G, and mercuric chloride. However, medium containing yeast extract (0.5% w/v) and glycerol (1.5% v/v), and supplementation of *M. piperita* (1.5% v/v) at log phase of strain MANF2 revealed maximum protein content of 9.4±0.4 mg/mL using CCD of RSM. The protein content from bacteria can be enhanced by supplementing the particular doses of antimicrobials at specific growth period of bacteria. Most importantly, the experimental values of response variables showed a close concordance with the predicted responding values, thereby confirming the validation of model.

Further, the study represents the first report on the identification of anti-tubercular and anticancer protein from *S. hominis* under mild stress of *M. piperita*. The molecular mass of the most abundant peptide was observed as 2110.87 Da, which showed 100% homology with ProDH, thereby categorizing it as new class of ProDH- like protein in *S. hominis*. Also, the peptide was considered new due to the lack of homology of molecular mass with existing peptides previously reported from *Staphylococcus* spp., and thus this peptide was named as SMANF2. Protein purified from strain MANF2 under mild stress of antimicrobials can be used as ideal anti-tubercular and anticancer agents.

Chapter 6

In silico modelling of anti-tubercular and anticancer peptide SMANF2: Stereo-chemical, physiochemical, functional, and docking insight

1. Introduction

Currently, peptides derived from native proteins of bacteria are being investigated as pivotal therapeutic agents due to their broad-spectrum bioactivities and non-specific mechanism of actions. Most of the peptides are amphipathic, cationic, and constitutes short amino acids. Peptides are isolated from disparate sources such as plants, animals, amphibians, and microorganisms which suggest advantages over existing drugs (Xin *et al.*, 2017). However, bacteria associated peptides have been considered auspicious therapeutic agents against wide ranges of infectious and non-infectious diseases. In general, peptides isolated from bacteria are not only thermo-stable but also show low toxicity to normal cells, which makes them ideal agents for the development of effective drugs in future medicine (Upton *et al.*, 2012).

Physiochemical properties viz. charge, hydrophobicity, structure, and amphipaticity are crucial parameters in identifying the peptide of interest through *in silico* studies (Juretic *et al.*, 2009). The stereo-chemistry of peptides can be understood by studying various stereo-chemical properties. Molecular docking is used to model the interaction between the peptide and receptor which helps to characterize the nature of peptide in the binding site of receptor as well as to elucidate fundamental biochemical processes (Passarini *et al.*, 2018).

Bacteria synthesize new proteins/peptides under stress conditions. These proteins/peptides help to evade stress toxicity as one of the adaptational strategies for bacterial survival. Understanding the therapeutic role of these kinds of bacterial peptides (synthesized under mild stress of antimicrobial agents) through computational tools is not investigated yet. In fact, peptides synthesized under stress may be used as prominent therapeutic agents due to their unique mode of actions and the ability to bind non-specifically to the protein binding sites. Considering this, in this chapter, a significant attempt has been undertaken to predict the physiochemical, stereo-chemical, and functional properties of peptide (peptide SMANF2) synthesized under mild stress of antimicrobial agent in strain MANF2 (previously discussed in chapter 5). Further, molecular docking of peptide SMANF2 against targeted proteins of *M. tuberculosis* and cancer (lung and colon) was analyzed using docking software in order to suggest its pronounced therapeutics attributes at pre-clinical as well as clinical trials phases and design peptide-based drugs in future with high success rate.

2. Materials and methods

2.1. Peptide of interest

Peptide SMANF2 was used in this investigation to predict its structure, stereo-chemical parameters, physiochemical properties, and molecular docking insight. The amino acid residues of SMANF2 were obtained as 'LVSTHNEAGLTSSLNRLIGK', as mentioned in the previous chapter.

2.2. Structure prediction and model evaluation of peptide

The 3D conformations of peptide (20 amino acid residues) were predicted using online software PEP-FOLD (http://bioserv.rpbs.univ-paris-diderot.fr/services/PEP-FOLD3/) (Beaufays *et al*., 2012) and iCn3D (https://www.ncbi.nlm.nih.gov/Structure/icn3d/full.html). The quality of peptide structure model was evaluated by determining different stereo chemical parameters such as Verify 3D, ERRAT, and WHATCHECK using PROCHECK https://servicesn.mbi.ucla.edu/PROCHECK/) (Laskowski *et al*., 1993).

2.3. Physiochemical properties of peptide

The physiochemical parameters viz. number of amino acids, theoretical pI (isoelectric point), instability index, aliphatic index, and GRAVY were analyzed using ExPASy-ProtParam tool (http:// web.expasy.org/protparam) (Dunker *et al*., 2001).

2.4. Primary structure analysis of peptide

The amino acid composition of peptide SMANF2 was determined using ExPASy-ProtParam tool (http:// web.expasy.org/protparam) (Dunker *et al*., 2001).

2.5. Secondary structure analysis of peptide

Secondary structure of peptide was analysed using ExPASy SIB Bioinformatics SOPMA tool (http://npsa-prabi.ibcp.fr/cgi-bin/npsa_automat.pl?page=npsa_sopma.html) which determines number of α-helices, β-turn, extended strand, β-sheet, and coils. Sequences were submitted in FASTA format in order to utilize SOPMA. Ramachandran plot was constructed using PROCHECK (https://servicesn.mbi.ucla.edu/PROCHECK/) (Laskowski *et al*., 1993) to visualize energetically allowed regions for backbone dihedral angles ϕ against Φ of amino acid residues of peptide SMANF2.

2.6. Functional analysis of peptide

The membrane spanning or extracellular nature of peptide SMANF2 was analyzed using TMHMM tool (www.cbs.dtu.dk/services/TMHMM). A helical wheel diagram of the peptide was generated by Helical Wheel Projections (http://www.bioinformatics.nl/cgi-bin/emboss/pepwheel).

2.7. Molecular docking-

2.7.1. Ligands selection

The structure of peptide SMANF2 obtained using PEP-FOLD (http://bioserv.rpbs.univ-paris-diderot.fr/services/PEP-FOLD3/) was saved as PDB file and used for molecular docking. On the other hand, structure of rifampicin and doxorubicin were obtained from PubChem (https://pubchem.ncbi.nlm.nih.gov/) and were used for docking analysis too.

2.7.2. Targeted M. tuberculosis proteins

The 3D structures of receptors viz. alanine racemase, DNA gyrase, isocitrate lyase, LysA, and ribonucleotide reductase were retrieved from RCSB PDB (http://www.rscb.org/pdb). The complexes bound to the receptor, such as non-essential water molecules and any inhibitors were removed while docking.

2.7.3. Targeted lung and colon cancer proteins

For targeting lung cancer (A540 cell line), the 3D structures of Bcl-2, H-Ras, and EGFR tyrosine kinase were retrieved from RCSB PDB (http://www.rscb.org/pdb). The complexes bound to the receptor, such as non-essential water molecules and inhibitors were removed from the target receptors while docking.

Likewise, for targeting HT-29 cell line, Bcl-xL, CDK2, and CDK4 were retrieved from RCSB PDB (http://www.rscb.org/pdb). The complexes bound to the receptor, such as non-essential water molecules and inhibitors were removed from the target receptors while docking.

2.7.4. Peptide-protein docking and visualization

Molecular docking between ligands and targeted proteins of *M. tuberculosis* and cancer cell lines (A540 and HT-29) were analyzed and visualized using Hex 8.0.0 docking software (Macindoe *et al.*, 2010) which identified the ligand with the best score and calculates the ligand-receptor interaction with the lowest free energy value.

The docking was performed by adjusting following parameters/features:

Correlation type - Shape + Electrostatics

FFT Mode - 3D

Post Processing - MM Energies

Grid Dimension - 0.6

Receptor range - 180

Ligand range - 180

Twist range - 360

Distance Range - 40

The binding energy (KJ/mol) estimated after docking was tabulated.

3. Results

3.1. Structure prediction and model evaluation of peptide

Modelled predicted structures such as 'Lines', 'Cartoon', 'Ribbon', 'Ball and Stick', 'Sphere', and 'Stick and Surface' of peptide SMANF2 is shown in Figure 1.

The quality of modelled peptide was analyzed by Verify 3D, and 80% residues of modelled peptide showed a score ≥0.2. The overall quality factor and compatibility of the model with amino acid residues were evaluated using ERRAT which was calculated as 95. In general, the modelled peptide is considered good if the quality factor is >50. Further, WHATCHECK evaluated the accuracy of modelled peptide structure, thereby indicated that the peptide SMANF2 structure was of reasonably good quality (Table 1).

3.2. Physiochemical properties of peptide

Table 1 shows the physiochemical parameters of peptide SMANF2. The pI of the peptide SMANF2 (Total number of amino acids - 20) was calculated as 8.75. The instability index of the peptide was obtained as 26.73, thereby indicating its stability. Further, the aliphatic index and GRAVY of the peptide were calculated as 117.0 and -0.05, respectively.

3.3. Primary structure analysis of peptide

The amino acid composition of peptide SMANF2 is shown in Figure 2. The amino acids such as Leusine (20.0%) and Serine (15.0%) were predominant in the peptide. On the other hand, 10.0% of Asparagine, Glycine, and Threonine were present in the peptide. While, only 5.0% of Alanine, Arginine, Glutamic acid, Histidine, Isoleucine, Lysine, and Valine were available in the peptide.

3.4. Secondary structure analysis of peptide

Figure 3 shows the secondary structure of peptide SMANF2 which was dominated by α-helices (70.0%), extended sheet region (10.0%), and random coil (20.0%).

Percentage of residues in the most favourable regions, additionally allowed regions, generously allowed regions, and disallowed regions of Ramachandran plot is shown in Figure 4. About 87.5% of residues were falling in favoured region, indicating high stability of this peptide.

3.5. Functional analysis of peptide

The membrane spanning or extracellular nature of peptide SMANF2 was analyzed using TMHMM tool which indicated lack of transmembrane domain in the peptide, thereby confirming the production of peptide SMANF2 extracellularly. Further, the helical wheel prediction of peptide SMANF2 is shown in Figure 5 which shows the presence of hydrophilic and positively charged residues.

3.6. Molecular docking

Figure 6 shows structures of ligands used (peptide SMANF2, rifampicin, and doxorubicin) for docking analysis. RCSB PDB IDs and metabolic pathways of *M. tuberculosis* receptors are illustrated in Table 2A. Likewise, RCSB PDB IDs and metabolic pathways of cancer cells receptors are described in Table 2B.

Table 3A shows the binding affinities between peptide SMANF2 and targeted proteins of *M. tuberculosis* using Hex 8.0.0 docking software. The peptide exhibited the highest negative energy value (E-value) of -747.99 KJ/mol with LysA, followed by -735.43, -631.07, -549.28, and -285.06 KJ/mol with ribonucleotide reductase, alanine racemase, DNA gyrase, and isocitrate lyase, respectively (Figure 7). Furthermore, rifampicin showed E-values with *M. tuberculosis* proteins in the order of alanine racemase (-332.23 KJ/mol) > ribonucleotide reductase (-324.09 KJ/mol) > LysA (-316.08 KJ/mol) > DNA gyrase (-300.01 KJ/mol) > isocitrate lyase (-248.83 KJ/mol) (Table 3B and Figure 8).

Among targeted proteins of A540 cell lines, peptide SMANF2 revealed the highest docking score of -539.12 KJ/mol with Bcl-2 (Figure 9). On the other hand, the peptide showed highest negative E-value of -422.70 KJ/mol with Bcl-xL among targeted HT-29 cell lines (Table 4A and Figure 10). Molecular docking of doxorubicin with selected proteins of A540 and HT-29 cancer cells is shown in Figure 11 and Figure

12, respectively. Doxorubicin revealed the highest docking score of -288.36 and -308.7 KJ/mol with Bcl-2 and CDK4, respectively (Table 4B).

Table 1: Stereo-chemical and physiochemical parameters of peptide.

Peptide	Stereo-chemical and physiochemical parameters							
SMANF2	Verify 3D	ERRAT	WHATCHECK	Number of amino acids	Theoretical pI	Instability index	Aliphatic index	GRAVY
	80%	95	Good	20	8.75	26.73	117.0	-0.05

Table 2A: RCSB PDB IDs and metabolic pathways of *M. tuberculosis* targeted proteins.

S. No.	Proteins	RCSB PDB IDs	Metabolic pathways
1.	Alanine racemase	1XFC	Peptidoglycan biosynthesis
2.	DNA gyrase	3UC1	DNA synthesis
3.	Isocitrate lyase	1F8I	Replenishing of tricarboxylic acid cycle intermediates
4.	LysA	1HKV	Amino acid biosynthesis
5.	Ribonucleotide reductase	1UZR	DNA synthesis

Table 2B: RCSB PDB IDs and metabolic pathways of lung cancer (A540) and colon cancer (HT-29) proteins.

S. No.	Proteins	RCSB PDB IDs	Metabolic pathways
1.	Bcl-2	1G5M	Blocking apoptosis
2.	H-Ras	5P21	Signal transduction
3.	EGFR tyrosine kinase	1M17	Autophosphorylation and signal transduction
4.	Bcl-xL	1R2D	Anti-apoptosis
5.	CDK2	5IEY	Abnormal regulation of cell cycle
6.	CDK4	2W96	Phosphorylation of retinoblastoma gene product

Table 3A: Docking analysis of peptide SMANF2 with *M. tuberculosis* receptors.

S. No.	Proteins	RCSB PDB IDs	Docking E-value (KJ/mol)
1.	Alanine racemase	1XFC	-631.07
2.	DNA gyrase	3UC1	-549.28
3.	Isocitrate lyase	1F8I	-285.06
4.	LysA	1HKV	-747.99
5.	Ribonucleotide reductase	1UZR	-735.43

Table 3B: Docking analysis of rifampicin with *M. tuberculosis* receptors.

S. No.	Proteins	RCSB PDB IDs	Docking E-value (KJ/mol)
1.	Alanine racemase	1XFC	-332.23
2.	DNA gyrase	3UC1	-300.01
3.	Isocitrate lyase	1F8I	-248.83
4.	LysA	1HKV	-316.08
5.	Ribonucleotide reductase	1UZR	-324.09

Table 4A: Docking analysis of peptide SMANF2 with A540 and HT-29 cancer cells receptors.

S. No.	Proteins	RCSB PDB IDs	Docking E-value (KJ/mol)
1.	Bcl-2	1G5M	-539.12
2.	H-Ras	5P21	-455.95
3.	EGFR tyrosine kinase	1M17	-424.60
4.	Bcl-xL	1R2D	-422.70
5.	CDK2	5IEY	-363.20
6.	CDK4	2W96	-352.99

Table 4B: Docking analysis of doxorubicin with A540 and HT-29 cancer cells receptors.

S. No.	Proteins	RCSB PDB IDs	Docking E-value (KJ/mol)
1.	Bcl-2	1G5M	-288.36
2.	H-Ras	5P21	-263.49
3.	EGFR tyrosine kinase	1M17	-32.45
4.	Bcl-xL	1R2D	-275.38
5.	CDK2	5IEY	-274.11
6.	CDK4	2W96	-308.70

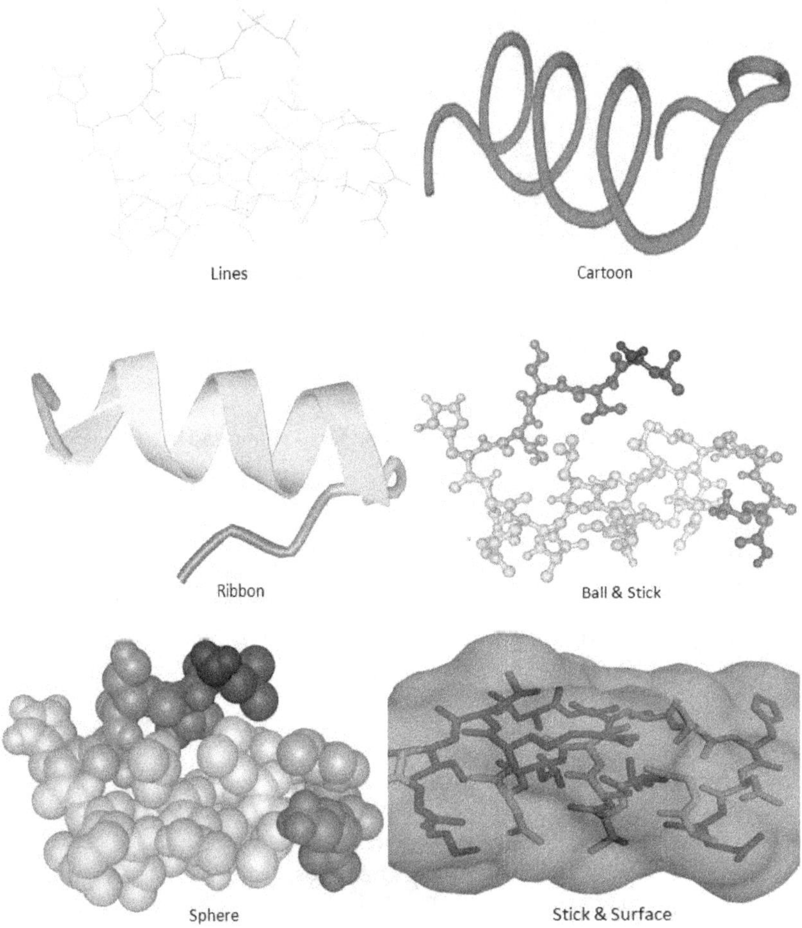

Figure 1: Structures of peptide SMANF2 obtained using PEP-FOLD and iCn3D.

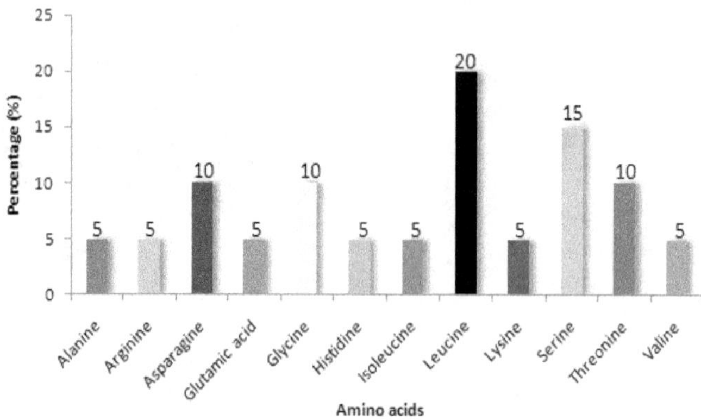

Figure 2: Amino acid composition (%) of peptide SMANF2.

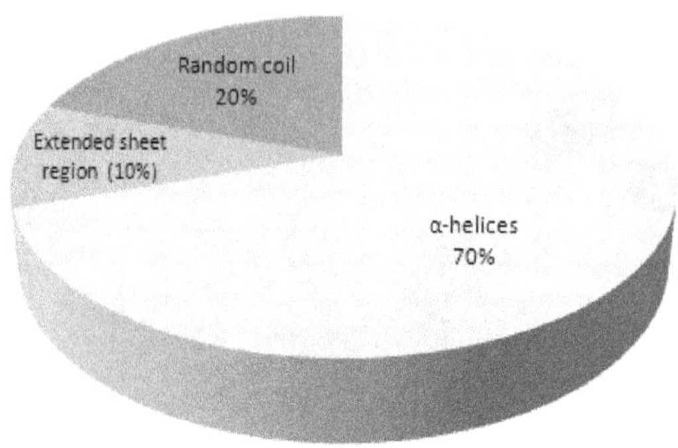

Figure 3: Secondary structure of peptide SMANF2. It was dominated by α-helices, extended sheet region, and random coil.

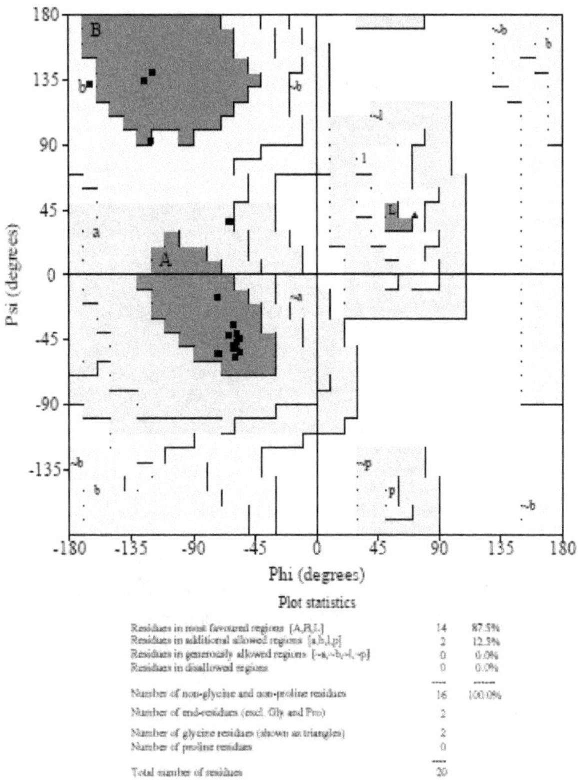

Figure 4: Ramachandran plot showing percentage of residues in the most favourable regions, additionally allowed regions, generously allowed regions, and disallowed regions.

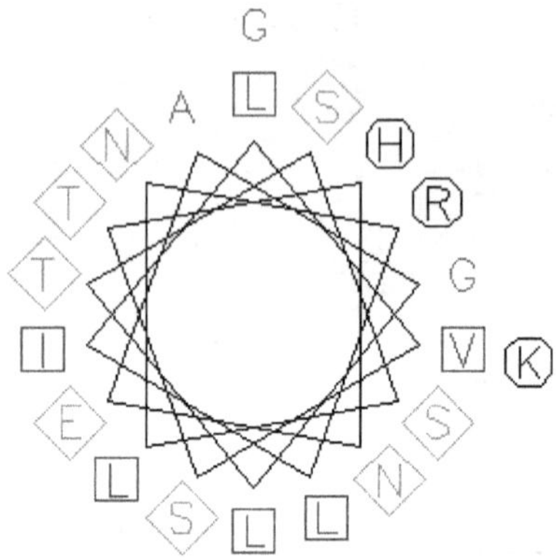

Figure 5: The helical wheel prediction of peptide SMANF2. Aliphatic residues are marked with squares, hydrophilic residues are marked with diamonds, and positively charged residues with octagons.

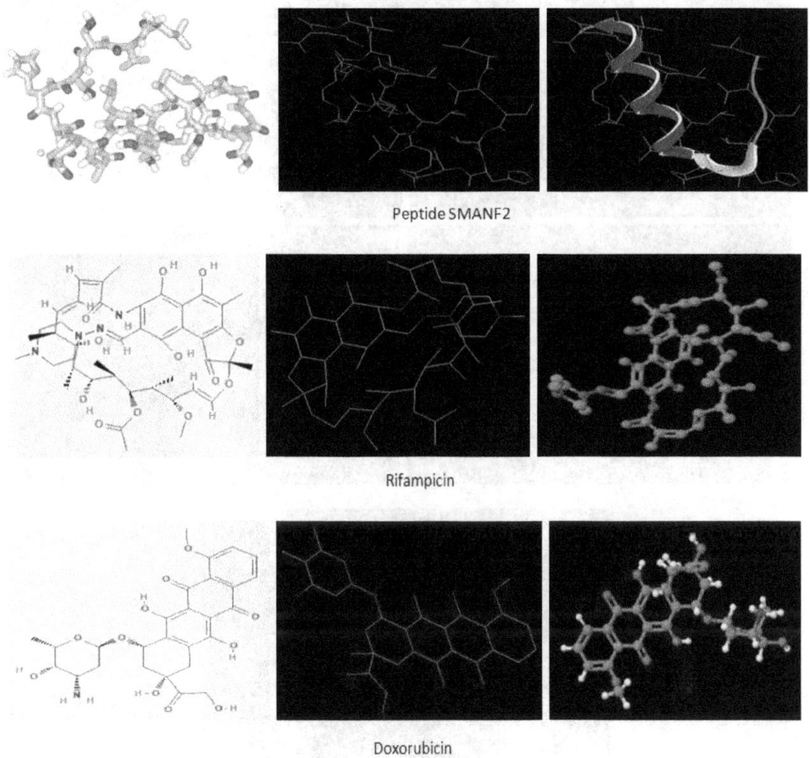

Figure 6: Different structures of ligands (peptide SMANF2, rifampicin, and doxorubicin).

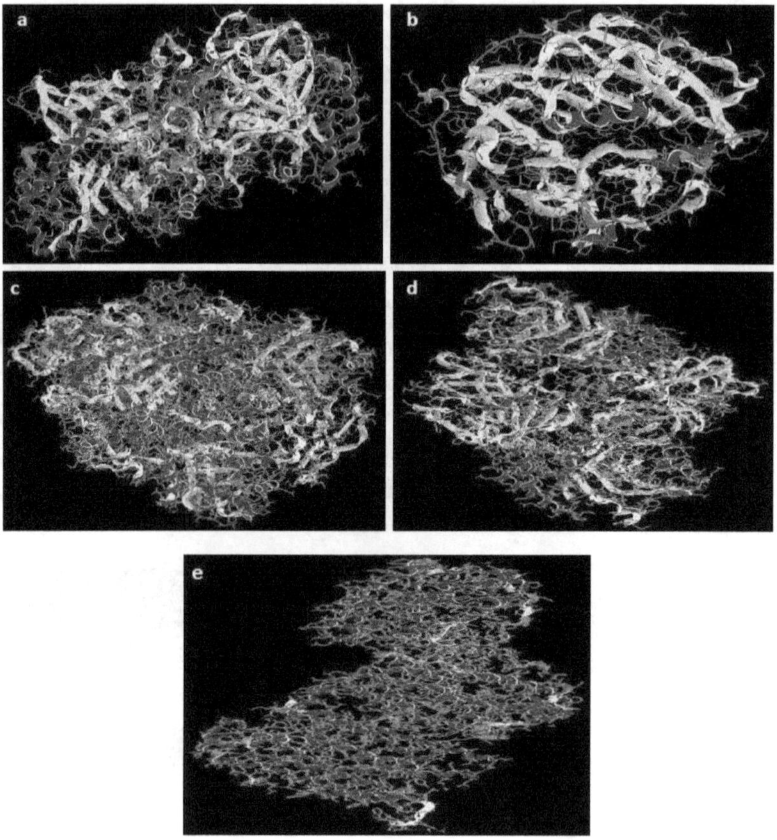

Figure 7: Molecular docking of peptide SMANF2 with (a) alanine racemase, (b) DNA gyrase, (c) isocitrate lyase, (d) LysA, and (e) ribonucleotide reductase.

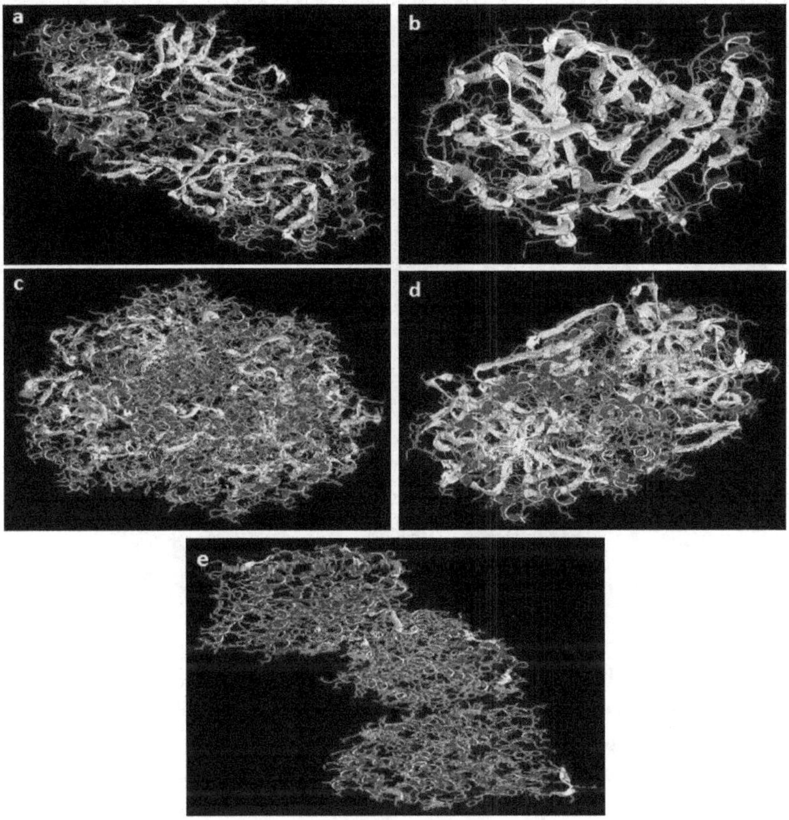

Figure 8: Molecular docking of rifampicin with (a) alanine racemase, (b) DNA gyrase, (c) isocitrate lyase, (d) LysA, and (e) ribonucleotide reductase.

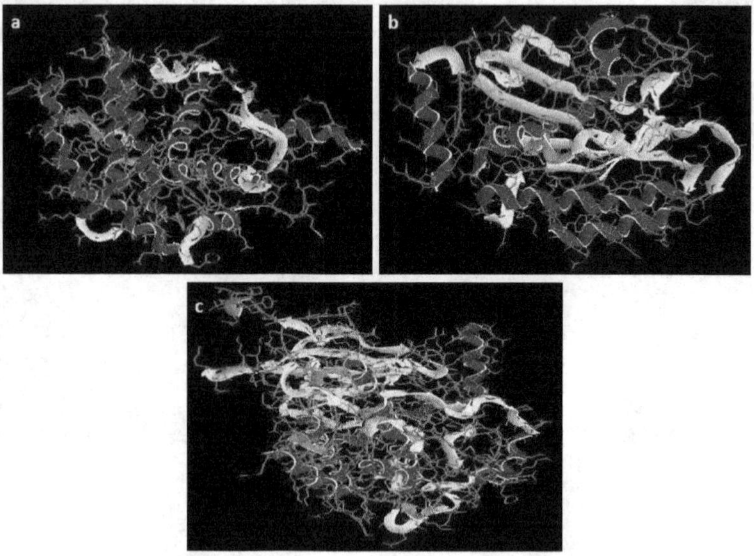

Figure 9: Molecular docking of peptide SMANF2 with (a) Bcl-2, (b) H-Ras, and (c) EGFR tyrosine kinase of A540 cell line.

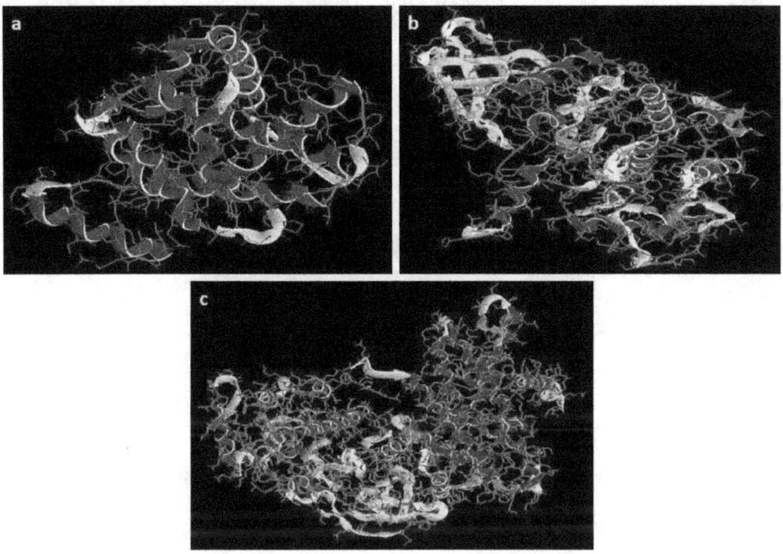

Figure 10: Molecular docking of peptide SMANF2 with (a) Bcl-xL, (b) CDK2, and (c) CDK4 of HT-29 cell line.

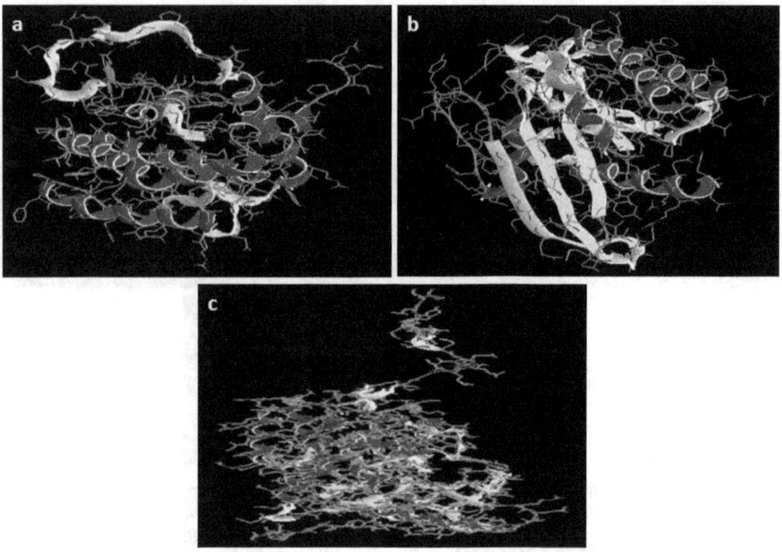

Figure 11: Molecular docking of doxorubicin with (a) Bcl-2, (b) H-Ras, and (c) EGFR tyrosine kinase of A540 cell line.

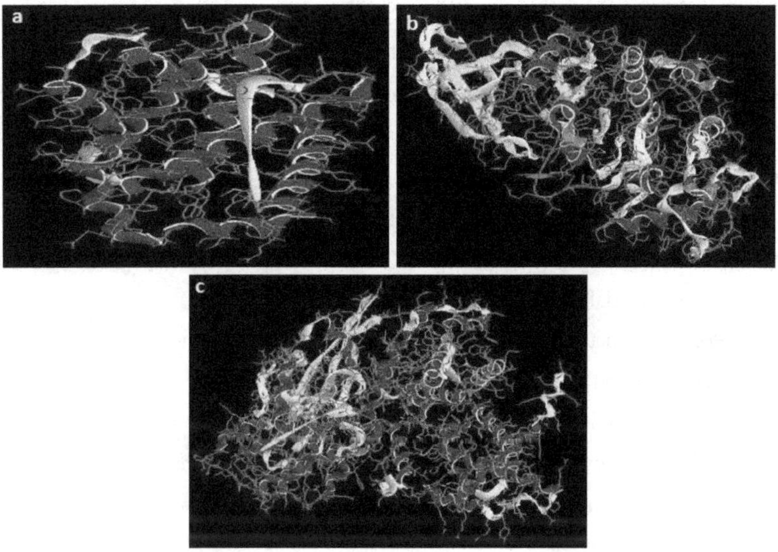

Figure 12: Molecular docking of doxorubicin with (a) Bcl-xL, (b) CDK2, and (c) CDK4 of HT-29 cell line.

4. Discussion

In the present study, Verify 3D showed 80% compatibility for the 3D model of peptide SMANF2. Similarly, ERRAT value of peptide SMANF2 is within the acceptable range. According to the report of Singh *et al.* (2016), any modelled structure exhibiting ERRAT score value of more than 50 is considered good. WHATCHECK predicts that the structure of peptide SMANF2 is of reasonably good quality. Similar observation was reported by Singh *et al.* (2016) too.

In this context, theoretical pI of peptide SMANF2 was determined alkaline in nature. The instability index value of peptide SMANF2 was calculated as 26.73, thereby indicating stability of this peptide. A high aliphatic index value more than 50 represents that the particular protein is temperature stable (Dutta *et al.*, 2018). In this study, peptide SMANF2 exhibited the aliphatic index value of 117.0, which indicates its thermal stability. Negative GRAVY value represents hydrophilic characteristics of peptide. In this study, the negative GRAVY value (-0.05) of peptide SMANF2 represents its potential interaction with water.

Primary structure analysis depicts the amino acid composition of peptides. Leusine (20.0%) and Serine (15.0%) were predominant in the peptide. Asparagine, Glycine, and Threonine were available in comparatively lower amount. Hydrophilic amino acids are known to seek contact with aqueous phase. In this study, the presence of Glycine indicates high flexibility to the peptide SMANF2, as previously suggested by Dutta *et al.* (2018) too.

Secondary structure of peptide SMANF2 was dominated by α-helices (70.0%), extended sheet region (10.0%), and random coil (20.0%). Thus, the finding illustrates that the peptide is stable in its structure as it is predominantly composed of α-helices. Ramachandran angles determine the rotation of the polypeptide backbone around the bonds between N-C_α (Φ) and C_α-C (ϕ) (Singh *et al.*, 2016). The higher residues in favoured region indicate more stability of the protein or peptide. In this study, about 87.5% of residues were falling in favoured region, indicating high stability of this peptide. The membrane spanning or extracellular nature of the peptide was analyzed using TMHMM tool which indicated extracellular production of peptide SMANF2. Further, the helical wheel prediction of peptide SMANF2 showed the presence of hydrophilic and positively charged residues, thus, supporting the findings of Xin *et al.* (2017).

Target proteins of *M. tuberculosis* were docked with the peptide SMANF2 and rifampicin using Hex 8.0.0 software in order to demonstrate their molecular interactions and binding energy. In the present investigation, peptide SMANF2 and rifampicin were reported as the most potent inhibitors against LysA and alanine racemase of *M. tuberculosis*, respectively, thereby showing higher E-values and strong interaction with receptors. Peptide SMANF2 exhibited higher docking score than rifampicin. This might be due to the fact that rifampicin had comparatively lower interaction with these selected targeted receptors. Likewise, peptide SMANF2 showed higher docking score with Bcl-2 and Bcl-xL of A540 and HT-29 cancer cells. Doxorubicin revealed higher docking score with Bcl-2 and CDK4 of A540 and HT-29 cancer cells. However, the E-values obtained due to the interaction with doxorubicin were reported to be lower than that of peptide SMANF2. This might also be due to the fact that doxorubicin had comparatively lower interaction with these targeted receptors.

In silico studies clearly showed the promising stereo-chemical, physiochemical, docking insight of peptide SMANF2. This peptide was synthesized in strain MANF2 under mild stress of *M. piperita* (discussed in chapter 5). Docking studies indicated the comparatively higher binding affinity of peptide SMANF2 against *M. tuberculosis* and cancer with respect to the peptide NMANF2 (as discussed in chapter 4), which was purified from bacteria under normal/non-stress conditions (discussed in chapter 3). Thus, our findings hypothesized that proteins or peptides synthesized in bacteria under mild stress of certain antimicrobials might be ideal agents for designing new therapeutic drugs with enhanced effectiveness and developing the possible new treatment strategies of TB and cancer (lung and colon) in few decades.

5. Conclusions

In a nutshell, *in silico* studies showed the promising stereo-chemical, physiochemical, and functional characteristics of peptide SMANF2. Further, the peptide showed the highest affinity with LysA, followed by ribonucleotide reductase, alanine racemase, DNA gyrase, and isocitrate lyase of *M. tuberculosis*. Among targeted proteins of A540 cell lines, peptide SMANF2 showed potential docking ability with Bcl-2. On the other hand, the peptide was reported to be potential inhibitor of Bcl-xL among targeted HT-29 cell line receptors.

Effect of *M. piperita* stress on some functional properties of *S. hominis* strain MANF2

1. Introduction

The ability of probiotic bacteria to resist sub-lethal stresses is achieved mainly by inducing diversified adaptive mechanisms. Surprisingly, the sub-lethal stress is known to alter the metabolic activities of the bacterium by repressing and inducing specific group of protein (Khusro *et al.*, 2014a).

The potentiality to resist acidic pH and bile salt, exhibit cell surface properties, show susceptibility to antibiotics, and produce bioactive components are the pivotal characteristics of probiotic bacteria. It is essential to maintain the functional characteristics of probiotic bacteria after exposure to disparate stress conditions. Probiotic bacteria are often exposed to heat, cold, oxidative, osmotic, acid, and bile while determining their promising probiotic and technological characteristics (Amund, 2016). Bacteria adapt varied strategies to these stresses response viz. protein folding, synthesis of oxygen-stress protective proteins, synthesis of cold induced proteins, extrusion of protein by F_0-F_1-ATPase, bile efflux pumps, variations in energetic metabolism etc. (Amund, 2016). Previously, Paradeshi *et al.* (2017) investigated impact of copper ions stress on probiotic properties of *Lactobacillus* sp. In another study, Haddaji *et al.* (2015) determined the cell surface properties of *Lactobacillus* sp. under heat shock treatment.

Despite the digestive system, metal ions, and physico-chemical stresses, the influence of antimicrobials, particularly medicinal plants at sub-lethal doses on the functional characteristics of probiotic bacteria is very limited, probably unavailable in fermented food associated coagulase-negative *Staphylococcus* spp. As discussed in previous chapter (chapter 5), strain MANF2 at log phase of its growth has unique ability to synthesize new therapeutic protein under mild stress condition of *M. piperita*, hence, it certainly emphasizes the necessity to investigate this very stress effect on other functional properties of bacterium too. In fact, it is essential to maintain the biological properties of bacteria after its exposure to stress environment for its colossal applications in various industries.

In view of this, a significant attempt was undertaken in this chapter to investigate the influence of *M. piperita* stress on growth and some key functional attributes of strain MANF2. In order to provide new insight regarding the adaptive strategies, hypothetical pathways for some of the functional properties studied under stress were also discussed.

2. Materials and methods

2.1. Bacterium of interest and growth conditions

Strain MANF2 was cultured in MRS broth (pH 6.5) at 30^{0}C and considered as control strain (CS). On the other hand, *M. piperita* (1.5% v/v) was supplemented at log phase of strain MANF2 and incubated at 30^{0}C to provide mild stress to the bacteria. Bacteria growing in the presence of *M. piperita* were considered as stressed strain (SS).

2.2. Growth profile of bacteria

The CS and SS cultures were prepared by growing into 250 mL of conical flasks containing 50 mL of MRS broth. Cultures were incubated at 30^{0}C for 48 h. One millilitre of culture was withdrawn from each flask aseptically every 6 h and the growth pattern was analyzed by reading absorbance at 600 nm using UV-Vis spectrophotometer.

2.3. Morphological analysis

The variations in the cellular morphology were observed by following the methodology of Khusro *et al.* (2014a). The CS and SS cultures were grown up to 48 h and then centrifuged at 8000 *g* for 15 min. Pellets were collected and washed with sterile distilled water. The suspension was centrifuged again at 8000 *g* for 15 min and pellets were re-suspended in 1 mL of sterile distilled water. An aliquot of each bacterial suspension was spread on clean glass slide and Gram staining was performed to observe the variations in the cellular morphology of CS and SS cultures. The stained cells were observed under light microscope (OLYMPUS: CH20i) at 100X magnification.

2.4. Acid tolerance

The acid tolerance properties of CS and SS culture were evaluated according to the methodology of Ramos *et al.* (2013) with minor modifications. The CS and SS culture were grown overnight at 30^{0}C and centrifuged at 8000 *g* for 10 min. Bacterial cells were re-suspended in MRS broth of diversified pH ranges and incubated at 30^{0}C up to 3 h. Bacterial suspensions were withdrawn and serially diluted in PBS after 0, 1,

2, and 3 h. Samples were plated on sterilized MRS agar plates and incubated at 30^{0}C for 48 h. Total cell viability was estimated by plate count method in terms of log cfu/mL.

2.5. Bile salt resistance

The survival of CS and SS cultures in the presence of bile salt was determined following the modified methodology of Kumar *et al.* (2011). Overnight grown CS and SS cultures were inoculated into MRS broth supplemented with oxgall (0.5% w/v) and incubated at 30^{0}C. After 24 h, aliquots of this suspension were withdrawn, serially diluted using saline, and plated on MRS agar plates. Viable cell colonies were enumerated after 24 h in a comparison with control culture (without oxgall).

2.6. *Cell surface hydrophobicity*

The adherence properties of CS and SS cultures to hydrocarbons were analyzed by employing the methodology of Mishra and Prasad (2005) with minor modifications. The CS and SS cultures were grown for 16-18 h, and centrifuged at 8000 *g* for 15 min. Pellets were collected and washed twice with PBS (pH 7.0). Pellets were re-suspended in the same buffer, vortexed, and absorbance of the cell suspension was read at 600 nm (A). Three millilitres of cell suspension were mixed with 1 mL of various hydrocarbons viz. chloroform, toluene, and ethyl acetate. The mixture was vortexed for 1 min, and incubated at 30^{0}C for 1 h in order to separate the aqueous and organic phase. The aqueous phase was carefully separated and decrease in absorbance was read at 600 nm (A_0). The cell surface hydrophobicity was calculated as follows:

$$\% \text{ Hydrophobicity} = [(A-A_0)/A] \times 100 \qquad \text{[Equation 1]}$$

2.7. Auto-aggregation

Cell auto-aggregation properties of CS and SS cultures were determined according to the methodology of Juarez Tomas *et al.* (2005) with slight modifications. Cultures were allowed to grow for 16-18 h and pellets were collected after centrifugation at 8000 *g* for 15 min. Cells were washed twice in PBS (pH 7.0) and adjusted to an absorbance of 0.5-0.6 at 600 nm (A). The cell suspension was further incubated at 30^{0}C for 24 h. The upper phase (1 mL) was carefully separated in order to measure the absorbance at 600 nm (A_0). Decrease in absorbance indicates the cell auto-aggregation property and auto-aggregation rate was calculated according to the following formula:

$$\% \text{ Auto-aggregation} = [(A-A_0)/A] \times 100 \qquad \text{[Equation 2]}$$

2.8. *Cell autolysis*

Autolysis of CS and SS cells was measured according to the methodology of Mora *et al.* (2003) with slight modification. Cultures were harvested at the exponential phase, washed in potassium phosphate buffer (0.1M, pH 6.5), re-suspended in the same buffer, and incubated at 30°C. The degree of autolysis was expressed as the percentage decrease in absorbance at 630 nm after 6, 12, and 24 h.

2.9. *Antibiotics susceptibility assay*

The susceptibility profile of CS and SS cultures to conventional antibiotics was determined by disc diffusion method (Bauer *et al.*, 1966). A homogeneous lawn of the exponentially phase grown CS and SS cultures was prepared on MRS agar plates. The standard antibiotic discs (HiMedia, India) such as streptomycin (10 µg), penicillin G (10 µg), chloramphenicol (30 µg), kanamycin (30 µg), gentamicin (10 µg), nalidixic acid (30 µg), and rifampicin (30 µg) were placed aseptically over the agar plates and incubated undisturbed at 30°C for 48 h. The diameter of the zone of bacterial growth inhibition was measured (in mm) after required period of incubation.

3. Results

3.1. *Growth profile of bacteria*

The growth of CS culture varied with respect to SS culture. The bacteria growing under mild stress of *M. piperita* showed increased growth with respect to the CS culture at regular interval of time (Figure 1).

3.2. *Morphological analysis*

The variations in cellular morphology of CS and SS cultures were observed under light microscope. Light microscopic observation of SS cells confirmed the heterogeneous nature of the cellular suspension as compared to CS cells. A drastic alteration in the morphology of SS cells was reported when observed at 100X magnification. Cells were separated apart with distortion in the shape from coccus to more or less round in shape (Figure 2).

3.3. *Acid tolerance*

Table 1 shows the acid tolerance abilities of CS and SS cultures at distinct pH values. A significant ($P<0.05$) reduction in the viabilities of SS culture were estimated as compared to CS culture from pH 2.0 to 5.0. However, the viabilities of SS culture were slightly increased as compared to CS culture at pH 6.5.

3.4. *Bile salt resistance*

The survival potentialities of SS culture with respect to CS culture were decreased due to the supplementation of bile salt. The viabilities of CS and SS cultures were estimated as 5.6±0.02 and 4.3±0.02 log cfu/mL, respectively at 24 h of incubation (Figure 3).

3.5. *Cell surface hydrophobicity and auto-aggregation*

Under mild stress of *M. piperita*, the SS culture showed significant increment in the hydrophobicity to chloroform (64.3±1.2%), toluene (73.3±1.1%), and ethyl acetate (69.2±2.2%) as compared to CS culture (Figure 4a). Likewise, percentage auto-aggregation of SS culture (74.1±1.3%) was increased with respect to CS culture (68.1±1.5%) (Figure 4b).

3.6. *Cell autolysis*

The autolysis abilities of SS culture were increased with respect to CS culture. The SS culture showed autolysis rate of 45.3±1.4, 49.3±1.5, and 66.6±1.5% at 6, 12, and 24 h of incubation, respectively (Figure 5).

3.7. *Antibiotics susceptibility assay*

Figure 6 shows the susceptibility patterns of CS and SS cultures to conventional antibiotics. The CS culture showed sensitivity towards the tested antibiotics in the order of penicillin G (32.3±0.3 mm) > gentamicin (31.3±0.4 mm) > rifampicin (30.3±0.5 mm) > kanamycin (22.3±0.6 mm) > chloramphenicol (21.3±0.5 mm) > streptomycin (13.3±0.4 mm). The CS culture was resistant to nalidixic acid. Likewise, SS culture showed more or less similar pattern of sensitivity towards rifampicin (30.6±0.5 mm), kanamycin (22.2±0.5 mm), and streptomycin (13.6±0.4 mm). Penicillin G and chloramphenicol showed increased activities against SS culture with diameter of zone of inhibition of 34.4±0.4 and 22.6±0.6 mm, respectively. On the other hand, gentamicin showed slight reduction in its activity against SS culture with diameter of zone of inhibition of 28.3±0.5 mm. The SS culture was observed resistant to nalidixic acid too, as similar to CS culture.

Table 1: Viable cell counts (log cfu/mL) of CS and SS cultures at various pHs.

pH	Time period	CS viable cell counts (log cfu/mL)	SS viable cell counts (log cfu/mL)
2.0	0	5.65±0.02[a]	5.6±0.03[a]
	1	5.6±0.02[a]	5.51±0.02[b]
	2	5.46±0.02[a]	5.32±0.02[b]
	3	5.25±0.01[a]	5.1±0.01[b]
3.0	0	5.92±0.03[a]	5.88±0.03[b]
	1	5.87±0.06[a]	5.8±0.06[b]
	2	5.77±0.03[a]	5.65±0.03[b]
	3	5.57±0.01[a]	5.45±0.01[b]
4.0	0	6.0±0.01[a]	5.98±0.01[b]
	1	5.96±0.01[a]	5.84±0.01[b]
	2	5.90±0.02[a]	5.80±0.02[b]
	3	5.85±0.02[a]	5.65±0.02[b]
5.0	0	6.04±0.03[a]	6.0±0.03[a]
	1	6.0±0.01[a]	5.86±0.01[b]
	2	5.94±0.05[a]	5.82±0.05[b]
	3	5.93±0.01[a]	5.73±0.01[b]
6.5	0	6.21±0.05[a]	6.23±0.05[b]
	1	6.21±0.03[a]	6.25±0.03[b]
	2	6.22±0.01[a]	6.28±0.01[b]
	3	6.2±0.01[a]	6.3±0.01[b]

Values represent mean±SD of experiments carried out in triplicate (n = 3).

[a,b]Means with different superscripts are significantly different ($P<0.05$).

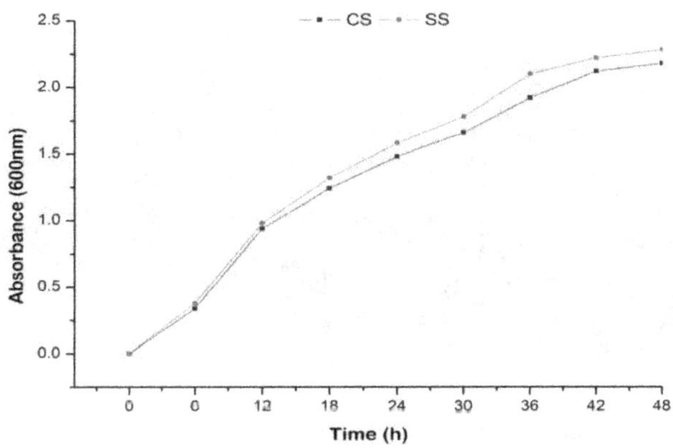

Figure 1: Growth response of CS and SS cultures.

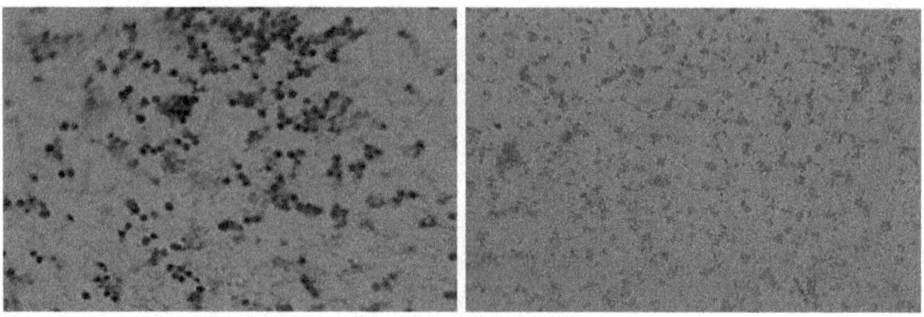

Figure 2: Morphological changes in CS and SS cultures, observed at 100X magnification of light microscope.

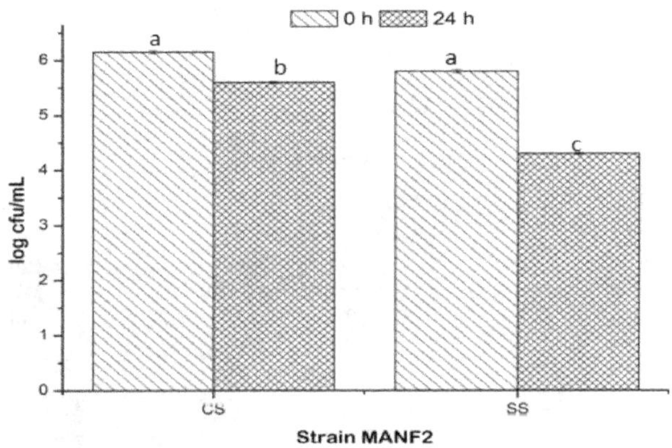

Figure 3: Bile salt tolerance of CS and SS cultures.

[Note: Values are represented as mean±SD of experiments carried out in triplicate (n = 3). [ab]Values with different letters are significantly ($P<0.05$) different.]

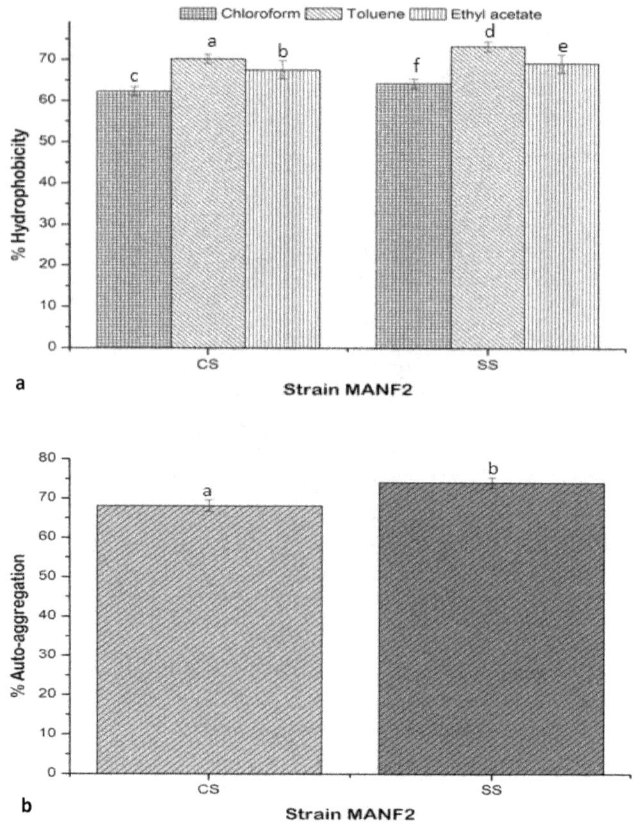

Figure 4: (a) Cell surface hydrophobicity and (b) auto-aggregation traits of CS and SS cultures.

[Note: Values are represented as mean±SD of experiments carried out in triplicate (n = 3). [abcdef]Values with different letters are significantly (P<0.05) different.]

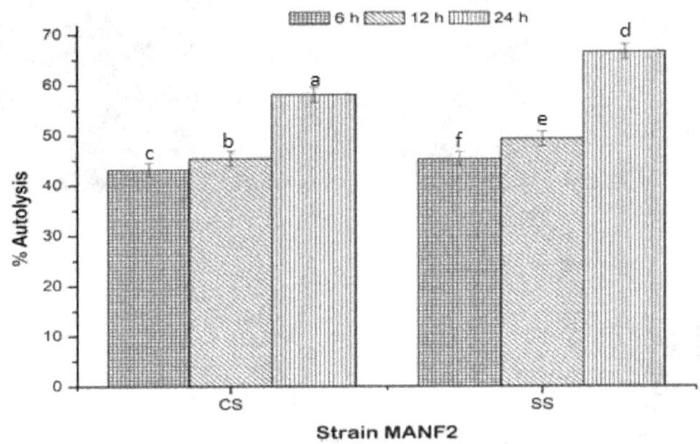

Figure 5: Autolysis abilities of CS and SS cultures.

[Note: Values are represented as mean±SD of experiments carried out in triplicate (n = 3).
[abcdef]Values with different letters are significantly ($P<0.05$) different.]

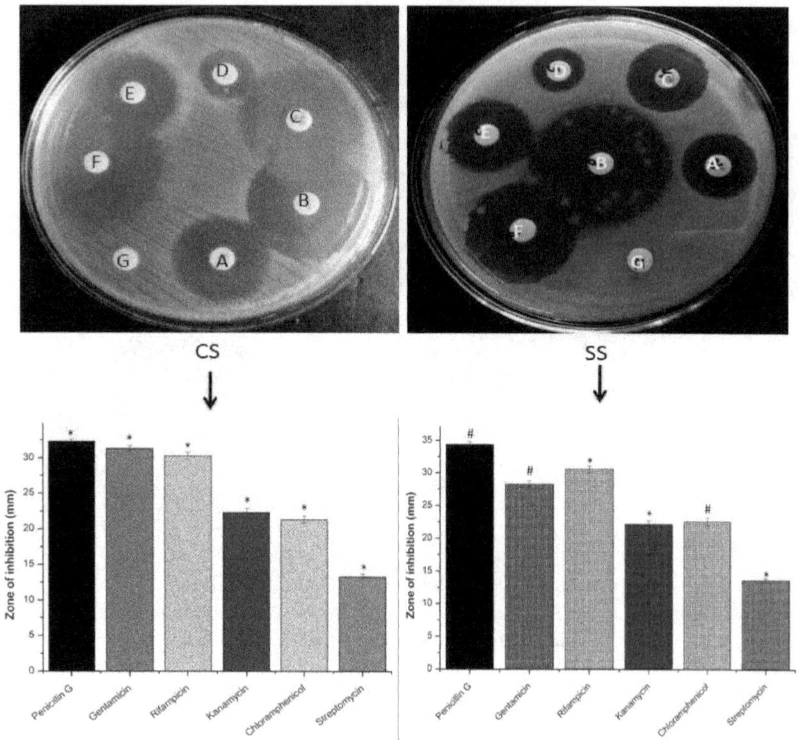

Figure 6: Antibiotic sensitivity test of CS and SS cultures.

[Note: A – Kanamycin, B – Penicillin G, C – Gentamicin, D – Streptomycin, E – Chloramphenicol, F – Rifampicin, and G – Nalidixic acid. Values are represented as mean±SD of experiments carried out in triplicate (n = 3). *Values differed significantly ($P<0.05$) with #values.]

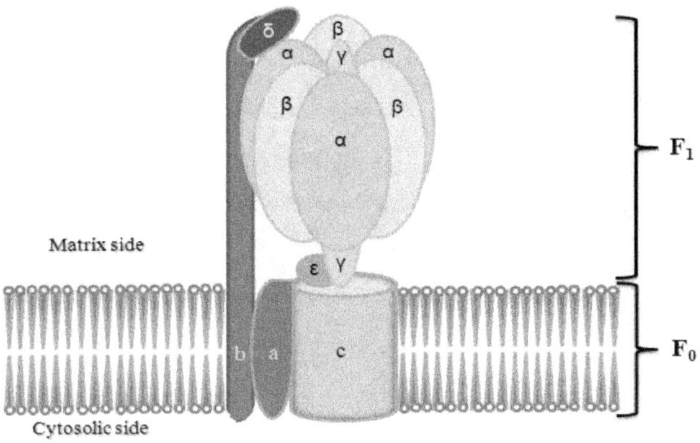

Figure 7: F_0F_1-ATPase consisting of a catalytic portion (F_1) incorporating α, β, γ, δ, and ε subunits for ATP hydrolysis and an integral membrane portion (F_0) including a, b, and c subunits.

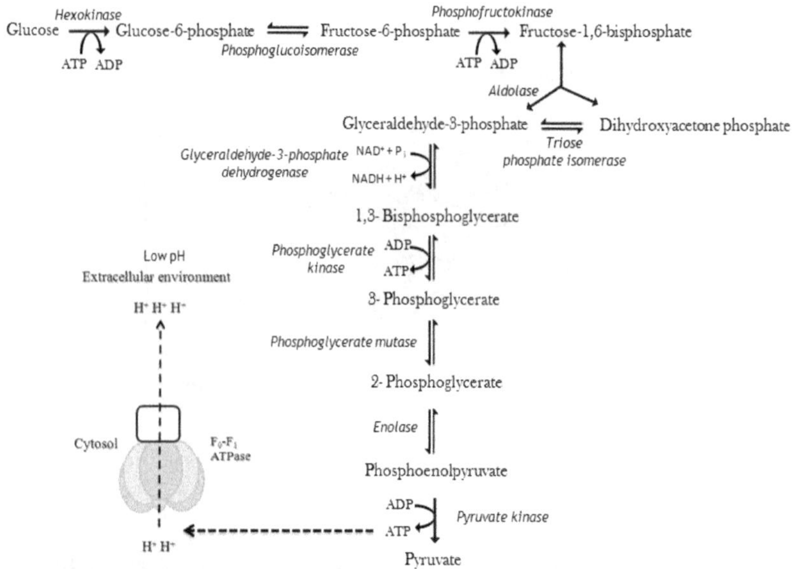

Figure 8: Acid tolerance pathway mechanism of CS culture. The F_0F_1-ATPase generates proton motive force by proton expulsion process in organisms devoid of a respiratory chain. The F_0F_1-ATPase increases the intracellular pH at low extracellular pH. The F_0F_1-ATPase is induced at low pH, and regulation appears to occur at the transcriptional level. The F_0F_1-ATPase requires ATP for expulsion of protons from the cell, thereby maintaining pH homeostasis and cell viability. ATP is obtained from the glycolysis process through step wise enzymatic mechanism.

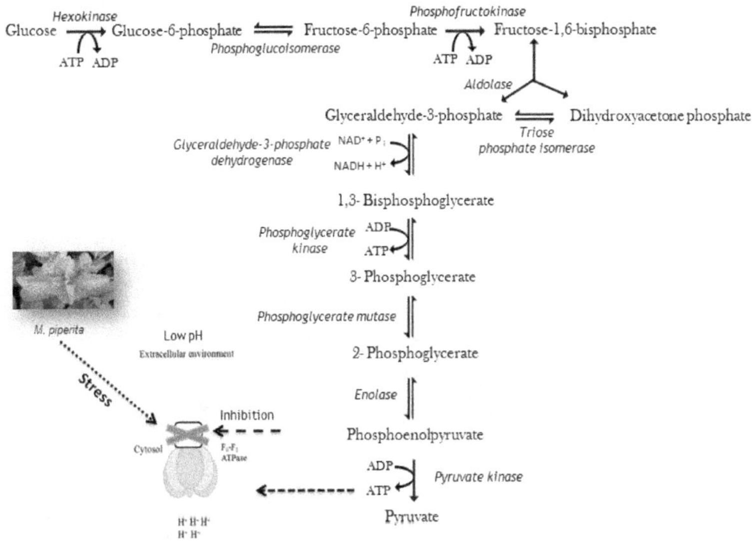

Figure 9: Hypothetical pathway for reduced viability of SS culture. The supplementation of *M. piperita* inhibited the F_0F_1-ATPase by covalent modification, as a result, ATPase did not pump out protons, thereby preventing proton translocation and causing reduced viability. The mild stress of *M. piperita* caused conformational variations in the F_0F_1-ATPase, leading to alterations in its metabolic activities, particularly disturbing the acid expulsion potentiality and thus, reducing resistivity to acidic pHs. The F_0F_1-ATPase requires ATP for expulsion of protons from the cell, thereby maintaining pH homeostasis and cell viability. The ATP is accumulated due to glycolysis. This hypothetical mechanism established a link between glycolysis, ATP synthesis, and inhibition of F_0F_1-ATPase activity due to *M. piperita* stress.

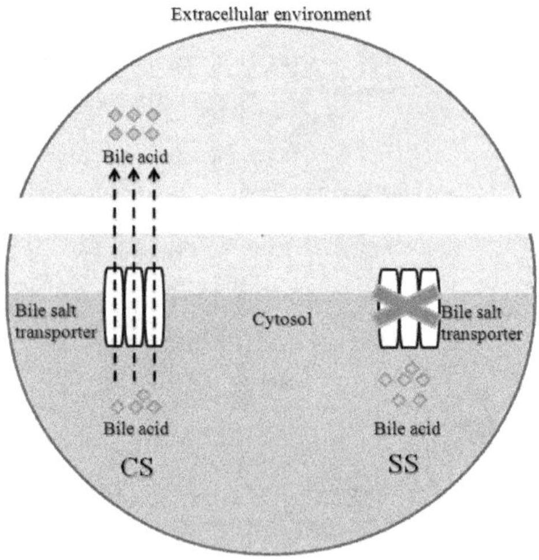

Figure 10: Hypothetical pathway mechanism revealing the viabilities of CS and SS cultures in the presence of bile salt. The sub-lethal dose of *M. piperita* in the cytoplasm might have affected the expression of varied membrane proteins that may inhibit bile transporter mechanism of strain MANF2, representing ATP-binding cassette.

4. Discussion

Stress is known to alter the growth and metabolism of bacteria. In the present investigation, strain MANF2 growing under mild stress of *M. piperita* (SS culture) showed increased growth with respect to CS culture at different time periods. Similar observations were reported by Khusro *et al.* (2014b) too who exhibited increased growth of *Bacillus* sp. under mild stress of metal ions as compared to the control strain. The increased growth of SS culture might be due to the reason that strain MANF2 received an alarm after sensing *M. piperita* stress and the mechanism within them start working overtime to neutralize the stress as well as to repair damaged components in the cell. Accumulation of active constituents of *M. piperita* in the bacterial cells and in their cell wall may be one of the reasons for the bacterial rapid growth compared to control because bacteria divide more in order to release the toxicity. In another study, Paradeshi *et al.* (2017) demonstrated reduction in the growth of *Lactobacillus* sp. under the mild stress of copper ions.

Variations in the morphology of microorganisms due to stress are an indicator of their adaptation. The alterations in the morphology of bacteria as an adaptive response to adverse situations have been demonstrated in previous studies (Ritz *et al.*, 2001; Khusro *et al.*, 2014a). In the present context, the cellular morphology of strain MANF2 under mild stress of *M. piperita* was altered with significant reduction in size and distortion of their shape. The microscopic image provided strong evidence that *M. piperita* at sub-lethal concentration is stressful for the strain MANF2, thereby changing their shape and size from cocci to more or less round shape as an adaptive response. In general, morphological changes are induced when the bacterial cells are incubated with sub-inhibitory concentrations of antimicrobials (Khusro *et al.*, 2014a).

The ability to resist acidic conditions is one of the most important qualities of probiotic bacteria. In the present study, CS and SS cultures showed survival potentialities at low pH. However, the ability to resist acidic pH was comparatively lower for SS culture with respect to CS culture. Similar observations were reported by Paradeshi *et al.* (2017) who estimated reduced acidic pH resistance ability of probiotic bacteria grown under copper ions stress.

The low pH resistivity trait of gram (+) bacteria is attributed to the presence of a constant gradient between extracellular and cytoplasmic pH. The metabolic activities of cells are inhibited when the internal pH reaches a threshold value, and thus, bacteria lose the viability (Kashket, 1987). Gram positive bacteria tolerate the acidic environment by stimulating F_0F_1-ATPase mechanism (Cotter and Hill, 2003). The F_0F_1-ATPase is a multiple-subunit enzyme consisting of a catalytic portion (F_1) incorporating α, β, gama (γ), delta (δ), and epsilon (ε) subunits for ATP hydrolysis and an integral membrane portion (F_0) including a, b, and c subunits (Figure 7), which function as a membranous channel for proton translocation (Sebald *et al.*, 1982). The F_0F_1-ATPase generates proton motive force by proton expulsion process in organisms devoid of a respiratory chain. As a result, F_0F_1-ATPase increases the intracellular pH at low extracellular pH (Figure 8). The F_0F_1-ATPase is induced at low pH, and regulation appears to occur at the transcriptional level (Fortier *et al.*, 2003).

In this study, we suggested the plausible inhibition of F_0F_1-ATPase due to *M. piperita* stress and thus subsequent reduction in the viability of strain MANF2. In general, the F_0F_1-ATPase was up-regulated in CS culture as a result of low acidic pH. On the other hand, the supplementation of *M. piperita* inhibited the F_0F_1-ATPase by covalent modification, as a result, ATPase did not pump out protons, thereby preventing proton translocation and causing reduced viability. Based on the outcomes of this study, it was hypothesized that mild stress of *M. piperita* caused conformational variations in the F_0F_1-ATPase, leading to alterations in its metabolic activities, particularly disturbing the acid expulsion potentiality and thus, reducing resistivity to acidic pHs. The F_0F_1-ATPase requires ATP for expulsion of protons from the cell, thereby maintaining pH homeostasis and cell viability. The ATP is accumulated due to glycolysis. This hypothetical mechanism established a link between glycolysis, ATP synthesis, and inhibition of F_0F_1-ATPase activity due to *M. piperita* stress (Figure 9).

The tolerance to bile salt is another pivotal functional property of probiotic bacteria. In this study, the viability of SS culture reduced significantly as compared to CS culture in the presence of bile salt, thereby indicating reduction in the bile salt tolerance ability of stressed bacteria with respect to non-stressed bacteria. Similar observations were reported by Paradeshi *et al.* (2017) who demonstrated reduced resistivity trait of metal ions-stressed probiotic bacteria toward bile salt. The hypothetical mechanism behind the reduced viability of SS culture in the presence of bile salt is shown in Figure 10. In a nutshell, the sub-lethal dose of *M. piperita* in the cytoplasm might have affected the expression of varied membrane proteins that may inhibit bile transporters representing ATP-binding cassette.

Stress is known to alter the bacterial surface characteristics such as hydrophobicity. Under mild stress of *M. piperita*, bacteria showed significant increment in the hydrophobicity levels to toluene, followed by ethyl acetate and chloroform. This might be due to the weak attractions of stressed cells with toluene and comparatively weak repulsion with ethyl acetate and chloroform. Observations confirmed that changes in the cell surface hydrophobicity occurred due to the adaptative response of bacteria to *M. piperita* stress. In previous study, Haddaji *et al.* (2015) estimated increased hydrophobicity trait of probiotic bacteria under heat shock stress.

Auto-aggregation is a crucial factor to evaluate bacterial adhesion characteristic to the intestinal cell line. In this study, the auto-aggregation property of SS culture was increased as compared to CS culture. Our findings were found to be in complete agreement with the study of Paradeshi *et al.* (2017) who revealed enhanced auto-aggregation characteristic of probiotic bacteria under copper stress. Likewise, the autolysis abilities of SS culture were increased with respect to CS culture. There is no study reported earlier assessing the role of any kind of stress on the autolysis nature of probiotic bacteria. Hence, comparative analysis of our results with previous finding is not discussed here. However, Khusro *et al.* (2014b) suggested that bacteria under stress adapt themselves by activating autolysis mechanisms.

The susceptibility of strain(s) to wide ranges of antibiotics is essential for its colossal applications in food and pharmaceutical industries. The lack of transferable antibiotic resistance genes is one of the desirable characteristics of probiotic bacterium. In the present context, similar to CS culture, the SS culture was observed susceptible to most of the antibiotics tested, thereby exhibiting its putative probiotic attributes. On the other hand, the SS culture was resistant to nalidixic acid, similar to CS strain. Findings indicated that despite the growth under sub-lethal concentration of *M. piperita*, the susceptibility nature of bacteria to tested antibiotics was found to be unaltered. Similar observations were demonstrated by Paradeshi *et al.* (2017) too.

5. Conclusions

Strain MANF2 growing under mild stress of *M. piperita* (SS culture) showed increased growth with respect to the CS culture at regular interval of time. The cellular morphology of strain MANF2 was distorted under mild stress of *M. piperita*, as observed under light microscope. The viabilities of SS culture were reduced as compared to CS culture at low pHs. In like manner, the survival abilities of SS culture with respect to CS culture were decreased too due to the supplementation of bile salt. On the other hand, the SS culture showed significant increment in the hydrophobicity, auto-aggregation, and autolysis properties as compared to CS culture. The SS culture showed more or less similar pattern of sensitivity towards rifampicin, kanamycin, and streptomycin. Penicillin G and chloramphenicol showed increased activities against SS culture. On the other hand, gentamicin showed slight reduction in its activity against SS culture.

Chapter 8

Bioconjugation of synthesized anisotropic gold nanoplates with purified protein for enhanced anti-tubercular and anticancer properties

1. Introduction

Among disparate nanomaterials, AuNPs have gained immense interest as therapeutics due to their unique physical, chemical, optical, magnetic, and thermal characteristics (Augustine *et al.*, 2014). The synthesis of AuNPs relies on diversified conventional methods which uses synthetic chemicals. Unfortunately, those chemicals are not only expensive but also toxic which may be serious threat to the human health and ecosystem. The use of microbes, particularly bacteria as reducing agents are considered promising environment friendly alternatives to the toxic chemicals used in the conventional methods of synthesis (Abboud *et al.*, 2013).

Currently, microwave heating is being adapted as an emerging technique for synthesizing a variety of nanomaterials from diversified groups of bacteria. Microwave assisted synthesis of nanoparticles is rapid, simple, and energy efficient process as compared to the conventional methods. Most importantly, the chemical reaction products are unaltered after microwave heating (Das *et al.*, 2012). It also provides improved reaction kinetics, short reaction time, and uniform volumetric heat distribution in a container (Arshi *et al.*, 2011). The interaction between the dipole moment of molecules and high frequency electromagnetic radiation result into the thermal process. Water is considered as an ideal solvent for microwave heating due to its high dipole moment. Since, a commercial microwave instrument has a built-in heat controlling system; hence, microwave irradiation can be a convenient process to explore the heating impact towards nanoparticle synthesis (Augustine *et al.*, 2014).

Over the past few years, statistical modelling tools are being used as an alternative to the traditional methods of optimization in order to enhance the concentrations of nanoparticles during biosynthesis process. Among varied designs of RSM, BBD is widely used to predict the inter-dependent relationship between input variables. However, despite the effectiveness of RSM-based modelling, it can not be implied for non-linear process. In order to overcome this issue, artificial intelligence-based optimization, particularly artificial neural network (ANN) is being considered in various fields. The ANN is a powerful simulation modelling computational program which is designed similar to the human brain processing (Nazar and Mozafar, 2012). The structure of ANN is influenced by the information which travels from the network because input and output datasets determine the variations in the network. In order to estimate the output data from the input datasets, ANN uses back propagation process through the learning mechanism (Shabanzadeh *et al.*, 2015). Artificial neuron or 'nodes' is the principal processing elements of ANN. Signals are transferred between neurons in the sequence through each synapse or 'connection' (Rostamizadeh and Rizi, 2012). In general, a neuron receives input data from sources, alters activation performances based on the input values, combines them, performs a non-linear operation on the results, and then outputs the final data based on learning and activation process (Shabanzadeh *et al.*, 2015). Three layers ('input', 'hidden', and 'output') design the architecture of ANN and also contains 'nodes' in each layer (Shabanzadeh *et al.*, 2015). For receiving the information, signals travel from the first layer to the last layer. Each unit takes its net input and activates it. The hidden layer can develop a similar layer structure as a neuron (Bezerra *et al.*, 2008).

Researchers are using the idea of efficient neural networking into various fields viz. system identification, data handling process, sequence recognition, spectral analyses, medical diagnosis, pharmaceutics etc. (Bingol *et al.*, 2012). Artificial neurons, connected with weights are used for developing an ANN. This computational modelling solves complex relationships between input and output factors by biological neurone processing (Thapliyal *et al.*, 2018). Recently, ANN has been implemented in nanotechnology by exhibiting non-linear relationships between the predicted and actual data sets (Shabanzadeh *et al.*, 2015; Thapliyal *et al.*, 2018). In fact, the use of ANN models would save time and cost by predicting the optimum conditions which can affect the variable response (Sadrzadeh *et al.*, 2008).

The synthesis of metallic nanoparticles of varying geometrical symmetry through controlled mechanism is an attractive area of investigation for the researchers worldwide. In general, the physiochemical and optical properties of nanoparticles are significantly affected by the shape, size, and composition. As a matter of fact, anisotropic nanoparticles play tremendous role in bionanotechnology. Among diversified metal nanoparticles, anisotropic AuNPs exhibit distinctive properties and colossal applications in medical diagnostics and therapeutics. The AuNPs of varying shapes such as spherical, triangular, squares, cubes, pentagonal, hexagonal, rods, and tadpoles have been successfully synthesized in recent years (Huang *et al.*, 2014). Surprisingly, very less attention has been paid towards synthesizing another kind of anisotropic AuNPs, particularly gold nanoplates. Gold nanoplates are considered highly suitable for biological applications and could show anisotropic electrical conductivity too. Previous studies showed the synthesis of triangular and hexagonal gold nanoplates through chemical processes (Zhu *et al.*, 2011; Huang *et al.*, 2014). However, rapid synthesis of polygonal gold nanoplates using bacteria as reducing agents in a single system is not investigated yet. In view of this, in the present chapter, microwave assisted AuNPs were primarily synthesized using strain MANF2 as reducing agent, and then conditions were optimized using BBD, followed by ANN. Further, the anti-tubercular as well as anticancer efficiency of synthesized polygonal gold nanoplates bioconjugated with purified proteins of strain MANF2 under stress were determined.

2. Materials and methods

2.1. Chemicals and glassware

Tetrachloroauric acid ($HAuCl_4.3H_2O$) was obtained from Sigma-Aldrich, India. Aqueous solution of $HAuCl_4.3H_2O$ (1mM) was prepared freshly using sterile double-distilled water. All glassware used in this study were sterilized and thoroughly rinsed with sterilized double-distilled water for experimental purposes.

2.2. Preparation of reducing agent

Strain MANF2 was inoculated into 50 mL of freshly prepared MRS broth (pH 6.5) and incubated at 30°C for 48 h. After required period of incubation, the broth culture was centrifuged at 8000 *g* for 10 min at 4°C and the supernatant was collected. pH of the supernatant was adjusted to 8.0 using 1M NaOH solution. This cell-free supernatant was used as reducing agent.

2.3. Biosynthesis of AuNPs

The potentiality of strain MANF2 to reduce Au^{3+} ions to Au^0 was determined by mixing cell-free supernatant and 1mM $HAuCl_4.3H_2O$ solution in a ratio of 1:1 in a small glass vial. The solution containing vial was kept in the centre of microwave oven (Model - SAMSUNG: M183DN) and irradiated for 30 sec. During the heat reduction process, the solution turned into purple colour, thereby indicating synthesis of AuNPs. The successful synthesis of AuNPs was further confirmed by recording absorption spectra in the wavelength range of 400-800 nm using UV-Vis spectrophotometer. The synthesis of AuNPs was further optimized via BBD followed by ANN, and confirmed by various characterization techniques.

2.4. *Optimization and modelling-*

2.4.1. *Data sets and BBD*

Three variables (irradiation time, $HAuCl_4.3H_2O$ concentration, and reducing agent concentration) were optimized adopting BBD at three different levels (-1, 0, +1). The coded values -1 and +1 indicate low and high levels of the variables studied. All variables were set at a central coded value of zero. According to the present experimental design, the total number of treatment combinations is $2^k + 2k + n$, where "k" is the number of independent variables and "n" is the number of repetition of experiments at the central point.

The dependent variable i.e. absorbance values of synthesized AuNPs were represented as *Y*. The impacts of factors to the response were analyzed using a second-order polynomial equation as mentioned below:

$Y = \beta_0 + \beta_1 A + \beta_2 B + \beta_3 C + \beta_{11} A^2 + \beta_{22} B^2 + \beta_{33} C^2 + \beta_{12} AB + \beta_{13} AC + \beta_{23} BC$ [Equation 1]

where, Y = Dependent variables; β_0 = Intercept; β_1, β_2, and β_3 = Linear coefficients; β_{11}, β_{22}, and β_{33} = Squared coefficients; β_{12}, β_{13}, and β_{23} = Interaction coefficients; A, B, C, A^2, B^2, C^2, AB, AC, and BC = Levels of independent variables.

The goodness of fit of the polynomial equation was expressed by R^2 and its statistical significance level was checked by F test, maintaining the desirability at maximum. The statistical optimization was validated by carrying out the experiments using optimized parameters.

2.4.2. *Artificial neural networks*

The BBD containing 17 experiments were used in ANN. In this modelling tool, data were sub-divided randomly into 3 sets - 'training', 'validation', and 'test' as 10-3-4 pattern. The structure of ANN is designed using the training data set. The correlation between input and output data is corrected using validation data set. The performance of unknown data set is determined by test data.

A multilayer perceptron (MLP) neural network was implemented in this study. The modelling of AuNPs synthesis was constructed by feed forward neural network using error back propagation learning algorithm (BPNN). The network contains an input layer, a hidden layer, and an output layer. These layers are connected by 'weights' which play a crucial role in data optimization. Input layer represents the variables' conditions, while the output layer represents the absorbance value. Trial and error method was used to optimize the total numbers of neurons in the hidden layer. Data were propagated through the input layer followed by its propagation to the hidden layer, and finally to the targets. Every node in input and hidden layer is connected to the nodes in the subsequent layer. Each neuron in the hidden and output layer acts as a junction, which combines and modifies the inputs from the previous layer using the following equation:

$$Y_i = \sum_{j=1}^{n} x_i w_{ij} + b_j \qquad \text{[Equation 2]}$$

where, Y_i = Net input to node j in hidden or output layer

x_i = Outputs of previous layer

w_{ij} = Weights between the ith node and j^{th} node

n = Number of neurons

b_j = Bias associated with node j

In order to avoid error between experimental and predicted data, sigmoid transfer function was used for the hidden layer, while linear transfer function was used for the output layer. The network was trained using Marquardt-Levenberg algorithm. In subsequent training steps, the weights and biases in hidden and output layers were adjusted in accordance with a convergence criterion to get the similarity in training and testing experimental data. The performance of ideal neural network model is dependent on two statistical parameters, R^2, and mean squared error (MSE).

The R^2 was determined to validate the ANN output error by estimating the variance in the modelled variables as per the formula given below. The R^2 value close to 1 indicates the model to be fit. The R^2 was calculated as per the equation given below:

$$R^2 = 1 - \frac{\sum_{i=1}^{n}(x_{pi} - x_{ai})2}{\sum_{i=1}^{n}(x_{pi} - x_m)2} \qquad \text{[Equation 3]}$$

where, n = Number of experiments

x_{pi} = Predicted value

x_{ai} = Actual value

x_m = Average of the real values.

Mean squared error represents the estimation of the standard deviation of the data component. The MSE value close to 0 indicates a good fit, which is calculated as per the formula mentioned below:

$$\text{MSE} = \frac{1}{r}\sum_{i=1}^{n}\left(x_{pi} - x_{ai}\right)2 \qquad \text{[Equation 4]}$$

where, n = Number of experiments

x_{pi} = Predicted value

x_{ai} = Actual value

2.5. *Characterization of AuNPs-*

2.5.1. *UV-Vis spectroscopy*

After optimization, the synthesis of AuNPs was confirmed again by recording absorption spectra in the wavelength range of 400-800 nm using UV-Vis spectrophotometer.

2.5.2. *Fourier transform-infrared spectroscopy*

The FT-IR spectrum of AuNPs was performed to determine the presence of distinct functional groups. The analysis was carried out using Nicolet 5700 instruments (Nicolet Instrument, Thermo Company, USA) with KBr pellet method. Each KBr disk was scanned over a wave number region of 500-4000 cm^{-1}.

2.5.3. *Zeta potential*

Zeta potential determines the repulsive force between particles and estimates its stability. It is calculated from the electrophoretic mobility of particles in stationary conducting liquid phase due to the external electric field applied. The zeta potential of AuNPs was determined using zeta potential analyzer (90 Plus Particle Size Analyzer, Brookhaven Instruments Corporation, using Zeta Plus software). Briefly, 100 μL of AuNPs solution was diluted to 1 mL using deionized water. The electrophoretic mobility of the nanparticles was calculated by applying electric field of 150 mV. Zeta potential of the particle is calculated using Smoluchowski's formula as given below:

$$\text{Zeta potential (mV)} = \frac{4\pi\eta}{\varepsilon} \times \text{U} \times 300 \times 300 \times 1000 \qquad \text{[Equation 5]}$$

where, η = Viscosity of solution

ε = Dielectric constant

U = Electrophoretic mobility ($U = \frac{v}{V/L}$)

v = Particle speed

V = Voltage

L = Electrode distance

2.5.4. *Dynamic light scattering (DLS)*

Dynamic light scattering is used to determine the size of the nanoparticles in the solution by scattering the light from the particle undergoing Brownian motion. For determining the size distribution and average size, 100 μL of AuNPs solution was diluted to 1 mL using deionized water and analyzed using particle size analyzer (90 Plus Particle Size Analyzer, Brookhaven Instruments Corporation). Size of the particle is analyzed using the equation as given below:

$$D = \frac{Tk_B}{3\pi\eta D_r} \quad \text{[Equation 6]}$$

where, D = Particle size

T = Absolute temperature in degrees Kelvin

k_B = Distribution Boltzmann constant

η = Viscosity of the solvent

r = Radius of particles.

2.5.5. *X-ray Diffraction (XRD)*

X-ray Diffraction of nanoparticles describes not only the phase composition to the crystalline size of nanoparticles but also crystallographic orientation. The area of the peak quantifies the each phase present in the sample. In fact, XRD of any substance is the fingerprint of that substance. The AuNPs were centrifuged at 10000 *g* for 10 min and pellets were washed thrice using sterile deionized water. Sample was freeze-dried and XRD measurement was taken by diffractometer (Model - Philips PW 17291) with a voltage of 40 kilovolt (kV) at 25 milliampere (mA). The scanning rate employed was 10 min^{-1} over a 2θ range of 10-80^0 using the equation as given below.

$$n\lambda = 2d\sin\theta \quad \text{[Equation 7]}$$

where, n = Integer

λ = Wavelength of the beam

d = Space between diffracting planes

θ = Angle of incidence

2.5.6. *Scanning electron microscopy (SEM) analysis*

Scanning electron microscopy was used to define the morphology and geometry of AnNPs synthesized. The sample was placed on a polycarbonate substrate and the excess water was dried at room temperature. Further, it was dried in a critical point dryer using carbon dioxide, and sputter coated with gold in a metallizer. The AuNPs were examined under SEM (Model - JSM5600LV, JEOL, Japan) operated at 20 kV.

2.5.7. Energy-Dispersive X-ray (EDX) Spectroscopy

Energy-Dispersive X-ray Spectroscopy was used to determine the accurate elemental composition analysis of AuNPs. The AuNPs solution was diluted 100-fold in deionized water and then 10 μL of diluted sample was placed on a carbon stub and air dried. The EDX spectrum was recorded at 20 kV.

2.6. Bioconjugation of purified protein with anisotropic gold nanoplates

The bioconjugation of polyglonal gold nanoplates with purified proteins of strain MANF2 (as discussed in chapter 5) was carried out according to the methodology of Gomaa (2018). Purified protein was dissolved in 0.1M sodium phosphate buffer (pH 7.0). This solution was added into 9 mL stock solution of gold nanoplates in a drop-wise manner and stirred for 2 h using a magnetic stirrer. The reaction mixture was incubated further under shaking conditions for 24 h at room temperature. After required period of incubation, the mixture was centrifuged at 8000 *g* for 10 min to remove proteins which were not conjugated with gold nanoplates. The protein/gold nanoplates bioconjugate was used for further anti-tubercular and anticancer studies.

2.7. Anti-tubercular activity of protein/gold nanoplates bioconjugate

The anti-tubercular activities of protein/gold nanoplates bioconjugate were determined against *M. tuberculosis* H37Rv and drug resistant strain of *M. tuberculosis* (resistant to isoniazid and rifampicin). *M. tuberculosis* strains were grown in the presence of various concentrations (10-50 μg/mL) of protein/gold nanoplates bioconjugate and the anti-tubercular activities were estimated according to the methodology as mentioned in chapter 1.

2.8. Anticancer activity of protein/gold nanoplates bioconjugate

Anticancer activities of protein/gold nanoplates bioconjugate (10-50 μg/mL) against lung cancer (A549) and colon cancer cells (HT-29) were evaluated using MTT assay (Mosmann, 1983) as described in chapter 3. Doxorubicin (Sigma) was used as positive control. The absorbance value was used to calculate the percentage of viability using the following formula.

$$\%\ \text{viability} = \frac{\text{Absorbance of sample}}{\text{Absorbance of control}} \times 100 \qquad \text{[Equation 8]}$$

The minimum concentration of protein/gold nanoplates bioconjugate required for 50% inhibition of cell viability (IC_{50}) was calculated using linear regression curve statistics.

2.9. Statistical analyses and softwares used

Experiments were carried out in triplicate and values were expressed in terms of mean±SD. Statistical optimization process was interpreted using Design Expert Version 11.0.0 (Stat-Ease Inc., Minneapolis, Minnesota, USA) software. Artificial neural networking was performed using MATLAB R2019a (The Mathworks USA). Data were validated using ANOVA and values $P \leq 0.05$ were considered statistically significant.

3. Results

3.1. Biosynthesis of AuNPs

The synthesis of AuNPs using strain MANF2 as reducing agent was evident by change in the colour of the solution from light yellow to purple (Figure 1). Initially, Au^{3+} ions were reduced to Au^{+} ions as mentioned below, resulting into a transparent colouration.

$$Au^{3+} + 2e^{-} \longrightarrow Au^{+}$$

Further, Au^{+} ions were reduced to Au^{0} as per the equation mentioned below, thereby changing the colour into purple.

$$Au^{+} + e^{-} \longrightarrow Au^{0}$$

The synthesis of AuNPs was confirmed by observing SPR peak (λ_{max}) at 530 nm using UV-Vis spectrum (Figure 1).

3.2. Optimization and modelling

The influence of three effective variables (irradiation time, $HAuCl_4.3H_2O$ concentration, and reducing agent concentration) on SPR (absorbance at 530 nm) was investigated and optimized using BBD of RSM at three different levels (Table 1). The synthesis of AuNPs during each run is shown in Figure 2. Run no. 4 showed maximum production of AuNPs (λ_{max} - 3.18) under the conditions of 1mM of $HAuCl_4.3H_2O$, 1 mL of reducing agent, and irradiation period of 45 s (Table 2). It was reported that the observed values for AuNPs production were in good agreement with predicted response values (Table 2), thereby representing closeness to the diagonal lines (Figure 3).

ANOVA was determined for validating as well as evaluating the significance of the quadratic regression model, and the results for AuNPs yield using BBD have been depicted in Table 3. The Model F-value of 422.14 implies that the model is significant. Values of "Prob>F"<0.05 indicate model terms are significant. In this case A, B, C, AB, AC, BC, A^2, B^2, and C^2 were observed to be statistically significant (P<0.05). The R^2 value (0.9982) of this model was close to the "Adj R^2" value (0.9958). The "Pred R^2" of

0.9425 is in reasonable agreement with the "Adj R^2" value. "Adeq Precision" measures the signal to noise ratio. In the present model, a ratio of 71.457 indicates an adequate signal. The Lack of Fit F-value of 47.46 implies the Lack of Fit is not significant relative to the pure error. Non-significant lack of fit is good. The C.V. (3.21%) indicated the reliability of the experiments. Thus, this model can be used to navigate the design space. The model equation for AuNPs production can be written as given below:

SPR λ_{max} at 530 nm (Y) = 1.56 + 0.6956A + 0.3050B + 0.0928C - 0.1375AB + 1.11AC - 0.1225BC + 0.8197A^2 - 0.9116B^2 + 0.279C^2 [Equation 7]

The 3D response surface plots revealed the interdependent interaction between two variables for AuNPs yield (Figure 4). The AuNPs yield was determined by interacting irradiation time and $HAuCl_4.3H_2O$ concentration (Figure 4a), $HAuCl_4.3H_2O$ concentration and reducing agent concentration (Figure 4b), and irradiation time and reducing agent concentration (Figure 4c). Plots indicated the profound influence of all three variables on AuNPs yield. Further, perturbation graph also showed that irradiation time, $HAuCl_4.3H_2O$ concentration, and reducing agent concentration significantly ($P \leq 0.05$) enhanced the AuNPs yield (Figure 5). Box-Cox Plot for the Power Transforms is represented in Figure 6 which showed the best Lambda at 0.78. The normal probability plot compared the distribution of the residuals to a normal distribution (the straight line). The optimized variables selected through BBD were further used for the authentication experiment based on the methodology described earlier. The observed response values (~3.18) were estimated to be very much close to the predicted response values (3.08), thereby indicating the validation of model towards AuNPs yields.

Data obtained were further modelled using ANN. Selected variables were used for constructing the network. Figure 7 shows the constructed neural network topology "3-8-1" neurons in input, hidden, and output layers, depicting the best fitness function. The R^2 and MSE were used to determine the standard error of regression fitting and the performance of mathematical model by training, validation, and testing data sets. The R^2 values for training, validation, and testing datasets were obtained as 0.99468, 0.99818, and 0.99689, respectively. On the other hand, overall R^2 was calculated as 0.99408 (Figure 8). Figure 9 shows the errors histogram of training, validation, and testing sets. Results showed that the actual experimental data have been fit to the predicted values with high accuracy using the obtained ANN model. The MSE of training, test, and validation datasets for 7 epochs (repetition) is shown in Figure 10. The best validation performance obtained is 0.00058959 at epoch 4 (iteration).

3.3. *Characterization of AuNPs*

After statistical optimization, the synthesis of AuNPs in the solution was ascertained again by observing SPR peak (λ_{max}) at 530 nm using UV-Vis spectrum (Figure 11). The FT-IR spectrum of the synthesized AuNPs is shown in Figure 12. Peaks observed at 3878.44, 3609.57, 3587.07, 3544.75, 3520.41, 3471.02, 3426.10, 3381.49, 3339.71, and 3286.01 cm^{-1} denote the strong O-H groups. On the other hand, shifts in the peaks at 1637.02 and 845.95 imply C=N stretching vibration and strong =C-H bending for alkene, respectively. The zeta potential value of the AuNPs was estimated as 32.8 mV, indicating the high stability of nanoparticles synthesized (Figure 13a). Figure 13b shows the DLS analysis of AuNPs in terms of size distribution Vs intensity. The graph depicts that the size of the highest percentage (25%) of AuNPs synthesized was 100 nm. The diffraction peaks pattern of AuNPs synthesized is shown in Figure 13c which revealed the face-centred cubic (fcc) structure of atomic gold crystals. The Bragg reflections with 2θ values of 38.27^0, 44.37^0, 64.54^0, and 77.80^0 were observed which corresponded to (111), (200), (220), and (311) lattice planes of fcc gold structure, respectively. No characteristic peaks of impurities were observed which exhibited good crystalline nature of the AuNPs. The elemental composition and stoichiometry of the synthesized AuNPs were determined using EDX. The presence of strong peak at 3.1 kiloelectron volts (keV) in the spectrum represents the presence of gold. The carbon peak present in the spectrum was attributed to the carbon tape used in the spectrum analysis. The EDX spectrum showed that the weight of gold was 73.18% (Figure 13d). The surface morphology of synthesized AuNPs was observed using SEM. The SEM image of nanoparticles revealed the new anisotropic structure of nanoparticles, particularly pentagonal and square-shaped nanoplates with sharp edges. Thus, these nanoparticles synthesized were categorized as anisotropic/polygonal gold nanoplates (Figure 14).

3.4. *Anti-tubercular activities of protein/gold nanoplates bioconjugate*

The anti-tubercular activities of protein/gold nanoplates bioconjugate against *M. tuberculosis* H37Rv were estimated to be increased in a concentration dependent manner (10-50 μg/mL) ranging from RLU reduction of 38.2±0.3 to 92.6±0.4% with respect to the standard (75.5±0.5 to 99.9±0.5%) (Figure 15a). On the other hand, protein/gold nanoplates bioconjugate showed anti-tubercular activities against drug resistance strain of *M. tuberculosis* too in the range of 36.2±0.9 to 85.6±0.9% (Figure 15b).

3.5. Anticancer activities of protein/gold nanoplates bioconjugate

The anticancer activities of protein/gold nanoplates bioconjugate against A549 cell line are shown in Figure 16. After treatment with protein/gold nanoplates bioconjugate at various concentrations, cell shrinkage followed by rounding of cells and reduction in cell counts occur. The viabilities of A549 cells were estimated (88.4±0.3-34.3±0.4%) to be reduced significantly ($P<0.05$) with increase in the protein/gold nanoplates bioconjugate concentrations. A similar morphological alteration was observed in HT-29 cells after treatment with protein/gold nanoplates bioconjugate (Figure 17). The viabilities of HT-29 cells were also estimated (90.3±0.3–38.3±0.4%) to be reduced significantly ($P<0.05$) with increase in the protein/gold nanoplates bioconjugate concentrations. The protein/gold nanoplates bioconjugate revealed comparatively higher anticancer activities against A549 cells with respect to HT-29 cells. The IC_{50} values of protein/gold nanoplates bioconjugate against A549 and HT-29 cells were calculated as 38.1 and 41.3 μg/mL, respectively. In contrary to this, doxorubicin exhibited pronounced anticancer activities with IC_{50} values of 7.4 and 9.6 μg/mL against A549 and HT-29 cells, respectively.

Table 1: Experimental range, level, and code of variables for BBD design.

Variables	Code	Unit	Range and Levels		
			-1	**0**	**+1**
Irradiation time	A	S	15	30	45
$HAuCl_4.3H_2O$ concentration	B	mM	0.5	1.0	2.0
Reducing agent concentration	C	mL	0.5	1.0	2.0

Table 2: Box-Behnken design for optimizing AuNPs yields.

Run order	A	B	C	Absorbance	
				Experimental	Predicted
1	15	2.0	1.0	1.23	1.22
2	30	1.0	1.0	1.56	1.56
3	30	0.5	0.5	0.44	0.40
4	45	1.0	1.0	3.18	3.08
5	15	0.5	1.0	0.34	0.33
6	15	1.0	2.0	0.95	0.94
7	45	0.5	1.0	1.96	2.0
8	30	1.0	1.0	1.56	1.56
9	30	2.0	0.5	1.29	1.26
10	30	1.0	1.0	1.54	1.56
11	30	1.0	1.0	1.54	1.56
12	45	2.0	1.0	2.30	2.33
13	45	1.0	0.5	2.12	2.15
14	15	1.0	0.5	2.96	2.99
15	30	0.5	2.0	0.84	0.84
16	30	1.0	1.0	1.56	1.56
17	30	2.0	2.0	1.20	1.21

Table 3: Analysis of variance (ANOVA) for optimizing AuNPs yields using BBD

Source	Sum of Squares	df	Mean Square	*F*-value	*P*-value	
Model	9.53	9	1.06	422.14	<0.0001	significant
A-A	3.25	1	3.25	1296.48	<0.0001	
B-B	0.7442	1	0.7442	296.58	<0.0001	
C-C	0.0484	1	0.0484	19.31	0.0032	
AB	0.0756	1	0.0756	30.14	0.0009	
AC	2.69	1	2.69	2.69	<0.0001	
BC	0.06	1	0.06	23.92	<0.0018	
A^2	2.61	1	2.61	1040.70	<0.0001	
B^2	3.14	1	3.14	1239.60	<0.0001	
C^2	0.2596	1	0.2596	103.46	<0.0001	
Residual	0.0176	7	0.0025			
Lack of Fit	0.0171	3	0.0057	47.46	0.0614	not significant
Pure Error	0.0005	4	0.0001			
Cor Total	9.55	16				

$R^2 = 0.9982$; Adjusted $R^2 = 0.9958$; Predicted $R^2 = 0.9425$; C.V.% = 3.21; Adeq precision = 71.457; df = degree of freedom; Highly significant = $P \leq 0.0001$; Significant = $P \leq 0.05$; Non- significant = $P > 0.05$

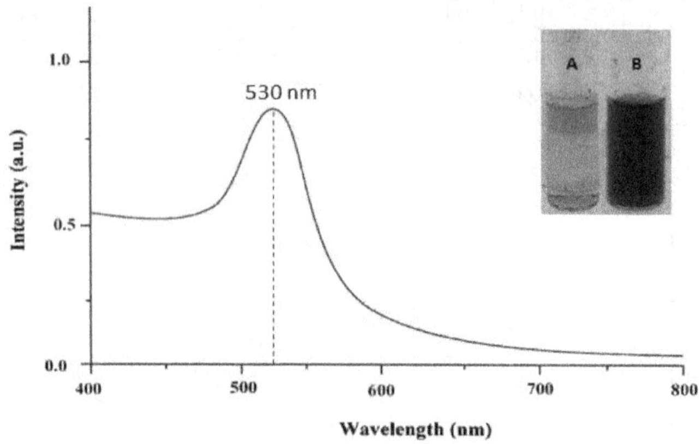

Figure 1: Synthesis of AuNPs using strain MANF2, as evident by change in the colour of the solution from light yellow (A) to dark purple (B) in colour. Synthesis of AuNPs was confirmed by observing SPR peak (λ_{max}) at 530 nm using UV-Vis spectrum.

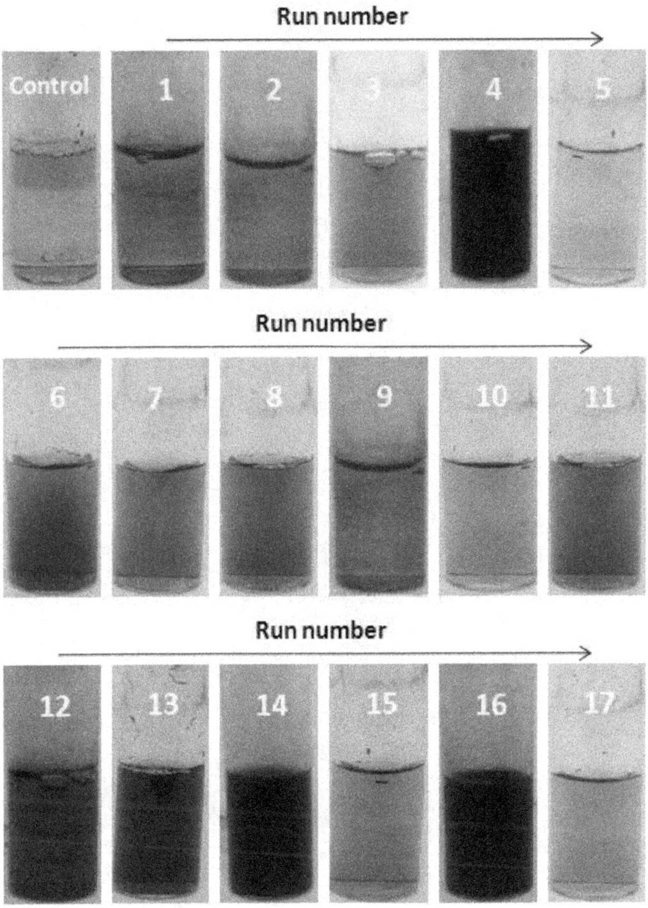

Figure 2: Synthesis of AuNPs during each run of BBD as indicated by colour change from light yellow (control) to light purple and deep purple.

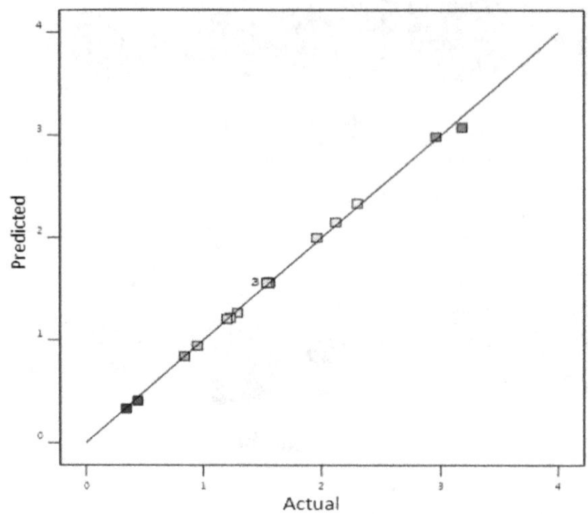

Figure 3: Actual Vs Predicted values of AuNPs yield, representing closeness to the diagonal lines.

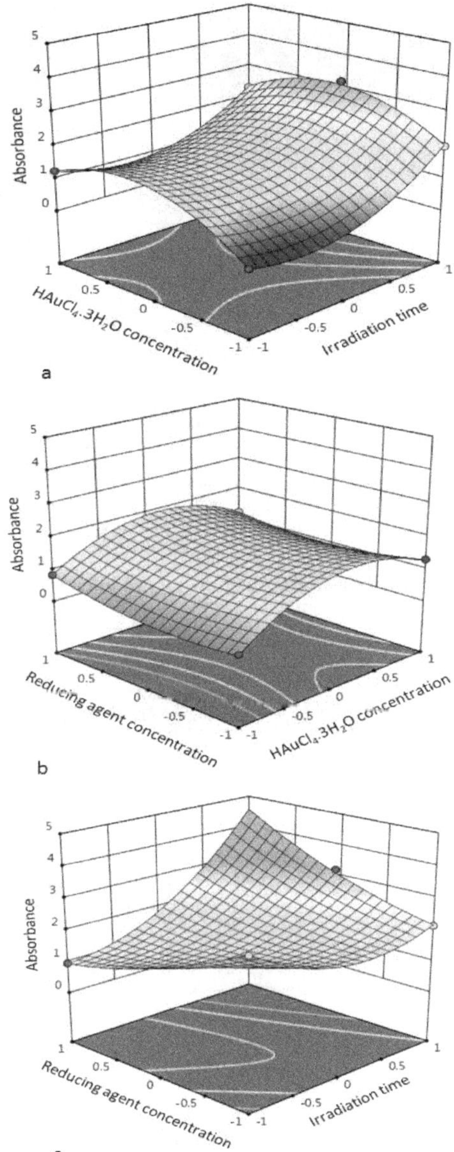

Figure 4: 3D response surface plots showing interdependent interaction between (a) irradiation time and $HAuCl_4.3H_2O$ concentration, (b) $HAuCl_4.3H_2O$ concentration and reducing agent concentration, and (c) irradiation time and reducing agent concentration.

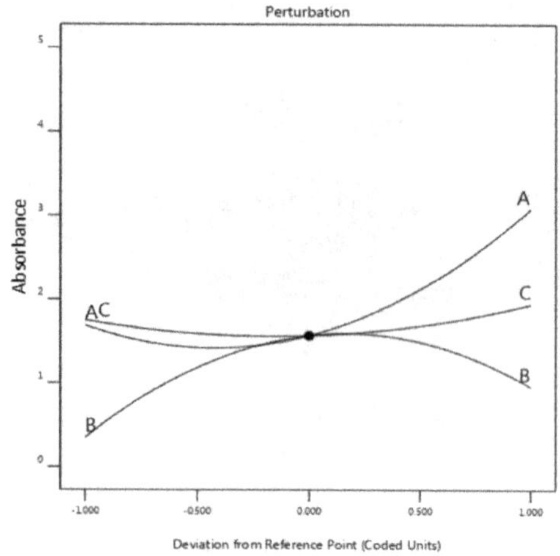

Figure 5: Perturbation graph showing enhanced AuNPs yield.

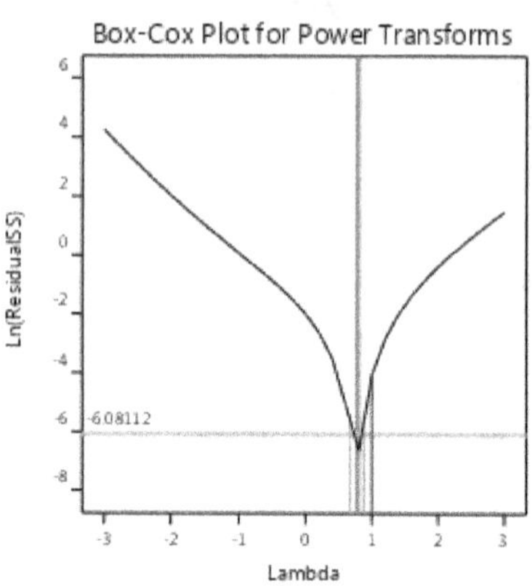

Figure 6: Box-Cox Plot for Power Transforms which showed the best Lambda at 0.78.

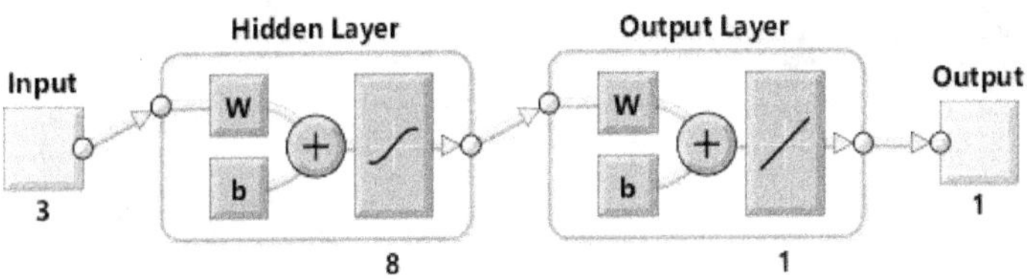

Figure 7: Constructed neural network topology "3-8-1" neurons in input, hidden, and output layers, depicting the best fitness function.

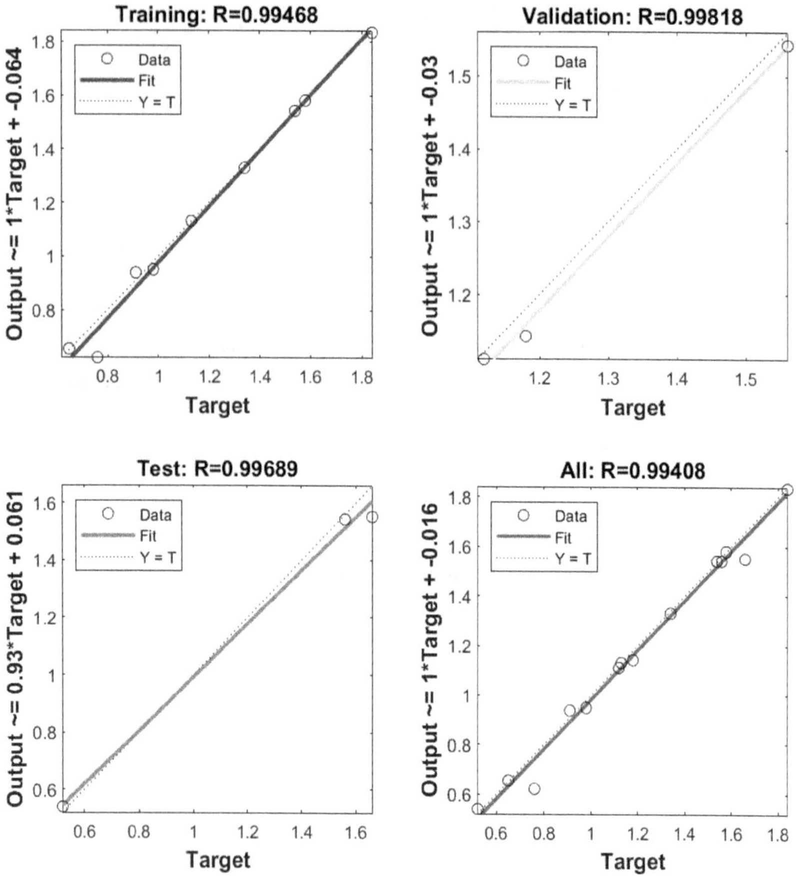

Figure 8: Standard error of regression fitting and the performance of mathematical model by training, validation, and testing data sets.

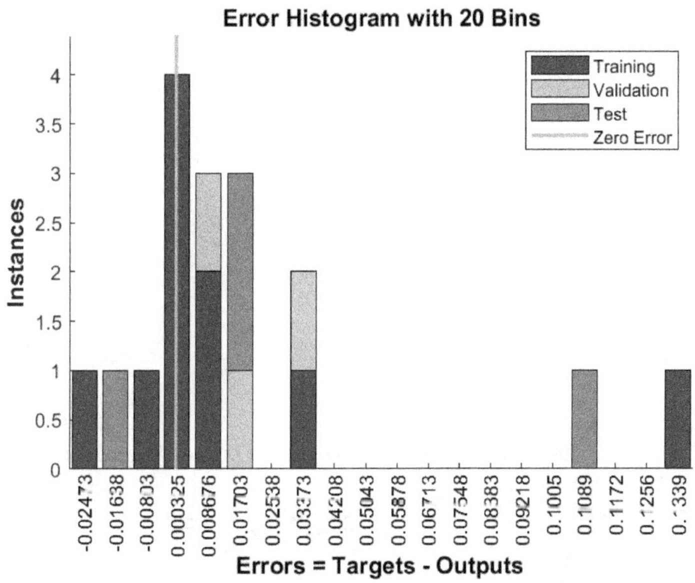

Figure 9: Errors histogram of training, validation, and testing sets generated after ANN modelling. It represents the instances Vs errors.

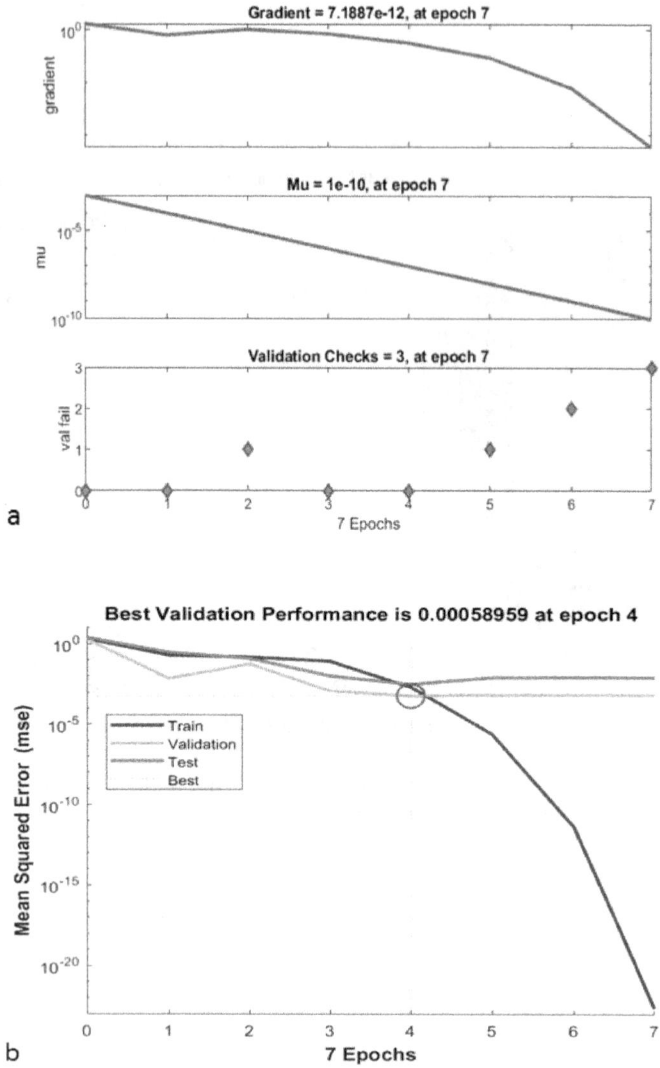

Figure 10: (a) MSE of training, test, and validation datasets for 7 epochs and (b) the best validation performance at epoch 4.

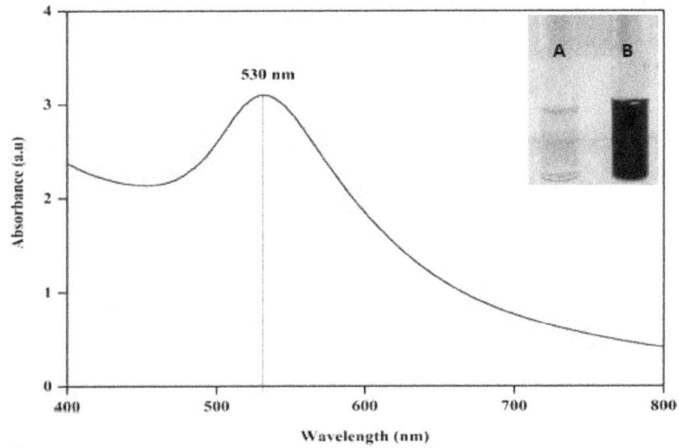

Figure 11: Synthesis of AuNPs after statistical optimization as evident by change in the colour of the solution from light yellow (A) to dark purple (B) in colour. Synthesis of AuNPs was confirmed again by observing SPR peak (λ_{max}) at 530 nm using UV-Vis spectrum.

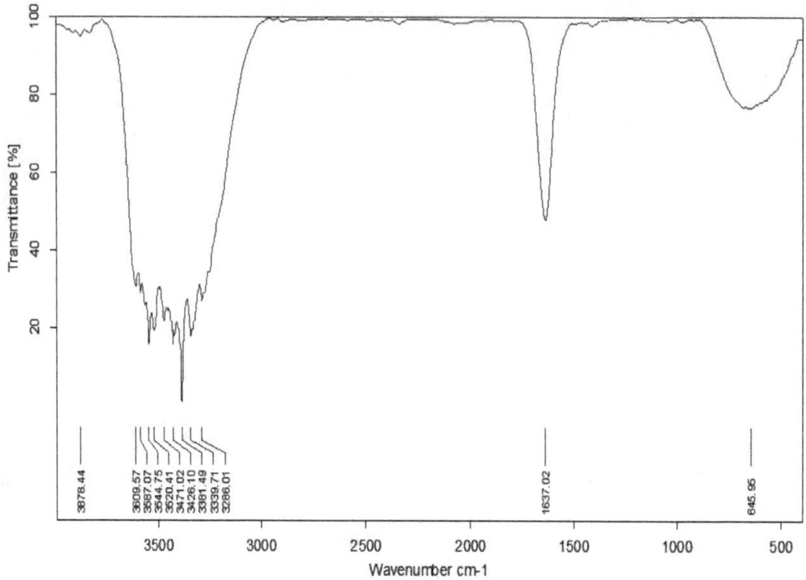

Figure 12: FT-IR spectrum of the synthesized AuNPs.

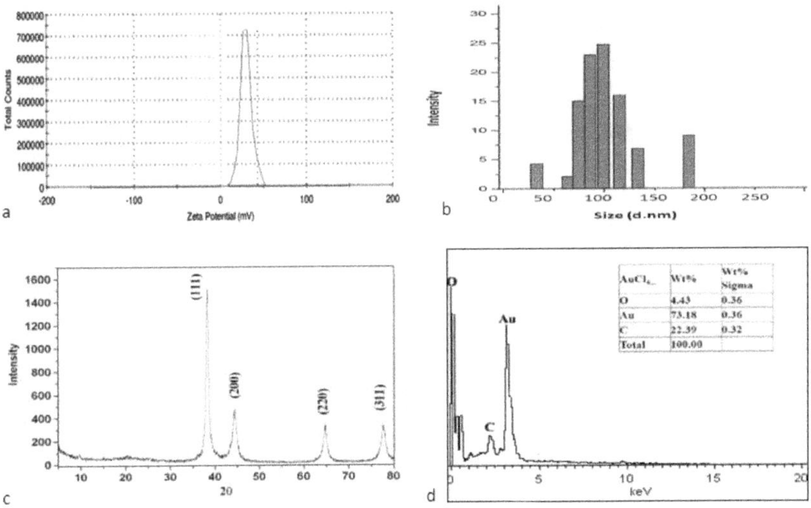

Figure 13: (a) Zeta potential, (b) DLS, (c) XRD, and (d) EDX analyses of AuNPs.

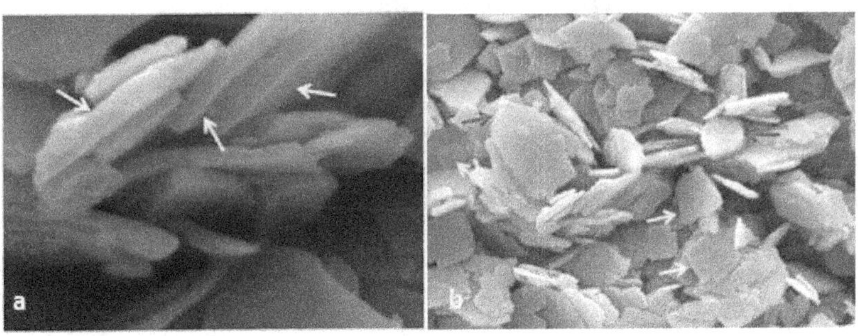

Figure 14: SEM image of (a) anisotropic gold nanoplates (yellow arrows), particularly (b) pentagonal (red arrows) and square-shaped (yellow arrows) nanoplates with sharp edges.

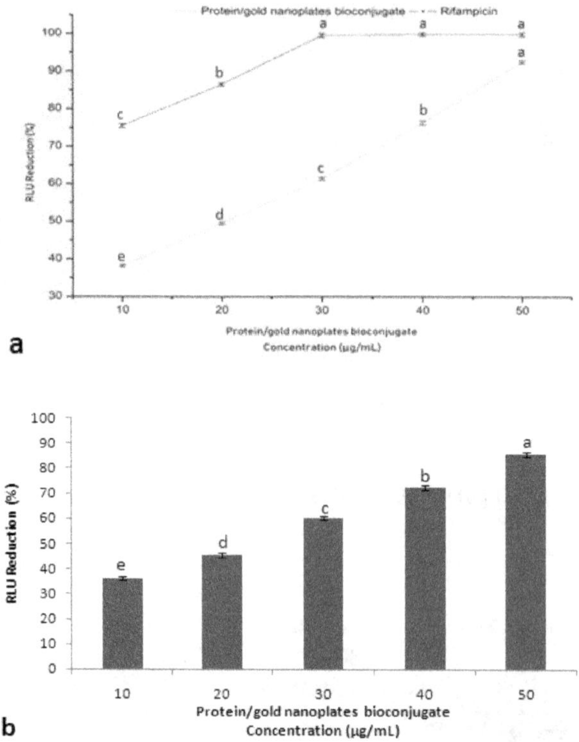

Figure 15: Anti-tubercular activities of protein/gold nanoplates bioconjugate and rifampicin at various concentrations (10-50 µg/mL) against (a) drug sensitive and (b) drug resistant strain of *M. tuberculosis.*

[Note: Values are represented as mean±SD of experiments carried out in triplicate (n=3) [abcde]Values with different letters are significantly (P<0.05) different.]

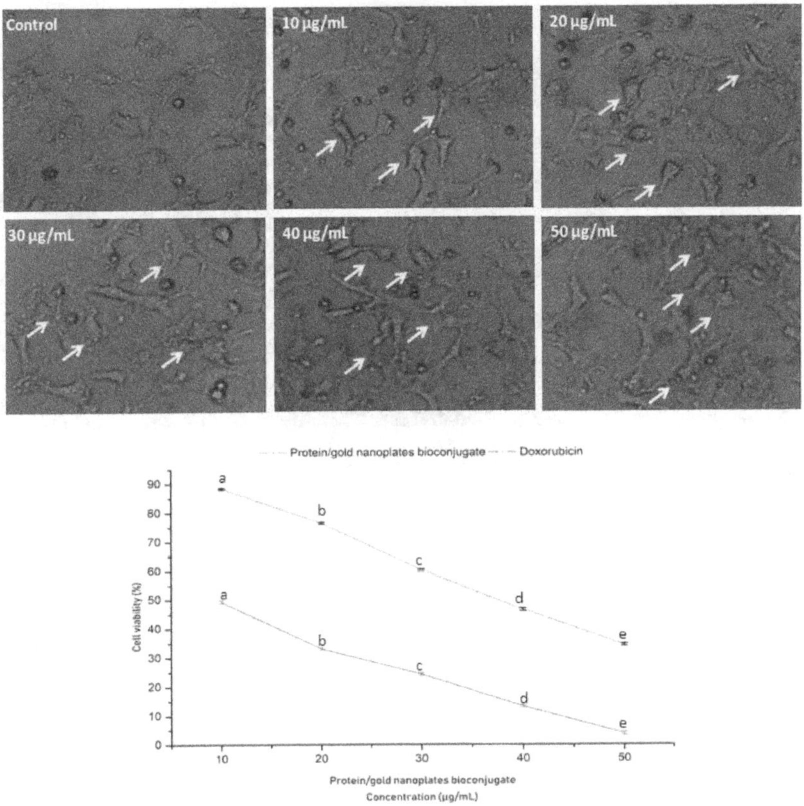

Figure 16: Morphological variations and reduction in the viabilities of A549 lung cancer cells in the presence of various concentrations (10-50 µg/mL) of protein/gold nanoplates bioconjugate. Yellow arrows indicate morphological changes in the cancer cells.

[Note: Values are represented as mean±SD of experiments carried out in triplicate (n = 3) ^{abcde}Values with different letters are significantly (P<0.05) different.]

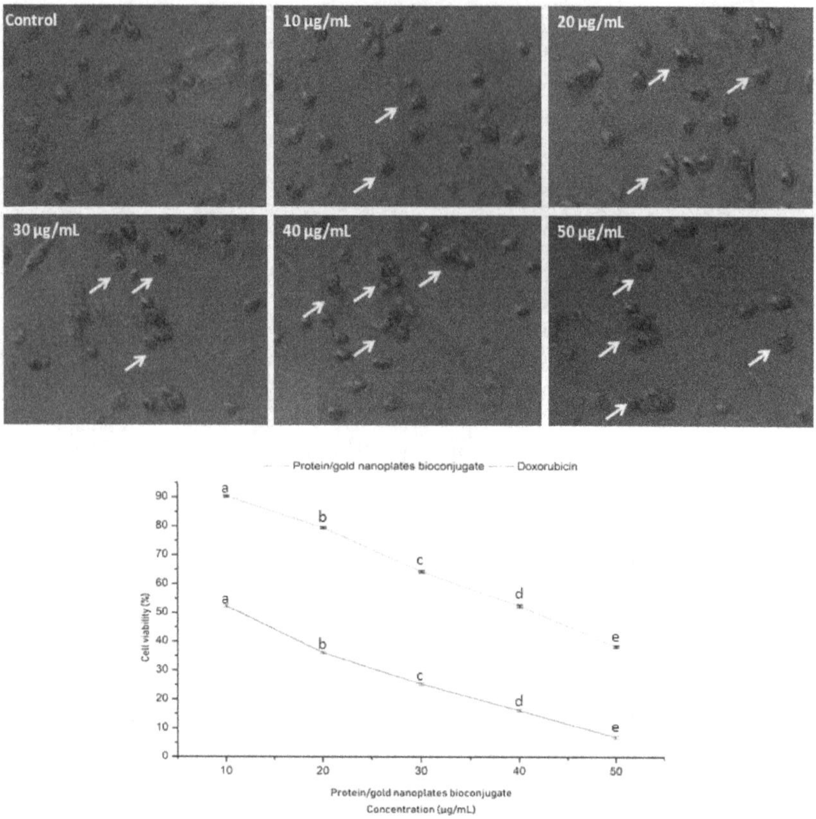

Figure 17: Morphological variations and reduction in the viabilities of HT-29 colon cancer cells in the presence of various concentrations (10–50 µg/mL) of protein/gold nanoplates bioconjugate. Yellow arrows indicate morphological changes in the cancer cells.

[Note: Values are represented as mean±SD of experiments carried out in triplicate (n = 3) [abcde]Values with different letters are significantly (P<0.05) different.]

4. Discussion

Bacteria have been recognized as natural factory for synthesizing AuNPs. Previously, plethora of studies has been investigated for synthesizing AuNPs using wide range of bacterial metabolites and cell biomass. Diverse group of bacteria viz. *Lactobacillus* sp. (Nair and Pradeep, 2002), *Shewanella alga* (Konishi *et al.*, 2007), *E. coli* (Du *et al.*, 2007), *Rhodopseudomonas capsulate* (He *et al.*, 2007), *Desulfovibrio desulfuricans* (Deplanche and Macaskie, 2008), *B. megaterium* (Wen *et al.*, 2009), and *W. confuse* (Adebayo-Tayo *et al.*, 2019) exhibited strong potentiality to synthesize AuNPs. In spite of few reports investigating nanoparticles synthesis from probiotic bacteria, the AuNPs synthesizing ability of fermented food associated coagulase-negative *Staphylococcus* sp. is undetermined yet. The present study represents the first report on the synthesis of AuNPs using *S. hominis* as reductant via microwave dielectric heating process. Microwave irradiation is an efficient heating processing technology which reduces the reaction period and enhances the yield without altering the composition of any product. In addition, this high frequency electromagnetic radiation based method shows homogeneous and rapid volumetric heating of the reaction mixture, leading to the easy nucleation of metallic naoparticles (Arshi *et al.*, 2011). Previous studies successfully demonstrated the immense role of microwave irradiation technique towards the rapid synthesis of AuNPs using disparate reducing agents (Arshi *et al.*, 2011; Das *et al.*, 2012; Augustine *et al.*, 2014).

The synthesis of AuNPs in the solution shows light to dark purple colour with characteristic absorption in the range of 520-560 nm (Reith *et al.*, 2009). The appearance of purple colour is mainly because of the excitation of surface plasmon vibrations, which is in fact an intrinsic trait of AuNPs formation (Das *et al.*, 2010). In this study, the synthesis of AuNPs using strain MANF2 was evident by observing dark purple colour solution and further confirmed by observing SPR peak (λ_{max}) too at 530 nm using UV-Vis spectrum. The broadened absorption of AuNPs might be due to the reason that the generated nanoparticles adsorbed the biomolecules on the surface exhibiting wide resonance peak (Das *et al.*, 2010). Additionally, the synthesis of AuNPs might also be because of the presence of enzymes, proteins, and other bioactive metabolites which reduced the gold cations into AuNPs (Aljabali *et al.*, 2018).

In order to attain greater stability, improved yield, and controlled size, it is essential to optimize varied factors used in the nanoparticles synthesis process. The traditional way of optimization is not only time consuming and laborious process but also misleads the outcomes of the bioprocessing researches. The application of statistical models to enhance certain responses is considered as successful alternatives to the classical strategy of optimization (Aarti *et al.*, 2017; Aarti *et al.*, 2018). In the present context, 3 effective variables (irradiation time, $HAuCl_4.3H_2O$ concentration, and reducing agent concentration) were optimized using BBD which showed significant (P<0.05) effect of parameters on AuNPs yield. The 3D plots indicated the profound influence of all 3 variables on AuNPs yields. Perturbation graph also showed that irradiation time, $HAuCl_4.3H_2O$ concentration, and reducing agent concentration significantly (P<0.05) increased the AuNPs synthesis. Further, the modelling of data using ANN showed the constructed neural network topology "3-8-1" neurons in input, hidden, and output layers, depicting the best fitness function. The R^2 and MSE revealed that the actual experimental data have been fit to the predicted values with high accuracy using the obtained ANN model. This study indicated the first report on the statistical optimization of AuNPs synthesis using BBD, followed by ANN of statistical modelling tools. Prior reports also showed the successful application of statistical tools (other than BBD and ANN) towards the optimization of nanoparticles yield (Biswas and Mulaba-Bafubiandi, 2016; Elsayed *et al.*, 2018).

The FT-IR spectrum demonstrates the availability of various functional groups of micro/macromolecules causing the gold ions reductions and stabilization of synthesized AuNPs (Preetam Raj *et al.*, 2016). In this study, FT-IR spectrum of the synthesized AuNPs revealed the presence of strong O-H groups, C=N stretching vibration, and strong =C-H bending for alkene. These functional groups might play crucial role in the reduction as well as stabilization of AuNPs synthesized. Zeta potential is a unique marker of colloidal particles stability. The value replicates the net charge on the outer surface of the particle that arises due to varied functional groups present on the surface (Aljabali *et al.*, 2018). In general, nanoparticles are considered stable colloids if the zeta potential values are estimated >25 mV or <-25 mV (Hiemenz and Rajagopalan, 1997). In this study, the zeta potential value obtained showed high stability of the synthesized AuNPs.

The DLS analysis of AuNPs in terms of size distribution vs. intensity demonstrated that the size of the highest percentage of AuNPs synthesized was 100 nm. The hydrodynamic diameter of AuNPs indicates the polydispersity distribution. The variations observed in the size of AuNPs may be due to the influence of micro/macromolecules which formed a covering on the nanoparticles synthesized (Wang *et al.*, 2015). The diffraction peaks pattern of AuNPs synthesized showed the fcc structure of atomic gold crystals. The lack of peaks of impurities depicted good crystalline nature of the nanoparticles. Findings of this investigation showed similarity with the peak values, planes, and fcc structures of AuNPs as demonstrated by Aljabali *et al.* (2018). Further, the EDX spectrum confirmed that the nanoparticles were primarily composed of gold, thereby showing lack of any kind of contaminants. Similar observation was reported by Aljabali *et al.* (2018) too.

Various size, shape, and composition of noble metallic nanoparticles are known to affect their physico-chemical characteristics (Oh and Lee, 2018). Controlling noble metal nanoparticles of desired morphologies are creating colossal attraction for diversified applications in nanomedicine. Among distinct gold nanostructures, 2D anisotropic gold nanoplates are of utmost interest not only due to their strong in-plane plasmon band in near infrared region but also decreased geometrical symmetry with sharp corners and edges (Oh and Lee, 2018). To date, uniform triangular, pentagonal, hexagonal, and rectangular gold nanoplates have been synthesized via chemical method of synthesis (Porel *et al.*, 2005; Huang *et al.*, 2014). The present investigation indicates the first report on the biological synthesis of anisotropic gold nanoplates, particularly pentagonal and square-shaped nanoplates with sharp edges. Thus, this study provided the great foundation for synthesizing polygonal gold nanoplates using probiotic bacteria, particularly *S. hominis* as ideal reducing agent through controlled mechanism.

Over the past few years, anisotropic AuNPs hold a colossal interest due to diversified therapeutic applications. Some of the recent studies demonstrated significant role of anisotropic AuNPs as antibacterial agents (Kumar *et al.*, 2012; Goyal *et al.*, 2019; Foliatini and Nurdiani, 2019). Additionally, anisotropic AuNPs have shown exemplary role in biosensing (surface enhanced Raman scattering, colorimetry, and fluorescence-based sensors), radiotherapy, and medical imaging (Kohout *et al.*, 2018) too. Surprisingly, there is dearth of research investigating anti-tubercular and anticancer attributes of anisotropic gold nanoplates synthesized using probiotic bacteria as effectual reducing agents. Currently, the conjugation of nanoparticles with proteins/peptides is an emerging area of research in order to achieve enhanced biological properties. However, the role of protein/gold nanoplates bioconjugate as therapeutic agents is undetermined yet. Considering this, a significant attempt was undertaken in this study to evaluate the therapeutic role of protein/gold nanoplates bioconjugate against *M. tuberculosis* (drug sensitive and drug resistant strains) and cancer cell lines (lung and colon) which exhibited noticeable anti-tubercular and anticancer traits of protein/gold nanoplates bioconjugate in a dose dependent manner. The protein/gold nanoplates bioconjugate revealed its potentiality to depict anti-tubercular activities against both drug sensitive and drug resistant strains of *M. tuberculosis*. Thus, the combination of bioactive proteins with gold nanoplates can certainly be used as potential anti-tubercular and tumoricidal agents in future. Unlike our findings, previous studies demonstrated antibacterial (Gomaa, 2018) and anticancer (Pal *et al*., 2016) role of bacteriocin/silver nanoparticles bioconjugate only.

5. Conclusions

In summary, microwave irradiation process was proved to be a rapid, non-toxic, and reproducible method to synthesize AuNPs using strain MANF2 as reductant. The BBD enhanced the yield of AuNPs under the conditions of 1mM of $HAuCl_4.3H_2O$, 1 mL of reducing agent, and irradiation period of 45 s. The modelling of data using ANN depicted the best fitness function. The R^2 and MSE revealed that the actual experimental data have been fit to the predicted values with high accuracy using the obtained ANN model. The synthesized AuNPs were crystalline in nature and morphologically distinct in structure. The SEM and DLS analyses revealed the synthesis of anisotropic gold nanoplates of 100 nm, particularly pentagonal and square-shaped nanoplates with sharp edges. The protein/gold nanoplates bioconjugate of varied concentrations depicted promising anti-tubercular (drug sensitive and drug resistant *M. tuberculosis* strains) and anticancer (A540 and HT-29 cancer cell lines) activities. Findings of this study clearly suggest the exemplary synergistic role of protein/gold nanoplates bioconjugate as ideal anti-tubercular and anticancer agents for the development of efficacious therapeutic drugs in future.

Dietary supplementation of *S. hominis* strain MANF2 towards gas production and fermentation kinetics in horses

1. Introduction

Over the past few years, plethoras of research are being focused to improve athletic performances as well as health of horses (Laghi *et al.*, 2018). Horses are non-ruminant herbivores whose hindgut is fermentative chamber for distinct microbiota (Shepherd *et al.*, 2012). Microbes ferment fibrous constituents of feed gradually and endow horses to prosper on starch rich forage. Horses obtain energy by fermenting these fibrous components of forage (Potter *et al.*, 1992). Unfortunately, reduced digestion of fibrous diets causes not only disorders viz. gastric ulceration, hindgut acidosis, endotoxemia, and colic in horses but also decreases energy utilization due to altered microbial counts (Rowe *et al.*, 1994). Hence, there is urgency to find new feed supplements which can improve the performances of horses by improving feed fermentative properties.

Probiotics are known to reduce varied disorders, particularly acidosis in horses (Ghorbani *et al.*, 2002). These direct-fed microbes exhibit beneficial impacts on animals by balancing microbial counts in intestine (Swyers *et al.*, 2008). Most importantly, probiotics improve the productivity of animals by enhancing the fermentation of feed, thereby estimating increased gas production (Garcia *et al.*, 2015). Surprisingly, most of the direct-fed microbes represent combinations of different genus of probiotic bacteria, which makes difficult to evaluate the potency of individual species (Swyers *et al.*, 2008). In view of this, a significant attempt was undertaken in this chapter to estimate not only the rate of gas production from horses but also fermentation kinetics via forage digestibility by supplementing varied doses of strain MANF2 into their diets.

2. Materials and methods

2.1. Ethical statement

This study was carried out as per the ethical standard laid down in the Declaration of Helsinki and its later amendments. Animals were treated and handled in accordance with the standard official protocols.

2.2. Bacterial inoculums preparation

The log phase grown culture of strain MANF2 was inoculated into 1 L of MRS broth medium and incubated for 48 h. After required incubation period, the culture was centrifuged at 10000 *g* for 20 min and supernatant was discarded. Cells were freeze-dried and stored at 4^0C for further experimental purposes.

2.3. Animals used

Azteca horses (age: 5 to 8 years, weight - 480 ±20.1 kg) were used in this study.

2.4. Diets used

Diets for animals were formulated as per the chemical composition mentioned in Table 1. Minerals included in the diet contains copper (21.18 ppm), iron (4950.5 ppm), zinc (343.7 ppm), calcium (9.91%), magnesium (0.25%), potassium (0.89%), sodium (1.3%), phosphorus (14.5%), and sulphur (3.1%). Diets were dried at 105^0C for 48 h in hot air oven (Bsco Hot air oven), ground to powder, and filtered using 1 mm sieve. The dried and powdered diets were termed as dry matter (DM) and stored in polyethylene bags.

2.5. Supplementation of strain MANF2

Substrate or diet was supplemented with two levels (1 and 3 mg/g of DM) of strain MANF2 and fed *ad libitum* to all the horses. Horses were divided into three treatments: 1) basal diet without bacterial culture (T0 - control), 2) basal diet with 1 mg/g of DM (T1), and 3) basal diet with 3 mg/g of DM (T2). Fresh water was provided to all the animals before faecal collection phase.

2.6. In vitro incubation-

2.6.1. Gas production

In vitro gas production from horses was estimated as per the methodology of Theodorou *et al.* (1994). Faecal samples (inoculum source) were collected from treated animals on clean straw-bedded floor and kept in a sterile polythene bags. Fifty millilitres of faecal buffer were prepared and added into bottles. Faecal buffer was prepared by diluting the faecal samples with the buffer solution (pH 7.0) in the ratio of 1:4 v/v (faeces: buffer) without trypticase. Bacterial cultures at two different concentrations (1 and 3 mg/g of DM) were added into each bottle. All the bottles were flushed with CO_2, sealed immediately using rubber stopper, and incubated at 39^0C. Total gas production was estimated up to 48 h using gas detector (AIR QUALITY MONITOR YesAIR, Critical Environment Technologies Canada Inc, Delta, British

Columbia, Canada). The kinetic parameters of gas production (mL/g of DM) were calculated according to the equation of France *et al.* (2000) as mentioned below using General Linear Model of Statistical Analysis System (SAS, 2002).

$$A = b \times (1 - e^{-c(t - Lag)})$$

where, A is the volume of gas production at time t; *b* is the asymptotic gas production (mL/g of DM); *c* is the rate of gas production (/h), and *Lag* (h) is the discrete lag time prior to gas production.

2.6.2. pH and degradable dry matter (DMD) determination

After required period of incubation, bottles were uncapped and the content was filtered under vacuum through glass crucibles with a sintered filter (coarse porosity no. 1, pore size 100 to 160 μm; Pyrex, Stone, UK). pH was measured using a digital pH meter (Conductronic pH 15.0, Puebla). The non-degradable residues of each bottle were dried at 65°C for 72 h for calculating DMD (Orskov and McDonald, 1979).

2.7. Statistical analyses

The responses for increasing doses of bacteria were estimated using linear and quadratic polynomial contrasts. All the experiments were performed in triplicate and the multiple comparisons among means were calculated using Turkey's test. Values representing $P \leq 0.05$ were considered significance.

3. Results

3.1. In vitro gas production

Figure 1a shows the asymptotic gas production at different doses of strain MANF2. The asymptotic gas production was increased (149.7±1.1 mL/g of DM) significantly ($P<0.05$) at high dose (3 mg/g of DM) with respect to control (128.4±1.1 mL/g of DM). The rate of gas production increased significantly ($P<0.05$) with respect to control, estimating 0.008±0.0002 gas production/h (Figure 1b). Likewise, the lag period was increased with increase in the doses of strain MANF2 (Figure 1c).

The supplementation of strain MANF2 revealed increased *in vitro* gas production at different incubation periods. Maximum gas production was estimated at 3 mg/g of DM ranging from 42.7 to 148.7 mL/g of DM at 8 and 48 h, respectively as compared to control (Figure 2).

3.2. pH and DMD determination

The inclusion of strain MANF2 showed slight non-significant ($P>0.05$) reduction in the pH values from 6.5 to 6.3 with respect to the control (6.5) (Figure 3a).

On the other hand, the DMD was increased at 1 (74.3±0.08) and 3 mg/g of DM (76.8±0.06) with respect to non-supplemented diet (72.9±0.06) (Figure 3b).

Table 1: Ingredients used as feed for horses.

Ingredients	Weight (g/kg of DM)
Ground corn	73.5
Soybean meal	9.0
Pastures	15.0
Organic matter	3.4
Crude protein	45.3
Ether extract	11.4
Acid detergent fibre	2.7
Neutral detergent fibre	4.7
Acid detergent lignin	2.1
Minerals	34.7

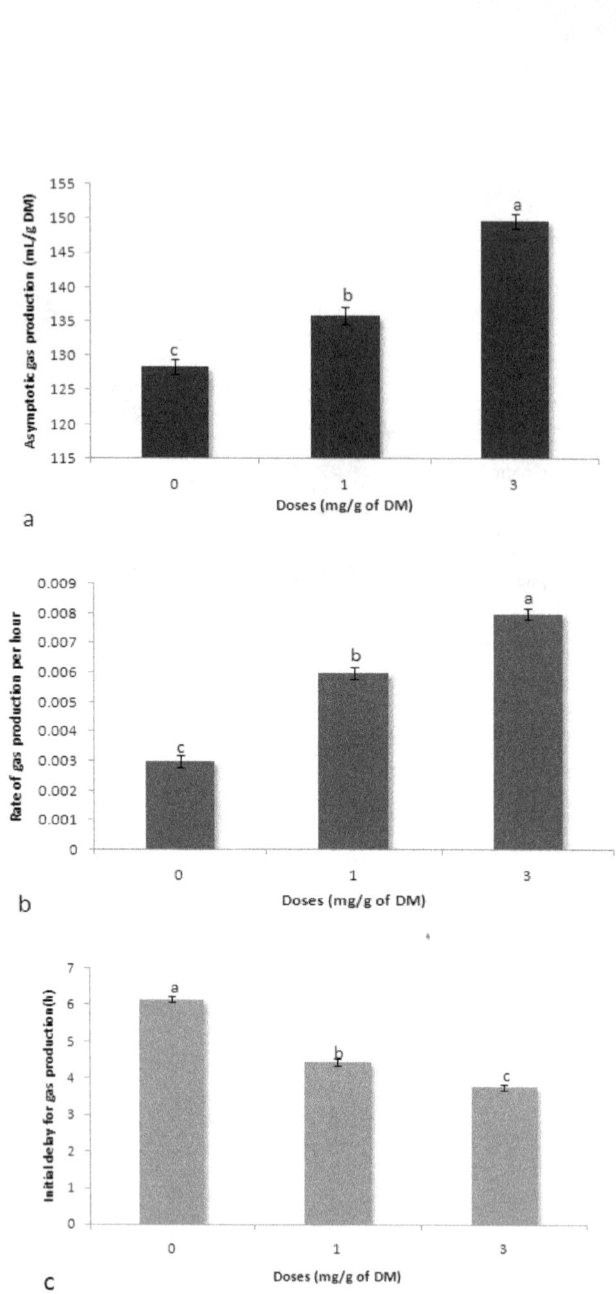

Figure 1: (a) asymptotic gas production, (b) rate of gas production, and (c) lag period in control (0 mg/g of DM) and strain MANF2 (1 and 3 mg/g of DM) supplemented diets.

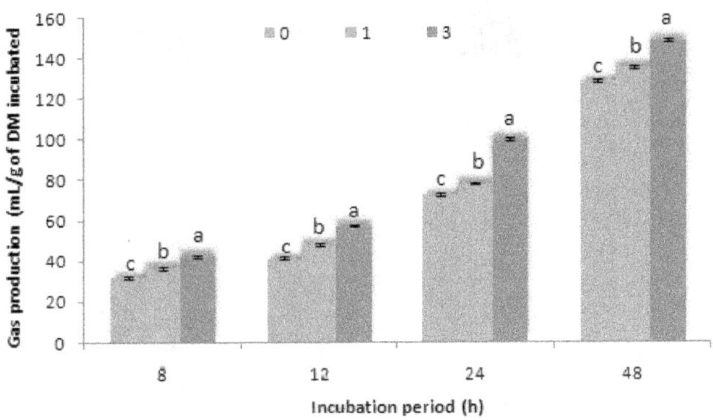

Figure 2: ***In vitro*** **gas production at various incubation periods in control (0 mg/g of DM) and strain MANF2 (1 and 3 mg/g of DM) supplemented diets.**

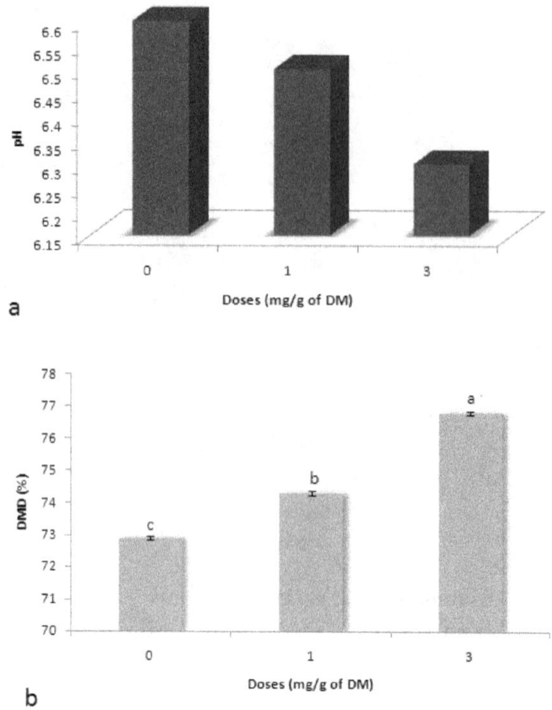

Figure 3: Effect of control (0 mg/g of DM) and strain MANF2 (1 and 3 mg/g of DM) supplemented diets on (a) pH and (b) DMD.

4. Discussion

Over the past few decades, veterinarians have focused to improve the athletics performances of horses by feeding high starch concentrates diets. The supplementation of direct-fed microbes into the animal's diets has reduced the risk of onset of health complications too. Probiotics are known to improve the intestinal microbiota in the host animals (Krehbiel *et al.*, 2003). Despite the role of commercial probiotics in prominent forage preparation, there is dearth of study investigating the efficacy of different groups of probiotic bacteria, particularly coagulase-negative *Staphylococcus* spp. towards nutrient digestion and fermentation kinetics in horses. Previous report assessed the influence of probiotic additive on fermentation kinetics and digestibility in horses fed high- and low-starch diets (Swyers *et al.*, 2008). In this investigation, we undertook a further pivotal attempt to evaluate the role of strain MANF2 as feed supplements towards the improvement of feed fermentation kinetics.

The supplementation of strain MANF2 at varied concentrations exhibited increased *in vitro* gas production from horse's faeces. It might be due to the fact that strain MANF2 contributed in the digestion of used substrate, thereby increasing faecal fermentation and thus, releasing increased gas production. Our findings were found to be in complete agreement with the report of Elghandour *et al.* (2014) who demonstrated improved digestion of feed due to the supplementation of direct-fed microbes into the horse's diet. In general, the increased gas production corresponds to the high fermentative characteristics of the feed used (Elghandour *et al.*, 2014).

pH is one of the most important fermentation parameters that indicates the acidity and alkalinity state in the gut (Faniyi *et al.*, 2019). pH is influenced by the types of forages consumed by livestock. In the present investigation, the inclusion of strain MANF2 reduced the fermentation pH. This might be due to the certain acid producing ability of bacteria during the fermentation process (Harlow *et al.*, 2017). On the other hand, in this study, the DMD of supplemented diet was increased with respect to the non-supplemented diet. In contrary to our results, Chen *et al.* (2017) estimated non-significant (P>0.05) effect of probiotics supplementation on DMD.

5. Conclusions

The supplementation of strain MANF2 showed increased *in vitro* gas production from horse's faeces at various incubation periods. Maximum gas production was estimated at 3 mg/g of DM. The inclusion of strain MANF2 showed non-significant

($P>0.05$) reduction in the pH values with respect to the control. The DMD was increased at 1 and 3 mg/g of DM with respect to non-supplemented diet. Thus, strain MANF2 can be utilized as ideal feed supplement towards improved digestibility and fermentation kinetics in horses.

Summary

A total of 56 bacteria were isolated from traditionally prepared various fermented foods of Tamil Nadu, India. '*Koozh*' associated 6 CNS strains showed anti-tubercular activities with high RLU reductions (92.4±0.3-97.7±0.4%). Among those isolates, strain MANF2 showed satisfactory probiotic attributes by exhibiting vast array of desirable characteristics. The strain demonstrated good technological characteristics as well as showed negative results towards *in vitro* haemolytic, DNase, and gelatinase tests, thereby revealing non-pathogenicity and safety aspect of this strain for possible development of functional food. As per statistical optimization tools (Taguchi OA design and BBD of RSM), MRS medium of pH 6.5 constituting yeast extract (0.5% w/v), magnesium sulphate (0.1% w/v), and glycerol (1.5% v/v), being further incubated at 30^{0}C showed increased anti-tubercular activity (98.7%) and approximately 4 fold improvement in the biomass yield (8.3 mg/mL) of strain MANF2 with respect to the traditional OFAT method. Anti-tubercular and anticancer protein of molecular mass 7712.3 Da was purified from strain MANF2, which showed sequence homology (95%) with Glyceraldehyde-3-phosphate dehydrogenase of *Staphylococcus* sp., suggesting a new Glyceraldehyde-3-phosphate dehydrogenase-like protein. The molecular mass of the most abundant peptide in the protein was observed as 1922.12 Da, and thus, this peptide was named as NMANF2. *In silico* tools indicated satisfactory stereo-chemical, physiochemical, and functional characteristics of peptide NMANF2. Further, the peptide showed strong affinity with various receptors such as DNA gyrase, ribonucleotide reductase, LysA, alanine racemase, and isocitrate lyase of *M. tuberculosis*. Similarly, among targeted proteins of A540 cell line, peptide NMANF2 revealed potential docking with Bcl-2. On the other hand, the peptide was reported as potential inhibitor of CDK4 among targeted HT-29 cell line receptors. Antimicrobial agents (*M. piperita*, penicillin G, and mercuric chloride) at sub-inhibitory concentration enhancedn total protein content of strain MANF2. The medium containing yeast extract (0.5% w/v) as well as glycerol (1.5% v/v), and supplementation of *M. piperita* (1.5% v/v) at log phase of strain MANF2 revealed maximum protein content of 9.4±0.4 mg/mL using CCD of RSM. Anti-tubercular and anticancer protein (molecular mass - 51293 Da) from strain MANF2 under mild stress of *M. piperita* was purified, which showed 100% homology with ProDH, thereby categorizing it as a new class of ProDH-like protein. The molecular mass of the most abundant peptide in this protein was observed as 2110.87 Da and thus, this peptide was named as SMANF2. *In silico* tools showed satisfactory stereo-chemical, physiochemical, and functional characteristics of peptide SMANF2. Further, the peptide showed the highest affinity with LysA, followed by ribonucleotide reductase, alanine racemase, DNA gyrase, and isocitrate lyase of *M. tuberculosis*. Among targeted proteins of A540 cell lines, peptide SMANF2 showed potential docking ability with Bcl-2. Likewise, the peptide was reported as potential inhibitor of Bcl-xL among targeted HT-29 cell line receptors. Further, some of the functional properties of strain MANF2 growing under mild stress of *M. piperita* varied with respect to the control strain. Statistical optimization tools such as BBD and ANN enhanced the production of microwave irradiation-based AuNPs, which was synthesized using strain MANF2 as reducing agent. The SEM and DLS analyses revealed the synthesis of anisotropic gold nanoplates of 100 nm, particularly pentagonal and square-shaped nanoplates with sharp edges. The protein/gold nanoplates bioconjugate of various concentrations exhibited promising anti-tubercular (against drug sensitive and drug resistant *M. tuberculosis* strains) and anticancer (A540 and HT-29 cancer cell lines) properties. The supplementation of strain MANF2 increased *in vitro* gas production from horse's faeces at different incubation periods. The inclusion of strain MANF2 showed non-significant ($P>0.05$) reductions in the pH values with respect to the control.

In a nutshell, findings of this research work suggested the exemplary biotechnological applications of strain MANF2 not only as auspicious anti-tubercular and anticancer agents for the development of efficacious therapeutic drug in future but also its pivotal role as ideal feed supplement towards improved digestibility and fermentation kinetics of horses.

References

Aarti C, Khusro A, Agastian P. Carboxymethyl cellulase production optimization from *Glutamicibacter arilaitensis* strain ALA4 and its application in lignocellulosic waste biomass saccharification. *Prep. Biochem. Biotechnol.* 2018; 48: 853-866.

Aarti C, Khusro A, Agastian P. Goat dung as a feedstock for hyper-production of amylase from *Glutamicibacter arilaitensis* strain ALA4. *Bioresour. Bioprocess.* 2017; 4: 43. doi.org/10.1186/s40643-017-0174-4.

Aarti C, Khusro A, Arasu MV, Agastian P, Al-Dhabi NA. Biological potency and characterization of antibacterial substances produced by *Lactobacillus pentosus* isolated from *Hentak*, a fermented fish product of North-East India. *SpringerPlus* 2016; 5: 1743. doi.org/10.1186/s40064-016-3452-2.

Abboud Y, Eddahbi A, El Bouari A, Aitenneite H, Brouzi K, Mouslim J. Microwave-assisted approach for rapid and green phytosynthesis of silver nanoparticles using aqueous onion (*Allium cepa*) extract and their antibacterial activity. *J. Nanostructure Chem.* 2013; 3: 84. doi.org/10.1186/2193-8865-3-84.

Adebayo-Tayo BC, Inem SA, Olaniyi OA. Rapid synthesis and characterization of gold and silver nanoparticles using exopolysaccharides and metabolites of *Wesiella confusa* as an antibacterial agent against *Esherichia coli. Int. J. Nano Dimens.* 2019; 10: 37-47.

Adeniyi BA, Adetoye A, Ayeni FA. Antibacterial activities of lactic acid bacteria isolated from cow faeces against potential enteric pathogens. *Afr. Health Sci.* 2015; 15: 888-895.

Aebi H. Catalase. In H. U. Bergmeyer (Ed.), Methods of Analytic Analysis. New York and London: Academic Press. 1974; 673-684. doi.org/10.1016/B978-0-12-091302-2.50032-3.

Agazzi A, Invernizzi G, Ferroni M, Fanelli A, Savoini G. Effect of live yeast (*Saccharomyces cerevisiae*) administration on apparent digestibility of horses. *Ital. J. Anim. Sci.* 2009; 8: 685- 687.

Albrecht AM, Evans CW, Raston CL. Green chemistry and the health implications of nanoparticles. *Green Chem.* 2006; 8: 417-432.

Alexandraki V, Tsakalidou E, Papadimitriou K, Holzapfel WH. Status and trends of the conservation and sustainable use of microorganisms in food processes.

Commission on Genetic Resources for Food and Agriculture. FAO. 2013; 65: 172.

Aljabali AAA, Akkam Y, Al Zoubi MS, Al-Batayneh KM, Al-Trad B, Abo Alrob O, Alkilany AM, Benamara M, Evans DJ. Synthesis of gold nanoparticles using leaf extract of *Ziziphus zizyphus* and their antimicrobial activity. *Nanomaterials* 2018; 8: 174. doi.org/10.3390/nano8030174.

Amund OD. Exploring the relationship between exposure to technological and gastrointestinal stress and probiotic functional properties of lactobacilli and bifidobacteria. *Can. J. Microbiol.* 2016; 62: 715-725.

Anandharaj M, Sivasankari B, Santhanakaruppu R, Manimaran M, Rani RP, Sivakumar S. Determining the probiotic potential of cholesterol-reducing *Lactobacillus* and *Weissella* strains isolated from gherkins (fermented cucumber) and South Indian fermented koozh. *Res. Microbiol.* 2015; 166: 428-439.

Anisha AHN, Anandham R, Kwon SW, Gandhi PI, Gopal NO. Evaluation of *Bacillus* spp. as dough starters for *Adhirasam* - A traditional rice based fermented food of Southern India. *Braz. J. Microbiol.* 2015; 46: 1183-1191.

Arshi N, Ahmed F, Kumar S, Anwar MS, Lu J, Koo BH, Lee CG. Microwave assisted synthesis of gold nanoparticles and their antibacterial activity against *Escherichia coli* (*E. coli*). *Curr. Appl. Phys.* 2011; 11: S360-S363.

Arumugam T, Kumar PS. Optimization of media components for production of antimicrobial compound by *Brevibacillus brevis* EGS9 isolated from mangrove ecosystem. *J. Microbiol. Methods* 2017; 142: 83-89.

Ashwini S, Varkey SP, Shantaram M. *In silico* docking of polyphenolic compounds against caspase 3-Hela cell line protein. *Int. J. Drug Dev. Res.* 2017; 9: 28-32.

Askary M, Talebi SM, Amini F, Bangan ADB. Effects of iron nanoparticles on *Mentha piperita* L. under salinity stress. *Biologija* 2017; 63: 65-75.

Augustine AK, Nampoori VPN, Kailasnath M. Rapid synthesize of gold nanoparticles by microwave irradiation method and its application as an optical limiting material. *Optik* 2014; 125: 6696-6699.

Awaisheh SS, Obeidat MM, Al-Tamimi HJ, Assaf AM, EL-Qudah JM, Al-khaza'leh JM, Rahahleh RJ. *In vitro* cytotoxic activity of probiotic bacterial cell extracts against Caco-2 and HRT-18 colorectal cancer cells. *Milk Sci. Int.* 2016; 69: 27-31.

Azam R, Ghafouri-Fard S, Tabrizi M, Modarressi MH, Ebrahimzadeh-Vesal R, Daneshvar M, Mobasheri MB, Motevaseli E. *Lactobacillus acidophilus* and *Lactobacillus crispatus* culture supernatants downregulate expression of cancer-testis genes in the MDA-MB-231 cell line. *Asian Pac. J. Cancer Prev.* 2014; 15: 4255-4259.

Baban BA, Vinod MP, Tanner JJ, Becker DF. Probing a hydrogen bond pair and the FAD redox properties in the proline dehydrogenase domain of *Escherichia coli* PutA. *Biochem. Biophys. Acta.* 2004; 1701: 49-59.

Badis A, Guetarni D, Moussa-Boudjemaa B, Henni DE, Tornadijo ME, Kihal M. Identification of cultivable lactic acid bacteria isolated from Algerian raw goat's milk and evaluation of their technological properties. *Food Microbiol.* 2004; 21: 343-349.

Bailey SR, Baillon ML, Rycroft AN, Harris PA, Elliott J. Identification of equine cecal bacteria producing amines in an *in vitro* model of carbohydrate overload. *Appl. Environ. Microbiol.* 2003; 69: 2087-2093.

Bajpai VK, Rather IA, Majumder R, Alshammari FH, Nam GJ, Park YH. Characterization and antibacterial mode of action of lactic acid bacterium *Leuconostoc mesenteroides* HJ69 from Kimchi. *J. Food Biochem* 2017; 41: e12290. doi.org/10.1111/jfbc.12290.

Balamurugan R, Chandragunasekaran AS, Chellappan G, Rajaram K, Ramamoorthi G, Ramakrishna BS. Probiotic potential of lactic acid bacteria present in home made curd in Southern India. *Indian J. Med. Res.* 2014, 140: 345-355.

Bao Y, Zhang Y, Zhang Y, Liu Y, Wang S, Dong X, Wang Y, Zhang H. Screening of potential probiotic properties of *Lactobacillus fermentum* isolated from traditional dairy products. *Food Control* 2010; 21: 695-701.

Bastos MCF, Ceotto H, Coelho MLV, Nascimento JS. Staphylococcal antimicrobial peptides: relevant properties and potential biotechnological applications. *Curr. Pharm. Biotechno.* 2009; 10: 38-61.

Bauer AW, Kirby WMM, Sherris JC, Turck M. Antibiotic susceptibility testing by a standardized single disk method. *Am. J. Clin. Pathol.* 1966; 45: 493-496.

Beaufays J, Lins L, Thomas A, Brasseur R. *In silico* predictions of 3D structures of linear and cyclic peptides with natural and non-proteinogenic residues. *J. Pept. Sci.* 2012; 18:17-24.

Berthelot G, Sedeaud A, Marck A, Antero-Jacquemin J, Schipman J, Saulière G, Marc A, Desgorces FD, Toussaint JF. Has Athletic Performance Reached its Peak? *Sports Med.* 2015; 45: 1263-1271.

Bezerra MA, Santelli RE, Oliveira EP, Villar LS, Escaleira LA. Response surface methodology (RSM) as a tool for optimization in analytical chemistry. *Talanta* 2008; 76: 965-677.

Bingol D, Hercan M, Elevli S, Kılıc E. Comparison of the results of response surface methodology and artificial neural network for the biosorption of lead using black cumin. *Bioresour. Technol.* 2012; 112: 111-115.

Biswas S, Mulaba-Bafubiandi AF. Optimization of process variables for the biosynthesis of silver nanoparticles by *Aspergillus wentii* using statistical experimental design. *Adv. Nat. Sci. Nanosci. Nanotechnol.* 2016; 7: 045005. doi.org/10.1088/2043-6262/7/4/045005.

Bizzini A, Beggah-Moller S, Moreillon P, Entenza JM. Lack of *in vitro* biofilm formation does not attenuate the virulence of *Streptococcus gordonii* in experimental endocarditis. *FEMS Immunol. Med. Microbiol.* 2006; 48: 419-423.

Borah D, Gogoi O, Adhikari C, Kakoti BB. Isolation and characterization of the new indigenous *Staphylococcus* sp. DBOCP06 as a probiotic bacterium from traditionally fermented fish and meat products of Assam state. *Egypt. J. Basic Appl. Sci.* 2016; 3: 232-240.

Borowicki A, Michelmann A, Stein K, Scharlau D, Scheu K, Obst U, Glei M. Fermented wheat aleurone enriched with probiotic strains LGG and Bb12 modulates markers of tumor progression in human colon cells. *Nutr. Cancer* 2011; 63: 151-160.

Bourdichon F, Casaregola S, Farrokh C, Frisvad JC, Gerds ML, Hammes WP, Harnett JM, Huys G, Laulund S, Ouwehand A, Powell IB, Prajapati JB, Seto Y, Schure ET, Boven AV, Vankerckhoven V, Zgoda A, Tuijtelaars S, Hansen EB. Food fermentations: Microorganisms with technological beneficial use. *Int. J. Food Microbiol.* 2012; 154: 87-97.

Bradford MM. A rapid and sensitive method for the quantitation of microgram quantities of protein utilizing the principle of protein-dye binding. *Anal. Biochem.* 1976; 72: 248-254.

Bruinsma J. Livestock Production. In: J. Bruinsma (Ed.) World Agriculture: Towards 2015/2030. An FAO perspective. Earthscan Publications Ltd, London. 2003.

Buchmeier N, Bossie S, Chen CY, Fang FC, Guiney DG, Libby SJ. SlyA- A transcriptional regulator of *Salmonella* Typhimurium is required for resistance to oxidative stress and is expressed in the intra cellular environment of macrophages. *Infect. Immun.* 1997; 65: 3725-3730.

Bulgasem BY, Hassan Z, Abdalsadiq NKA, Yusoff WMW, Musa EMT, Lani MN. Anti-adhesion activity of lactic acid bacteria supernatant against human pathogenic *Candida* species. *Biofilm. Health Sci. J.* 2015; 9: 1-9.

Carroll J, Draper LA, O'Connor PM, Coffey A, Hill C, Ross RP, Cotter PD, O'Mahony J. Comparison of the activities of the lantibiotics nisin and lacticin 3147 against clinically significant mycobacteria. *Int. J. Antimicrob. Agents* 2010; 36: 132-136.

Carroll J, O'Mahony J. Anti-mycobacterial peptides. Made to order with delivery included. *Bioeng. Bugs* 2011; 2: 241-246.

Casaburi A, Blaiotta G, Mauriello G, Pepe O, Villani F. Technological activities of *Staphylococcus carnosus* and *Staphylococcus simulans* strains isolated from fermented sausages. *Meat Sci.* 2005; 71: 643-650.

Cha MK, Lee DK, An HM, Lee SW, Shin SH, Kwon JH, Kim KJ, Ha NJ. Antiviral activity of *Bifidobacterium adolescentis* SPM1005-A on human papillomavirus type 16. *BMC Med.* 2012; 10: 72. doi.org/10.1186/1741-7015-10-72.

Chandra P, Shilpa VS. Molecular characterization and identification of bioactive peptides producing *Lactobacillus* sps. based on 16S rRNA gene sequencing. *Food Biotechnol.* 2018; 32: 1-14.

Charteris WP, Kelly PM, Morelli L, Collins JK. Development and application of an *in-vitro* methodology to determine the transit tolerance of potentially probiotic *Lactobacillus* and *Bifidobacterium* species in the upper human gastrointestinal tract. *J. Appl. Microbiol.* 1998; 84: 759-768.

Chauviere G, Coconnier MH, Kerneis S, Darfeuille-Michaud A. Competitive exclusion of diarrheagenic *Escherichia coli* (ETEC) from human enterocyte-like Caco-2 cells by heat killed *Lactobacillus*. *FEMS Microbiol. Lett.* 1992; 70: 213-217.

Chen L, Ren A, Zhou C, Tan Z. Effects of *Lactobacillus acidophilus* supplementation for improving *in vitro* rumen fermentation characteristics of cereal straws. *Ital. J. Anim. Sci.* 2017; 16: 52-60.

Chen YC, Sugiyama Y, Abe N, Kuruto-Nima R, Nozawa R, Hirota A. DPPH radical scavenging compounds from Dou-Chi, a soybean fermented food. *Biosci. Biotechnol. Biochem.* 2005; 69: 999-1006.

Chiu YH, Hsieh YJ, Liao KW, Peng KC. Preferential promotion of apoptosis of monocytes by *Lactobacillus casei* rhamnosus soluble factors. *Clin. Nutr.* 2010; 29: 131-140.

Choi SS, Kim Y, Han KS, You S, Oh S, Kim SH. Effects of *Lactobacillus* strains on cancer cell proliferation and oxidative stress *in vitro*. *Lett. Appl. Microbiol.* 2006; 42: 452-458.

Chung HJ, Montville TJ, Chikindas ML. Nisin depletes ATP and proton motive force in mycobacteria. *Lett. Appl. Microbiol.* 2000; 31: 416-420.

Cooper WA, Lam DC, O'Toole SA, Minna JD. Molecular biology of lung cancer. *J. Thorac. Dis.* 2013; 5: 479-490.

Costa M, Weese JS. 2012. The equine intestinal microbiome. *Anim. Heal. Res. Rev.* 2012; 13: 121-128.

Cotter PD, Hill C. Surviving the acid test: responses of gram positive bacteria to low pH. *Microbiol. Mol. Biol. Rev.* 2003; 67: 429-453.

Cousin FJ, Jouan-Lanhouet S, Dimanche-Boitrel MT, Corcos L, Jan G. Milk fermented by *Propionibacterium freudenreichii* induces apoptosis of HGT-1 human gastric cancer cells. *PLoS One* 2012; 7: e31892. doi.org/10.1371/journal.pone.0031892.

Craik DJ, Fairlie DP, Liras S, Price D. The future of peptide-based drugs. *Chem. Biol. Drug Des.* 2013; 81: 136-147.

Csonka LN. Proline over-production results in enhanced osmotolerance in *Salmonella* Typhimurium. *Mol. Gen. Genet.* 1981; 182: 82-86.

Das RK, Babu PJ, Gogoi N, Sharma P, Bora U. Microwave-mediated rapid synthesis of gold nanoparticles using *Calotropis procera* latex and study of optical properties. *ISRN Nanomater.* 2012; 2012, doi.org/10.5402/2012/650759.

David JK, Dhivya A, Janani D, Sukumar A, Subramaniam V. Comparison of the probiotic effect of *Lactobacillus acidophilus*, *Streptococcus thermophilus* and

Saccharomyces cerevisiae on staple south Indian fermented foods. *World J. Pharm. Res.* 2013; 2: 3229-3239.

De Rezende ASC, Trigo P, Lana AMQ, Santiago JM, Silva VP, Montijano FC. Yeast as a feed additive for training horses. *Cienc. Agrotechnol.* 2012; 36: 354-362.

De Vrese M, Stegelmann A, Richter B, Fenselau S, Laue C, Schrezenmeir J. Probiotics compensation for lactase insufficiency. *Am. J. Clin. Nutr.* 2001; 73: 421-429.

Delgado S, Leite AMO, Ruas-Madiedo P, Mayo B. Probiotic and technological properties of *Lactobacillus* spp. strains from the human stomach in the search for potential candidates against gastric microbial dysbiosis. *Front. Microbiol.* 2015; 5: 766. doi.org/10.3389/fmicb.2014.00766.

De-Oliveira SS, Abrantes J, Cardoso M, Sordelli D, Bastos MC. Staphylococcal strains involved in bovine mastitis are inhibited by *Staphylococcal aureus* antimicrobial peptides. *Lett. Appl. Microbiol.* 1998; 27: 287-291.

Deplanche K, Macaskie LE. Biorecovery of gold by *Escherichia coli* and *Desulfovibrio desulfuricans*. *Biotechnol. Bioeng.*2008; 99: 1055-1064.

Desrochers AM, Dolente BA, Roy MF, Boston R, Carlisle S. Efficacy of *Saccharomyces boulardii* for treatment of horses with acute enterocolitis. *J. Am. Vet. Med. Assoc.* 2005; 227: 954-959.

Devagaopalan H, Krishnaswamy H. Isolation and characterization of probiotic microorganism from milk and milk product. *Int. J. Chem. Stud.* 2018; 6: 2692-2695.

Donaghy JA, Totton NL, Rowe MT. The *in vitro* antagonistic activities of lactic acid bacteria against *Mycobacterium avium* subsp. *paratuberculosis*. Paratuberculosis. 2005; 8.

Drummond AJ, Ashton B, Buxton S, Cheung M, Cooper A, Duran C, Field M, Heled J, Kearse M, Markowitz S, Moir R, Stones-Havas S, Sturrock S, Thierer T, Wilson A. Geneious v5.6, 2012; Available from http://www.geneious.com.

Du L, Jiang H, Liu X, Wang E. Biosynthesis of gold nanoparticles assisted by *Escherichia coli* DH5α and its application on direct electrochemistry of haemoglobin. *Electrochem. Commun.* 2007; 9: 1165-1170.

Du Toit M, Dicks LMT, Holzapfe WH. Identification of heterofermentative lactobacilli isolated from pig faeces by numerical analysis of total soluble cell protein patterns and RAPD-PCR. *Lett. Appl. Microbiol.* 2003; 37: 12-16.

Dunker AK, Obradovic Z. The protein trinity-linking function and disorder. *Nat. Biotechnol.* 2001; 19: 805-806.

Dunne C, O'Mahony L, Murphy L, Thornton G, Morrissey D, O'Halloran S, Feeney M, Flynn S, Fitzgerald G, Daly C, Kiely B, O'Sullivan GC, Shanahan F, Collins JK. *In vitro* selection criteria for probiotic bacteria of human origin: Correlation with *in vivo* findings. *Am. J. Clin. Nutr.* 2001; 73: 386-392.

Dutta B, Banerjee A, Chakraborty P, Bandopadhyay R. *In silico* studies on bacterial xylanase enzyme: Structural and functional insight. *J. Genet. Eng. Biotechnol.* 2018; 16: 749-756.

Dykman L, Khlebtsov N. Gold nanoparticles in biomedical applications: Recent advances and perspectives. *Chem. Soc. Rev.* 2012; 41: 2256-2282.

Elghandour MMY, Vazquez Chagoyan JC, Salem AZM, Kholif AE, Martínez Castaneda JS, Camacho LM, Buendía G. *In vitro* fermentative capacity of equine fecal inocula of 9 fibrous forages in the presence of different doses of *Saccharomyces cerevisiae*. *J. Equine Vet. Sci.* 2014; 34: 619-625.

Eloff JN. A sensitive and quick microplate method to determine the minimal inhibitory concentration of plant extracts for bacteria. *Plant Med.* 1998; 64: 711-713.

Elsayed MA, Abdelmageed M. Hassan OMM, Elshafei AM. Optimization of silver nanoparticles biosynthesis mediated by *Aspergillus niger* NRC1731 through application of statistical methods: Enhancement and characterization. *3 Biotech* 2018; 8: 132. doi.org/10.1007/s13205-018-1158-6.

Escamilla J, Lane MA, Maitin V. Cell-free supernatants from probiotic *Lactobacillus casei* and *Lactobacillus rhamnosus* GG decrease colon cancer cell invasion *in vitro*. *Nutr. Cancer* 2012; 64: 871-878.

Eustis S, El-Sayed MA. Why gold nanoparticles are more precious than pretty gold: Noble metal surface plasmon resonance and its enhancement of the radiative and nonradiative properties of nanocrystals of different shapes. *Chem. Soc. Rev.* 2006; 35: 209-217.

Ezat AA, El-Bialy NS, Mostafa HIA, Ibrahim MA. Molecular docking investigation of the binding interactions of macrocyclic inhibitors with HCV NS3 protease and its mutants (R155K, D168A and A156V). *Protein J.* 2014; 33: 32-47.

Faniyi TO, Adegbeye MJ, Elghandour MMY, Pilego AB, Salem AZM, Olaniyi TA, Adediran O, Adewumi MK. Role of diverse fermentative factors towards microbial community shift in ruminants. *J. Appl. Microbiol.* 2019; 30: 1-10.

Fanning S, Hall LJ, Cronin M, Zomer A, MacSharry J, Goulding D, Motherway MO, Shanahan F, Nally K, Dougan G, Van Sinderen D. Bifidobacterial surface-exopolysaccharide facilitates commensal-host interaction through immune modulation and pathogen protection. *Proc. Natl. Acad. Sci.* 2012; 109: 2108-2113.

Farhad M, Kailasapathy K, Tamang JP. Health aspects of fermented foods. In Fermented Foods and Beverages of the World, Eds J.P. Tamang and K. Kailasapathy (New York, NY: CRC Press), 2010: 391-414.

Feitelson MA, Arzumanyan A, Kulathinal RJ, Blain SW, Holcombe RF, Mahajna J, Marino M, Martinez Chanter ML, Nawroth R, Sanchez Garcia I, Sharma D, Saxena NK, Singh N, Vlachostergios PJ, Guo S, Honoki K, Fujii H, Georgakilas AG, Bilsland AI, Amedei A, Niccolai E, Amin A, Ashraf S S, Boosani CS, Guha G, Ciriolo MR, Aquilano K, Chen S, Mohammed SI, Azmi AS, Bhakta D, Halicka D, Keith WN, Nowsheen S. Sustained proliferation in cancer: Mechanisms and novel therapeutic targets. *Semin. Cancer Biol.* 2015; 35: S25–S54.

Field SK. Bedaquiline for the treatment of multidrug-resistant tuberculosis: Great promise or disappointment? *Ther. Adv. Chronic Dis.* 2015; 6: 170-184.

Filion LG, Al-Ahdal MN, Tetro JA. Vaccines against *Mycobacterium tuberculosis*: Exploring alternate strategies to combat a near perfect pathogen. *J. Mycobac. Dis.* 2013; S1: 003. doi.org/10.4172/2161-1068.S1-003.

Foliatini F, Nurdiani N. One-step synthesis of anisotropic gold nanoparticles with the aid extract from wuluh starfruit (*Averrhoa bilimbi*) fruit as reducing and morphology controlling agent. *Orient. J. Chem.* 2019; 35: 1453-1462.

Fortier LC, Tourdot-Mare´chal R, Divie`s C, Lee BH, Guzzo J. Induction of *Oenococcus oeni* H^+-ATPase activity and mRNA transcription under acidic conditions. *FEMS Microbiol. Lett.* 2003; 222: 165-169.

Fosgerau K, Hoffmann T. Peptide therapeutics: current status and future directions. *Drug Discov. Today* 2015; 20: 122-128.

France J, Dijkstra J, Dhanoa MS, Lopez S, Bannink A. Estimating the extent of degradation of ruminant feeds from a description of their gas production profiles observed *in vitro*: Derivation of models and other mathematical considerations. *Brit. J. Nutr.* 2000; 83: 143-150.

Gad SA, AbdEi-Baky ARM, Ahmed ABF, Gad GFM. *In vitro* evaluation of probiotic potential of five lactic acid bacteria and their antimicrobial activity against some enteric and foodborne pathogens. *Afr. J. Microbiol. Res.* 2016; 10: 400-409.

Gao J, Xu B. Applications of nanomaterials inside cells. *Nano Today* 2009; 4: 37-51.

Garcia TR, de Rezende AS, Trigo P, Santiago JM, de Almeida FQ, Terra RA, Fonseca MG, Castejón F. Effects of supplementation with *Saccharomyces cerevisiae* and aerobic training on physical performance of Mangalarga Marchador mares. *Rev. Bras. Zootec.* 2015; 44: 22-26.

Gavrilova NN, Ratnikova IA, Sadanov AK, Bayakisheva K, Tourlibaeva ZJ, Belikova OA. Application of probiotics in complex treatment of tuberculosis. *Int. J. Eng. Res. Appl.* 2014; 4: 13-18.

Gerhardt P, Murry RGE, Willis AW, Krieg NR. Methods for general and molecular bacteriology. Phenotypic characterization. 1994; 623-624. doi.org/10.1002/food.19960400226.

Ghoneum M, Gimzewski J: Apoptotic effect of a novel kefir product, PFT, on multidrug-resistant myeloid leukemia cells via a hole-piercing mechanism. *Int. J. Oncol.* 2014; 44: 830-837.

Ghorbani GR, Morgavi DP, Beauchemin KA, Leedle JAA. Effects of bacterial direct fed microbials on ruminal fermentation, blood variables, and the microbial populations of feedlot cattle. *J. Anim. Sci.* 2002; 80: 1977-1985.

Gibson GR, McCartney AL, Rastall RA. Prebiotics and resistance to gastrointestinal infections. *Br. J. Nutr*. 2005; 93: 31-34.

Goh EB, Yim G, Tsui W, McClure J, Surette MG, Davies J. Transcriptional modulation of bacterial gene expression by subinhibitory concentrations of antibiotics. *Prod. Natl. Acad. Sci. U.S.A.* 2002; 99: 17025-17030.

Gomaa EZ. Synergistic antibacterial efficiency of bacteriocin and silver nanoparticles produced by probiotic *Lactobacillus paracasei* against multidrug resistant bacteria. *Int. J. Pep. Res. Ther.* 2018; 25. doi.org/10.1007/s10989-018-9759-9.

Götz F, Bannerman T, Schleifer KH. The genera *Staphylococcus* and *Macrococcus*. In: Dworkin, M. (Ed.). Procaryotes 2006; 4: 5-75.

Goyal D, Saini A, Saini GSS, Kumar R. Green synthesis of anisotropic gold nanoparticles using cinnamon with superior antibacterial activity. *Mater. Res. Express* 2019; 6: 075043. doi.org/10.1088/2053-1591/ab15a6.

Greenwood D, Eley A. Comparative antipseudomonal activity of some newer beta-lactam agents. *Antimicrob. Agents Chemother.* 1982; 21: 204-209.

Gronvold AR, L'abee-Lund TM, Sorum H, Skancke E, Yannarell AC, Mackie RI. Changes in fecal microbiota of healthy dogs administered amoxicillin. *FEMS Microbiol. Ecol.* 2010; 71: 313-326.

Gruber AR, Lorenz R, Bernhart SH, Neuböck R, Hofacker IL. The Vienna RNA websuite. *Nucleic Acids Res.* 2008; 36: 70-74.

Grześkowiak L, Collado MC, Salminen S. Evaluation of aggregation abilities between commensal fish bacteria and pathogens. *Aquaculture.* 2012; 356: 412-414.

Gu RX, Yang ZQ, Li ZH, Chen SL, Luo ZL. Probiotic properties of lactic acid bacteria isolated from stool samples of longevous people in regions of Hotan, Xinjiang and Bama, Guangxi, China. *Anaerobe* 2008; 14: 313-317.

Gualano G, Capone S, Matteelli A, Palmieri F. New antituberculosis drugs: From clinical trial to programmatic use. *Infect. Dis. Rep.* 2016; 8: 65-69.

Guisbiers G, Mejía-Rosales S, Deepak FL. Nanomaterial properties: size and shape dependencies. *J. Nanomater.* 2012; 2012: 1-2.

Haddaji N, Mahdhi AK, Krifi B, Ismail MB, Bakhrouf A. Change in cell surface properties of *Lactobacillus casei* under heat shock treatment. *FEMS Microbiol. Lett.* 2015; 362. doi.org/10.1093/femsle/fnv047.

Hale EM, Hinsdill RD. Characterization of a bacteriocin from *Staphylococcus aureus* strain 462. *Antimicrob. Agents Chemother.* 1973; 4: 634-640.

Hamon E, Horvatovich P, Izquierdo E, Bringel F, Marchionil E, Aoudé-Werner D, Ennahar S. Comparative proteomic analysis of *Lactobacillus plantarum* for the identification of key proteins in bile tolerance. *BMC Microbiol.* 2011; 11: 63. doi.org/10.1186/1471-2180-11-63.

Han K, Lee N, Park H, Paik H. Anticancer and anti-inflammatory activity of probiotic *Lactococcus lactis* NK34. *J. Microbiol. Biotechnol.* 2015; 25: 1697-1701.

Hanina MN, Hairul Shahril M, Ismatul NAI, Abdul Jalil AK, Salina MR, Maryam MR, Rosfarizan M. Extracellular protein secreted by *Bacillus subtilis* ATCC21332 in the presence of streptomycin sulfate. *World Acad. Sci. Eng. Technol. Int. J. Biol. Food Vet. Agric. Eng.* 2014; 8: 791-795.

Harding HP, Zhang Y, Bertolotti A, Zeng H, Ron D. Perk is essential for translational regulation and cell survival during the unfolded protein response. *Mol. Cell.* 2000; 5: 897-904.

Hards K, Robson JR, Berney M, Shaw L, Bald D, Koul A, Andries K, Cook GM. Bactericidal mode of action of bedaquiline. *J. Antimicrob. Chemother.* 2015; 70: 2028-2037.

Harlow BE, Lawrence LM, Harris PA, Aiken GE, Flythe MD. Exogenous lactobacilli mitigate microbial changes associated with grain fermentation (corn, oats, and wheat) by equine fecal microflora *ex vivo*. *PLoS One* 2017; 12: e0174059. doi.org/10.1371/journal.pone.0174059.

Havenaar R, Ten Brink B, Huis In't Veld JHJ. Selection of Strains for Probiotic Use. In: Fuller, R. (Ed.), Probiotics. The Scientific Basis. Chapman and Hall, London. 1992; 209-221.

He S, Guo Z, Zhang Y, Zhang S, Wang J, Gu N. Biosynthesis of gold nanoparticles using the bacteria *Rhodopseudomonas capsulate*. *Mater. Lett.* 2007; 61: 3984-3987.

He ZS, Luo H, Cao CH, Cui ZW. Photometric determination of hydroxyl free radical in Fenton system by brilliant green. *Am. J. Clin. Med.* 2004; 6: 236-237.

Herbst RS, Heymach JV, Lippman SM. Lung cancer. *N. Engl. J. Med.* 2008; 359: 1367-1380.

Heunis TDJ, Botes M, Dicks LM. Encapsulation of *Lactobacillus plantarum* 423 and its bacteriocin in nanofibers. *Probiotics Antimicrob. Proteins* 2010; 2: 1867-1906.

Hiemenz PC, Rajagopalan R. Principles of Colloid and Surface Chemistry, 3rd ed.; Marcel Dekker: New York, NY, USA, 1997; 3: 1-650.

Hill C, Guarner F, Reid G, Gibson GR, Merenstein DJ, Pot B, Morelli L, Canani RB, Flint HJ, Salminen S, Calder PC, Sanders ME. Expert consensus document: the international scientific association for probiotics and probiotics consensus statement on the scope and appropriate use of the term probiotic. *Nat. Rev. Gastroenterol. Hepatol.* 2014; 11: 506-514.

Hong G, Robinson JT, Zhang Y, Diao S, Antaris AL, Wang Q, Dai H. *In vivo* fluorescence imaging with AG2S quantum dots in the second near-infrared region. *Angew. Chem. Int. Ed. Eng.* 2012; 51: 9818-9821.

Hsu CA, Yu RC, Chou CC. Production of β-galactosidase by bifidobacteria as influenced by various culture conditions. *Int. J. Food Microbiol.* 2005; 104: 197-206.

Huang SY, Zou X. Advances and challenges in protein ligand docking. *Int. J. Mol. Sci.* 2010; 11: 3016-3034.

Huang Y, Ferhan AR, Gao Y, Dandapat A, Kim DH. High-yield synthesis of triangular gold nanoplates with improved shape uniformity, tunable edge length and thickness. *Nanoscale* 2014; 6: 6496-6500.

Hwang CC, Lee YC, Huang YR, Lin CM, Shiau CY, Hwang DF, Tsai YH. Biogenic amines content, histamine-forming bacteria and adulteration of bonito in tuna candy products. *Food Control* 2010; 21: 845-850.

Iqbal A, Ali SA, Abbasi A, Volter W, Rasool SA. Production and some properties of Bac201: a bacteriocin like inhibitory substance from *Staphylococcus aureus* AB201. *J. Basic Microbiol.* 2001; 41: 25-36.

Iravani S, Korbekandi H, Mirmohammadi SV, Zolfaghari B. Synthesis of silver nanoparticles: chemical, physical and biological methods. *Res. Pharm. Sci.* 2014; 9: 385-406.

Iravani S. Bacteria in nanoparticle synthesis: Current status and future prospects. *Int. Sch. Res. Not.* 2014; 2014. doi.org/10.1155/2014/359316.

Irlinger F. Safety assessment of dairy microorganisms: Coagulase-negative staphylococci. *Int. J. Food Microbiol.* 2008; 126: 302-310.

Ismail INA, Noor HM, Muhamad HS, Radzi SM, Kader AJA, Rehan MM, Mohamad R. Bioactive protein produced by *Lactobacillus plantarum* ATCC 8014 in the presence of *Allium sativum*. *Int. J. Med. Sci. Health Care* 2013; 1: 1-8.

Jeong D, Lee B, Her J, Lee K, Lee J. Safety and technological characterization of coagulase-negative staphylococci isolates from traditional Korean fermented soybean foods for starter development. *Int. J. Food Microbiol.* 2016; 236: 9-16.

Jha AK, Prasad K, Prasad K. Biosynthesis of Sb_2O_3 nanoparticles: A low-cost green approach. *BIOT Biotechnol. J.* 2009; 4: 1582-1585.

Jouany JP, Gobert J, Medina B, Bertin G, Julliand V. Effect of live yeast culture supplementation on apparent digestibility and rate of passage in horses fed a high-fiber or high-starch diet. *J. Anim. Sci.* 2008; 86: 339-347.

Juárez Tomás MS, Wiese B, Nader-Macías ME. Effects of culture conditions on the growth and auto-aggregation ability of vaginal *Lactobacillus johnsonii* CRL 1294. *J. Appl. Microbiol.* 2005; 99: 1383-1391.

Julliand V. Impact of nutrition on the gastrointestinal tract in horses. *Appl. Equine Nutr.* 2005; 1: 85-103.

Juretic D, Vukicevic D, Ilic N, Antcheva N, Tossi A. Computational design of high selective antimicrobial peptides. *J. Chem. Inf. Model.* 2009; 49: 2873-2882.

Kanmani P, Kumar RS, Yuvaraj N, Paari KA, Pattukumar V, Arul V. Probiotics and its functionally valuable products. A review. *Crit. Rev. Food Sci. Nutr.* 2013; 53: 641-658.

Kao T, Chen B. Functional components in soybean cake and their effects on antioxidant activity. *J. Agric. Food Chem.* 2006; 54: 7544-7555.

Kashket ER. Bioenergetics of lactic acid bacteria: cytoplasmic pH and osmotolerance. *FEMS Microbiol. Rev.* 1987; 46: 233-244.

Kaur S, Kaur S. Bacteriocins as potential anticancer agents. *Front. Pharmacol.* 2015; 6: 272. doi.org/10.3389/fphar.2015.00272.

Kavir-Kishor PB, Sangam S, Amrutha RN, Sri-Laxmi P, Naidu KA, Rao S, Reddy KJ, Sreenivasulu N. Regulation of proline biosynthesis degradation, uptake and transport in higher plants: Its implication in plant growth and abiotic stress tolerance. *Curr. Sci.* 2005; 88: 424-438.

Khalek FJ, Gallicano GI, Mishra L. Colon cancer stem cells. *Gastrointest. Cancer Res.* 2010; 1: S16–S23.

Kheadr E, Dabour N, Le Lay C, Lacroix C, Fliss I. Antibiotic susceptibility profile of bifidobacteria as affected by oxgall, acid, and hydrogen peroxide stress. *Antimicrob. Agents Chemother.* 2007; 51: 169-174.

Khusro A, Aarti C. Molecular identification of newly isolated *Bacillus* strains from poultry farm and optimization of process parameters for enhanced production of extracellular amylase using OFAT method. *Res. J. Microbiol.* 2015; 10: 393-420.

Khusro A, Preetam Raj JP, Panicker SG. Adaptational changes in cellular morphology of *Bacillus subtilis* strain KPA in response to certain antimicrobials. *Int. J. Chem. Tech. Res.* 2014a; 6: 2815-2823.

Khusro A, Preetam Raj JP, Panicker SG. Multiple heavy metals response and antibiotic sensitivity pattern of *Bacillus subtilis* strain KPA. *J. Chem. Pharm. Res.* 2014b; 6: 532-538.

Khusro A, Sankari D. Synthesis and estimation of total protein in *Bacillus subtilis* strain KPA under mild stress condition of certain antimicrobials. *Asian J. Pharm. Clin. Res.* 2015; 8: 86-90.

Khusro A, Barathikannan K, Aarti C, Agastian P. Optimization of thermo-alkali stable amylase production and biomass yield from *Bacillus* sp. under submerged cultivation. *Ferment.* 2017; 3: 7. doi.org/10.3390/fermentation3010007.

Kim JY, Woo HJ, Kim KH, Kim ER, Jung HK. Antitumor activity of *Lactobacillus plantarum* cytoplasm on teratocarcinoma-bearing mice. *J. Microbiol. Biotechnol.* 2002; 12: 998-1001.

Kim P, Sohng JK, Sung C, Joo HS, Kim EM, Yamaguchi T, Park D, Kim BG. Characterization and structure identification of an antimicrobial peptide, hominicin, produced by *Staphylococcus hominis* MBBL 2-9 *Biochem. Biophys. Res. Commun.* 2010; 399: 133-138.

Kim PI, Jung MY, Chang YH, Kim S, Kim SJ, Park YH. Probiotic properties of *Lactobacillus* and *Bifidobacterium* strains isolated from porcine gastrointestinal tract. *Appl. Microbiol. Biotechnol.* 2007; 74: 1103-1111.

Kim Y, Lee D, Kim D, Cho J, Yang J, Chung M, Kim K, Ha N. Inhibition of proliferation in colon cancer cell lines and harmful enzyme activity of colon bacteria by *Bifidobacterium adolescentis* SPM0212. *Arch. Pharm. Res.* 2008; 31: 468-473.

Kim Y, Oh S, Yun HS, Oh S, Kim SH. Cell-bound exopolysaccharide from probiotic bacteria induces autophagic cell death of tumour cells. *Lett. Appl. Microbiol.* 2010; 51: 123-130.

Knecht H Neulinger SC Heinsen FA, Knecht C, Schilhabel A, Schmitz RA, Zimmermann A, dos Santos VM, Ferrer M, Rosenstiel PC, Schreiber S, Friedrichs AK, Ott SJ. Effects of beta-lactam antibiotics and fluoroquinolones on human gut microbiota in relation to *Clostridium difficile* associated diarrhea. *PLoS One* 2014; 9: e89417. doi.org/10.1371/journal.pone.0089417.

Kohout C, Santi C, Polito L. Anisotropic gold nanoparticles in biomedical applications. *Int. J. Mol. Sci.* 2018; 19: 3385. doi.org/10.3390/ijms19113385.

Konishi Y, Tsukiyama T, Tachimi T, Saitoh N, Nomura T, Nagamine S. Microbial deposition of gold nanoparticles by themetal-reducing bacterium *Shewanella algae*. *Electrochem. Acta*. 2007; 53: 186-192.

Korbekandi H, Iravani S, Abbasi S. Optimization of biological synthesis of silver nanoparticles using *Lactobacillus casei* subsp. *casei*. *J. Chem. Technol. Biotechnol.* 2012; 87: 932-937.

Kotzamanidis C, Kourelis A, Litopoulou-Tzanetaki E, Tzanetakis N, Yiangou M. Evaluation of adhesion capacity, cell surface traits and immunomodulatory activity of presumptive probiotic *Lactobacillus* strains. *Int. J. Food Microbiol.* 2010; 140: 154-163.

Krehbiel CR, Rust SR, Zhang G, Gilliland SE. Bacteria direct-fed microbials in ruminant diets: performance response and mode of action. *J. Anim. Sci.* 2003; 81: 120-132.

Kubo Y, Rooney AP, Tsukakoshi Y, Nakagawa R, Hasegawa H, Kimura K. Phylogenetic analysis of *Bacillus subtilis* strains applicable to natto (fermented soybean) production. *Appl. Environ. Microbiol.* 2011; 77: 6463-6469.

Kumar H, Rangrez A, Dayananda K, Atre A, Patole M, Shouche Y. *Lactobacillus plantarum* (VR1) isolated from an Ayurvedic medicine (Kutajarista) ameliorates *in vitro* cellular damage caused by *Aeromonas veronii*. *BMC Microbiol.* 2011; 11: 152. doi.org/10.1186/1471-2180-11-152.

Kumar KM, Mandal BK, Sinha M, Krishnakumar V. *Terminalia chebula* mediated green and rapid synthesis of gold nanoparticles. *Spectrochimica. Acta A: Mol. Biomol. Spectros.* 2012; 86: 490-494.

Kumar RS, Varman DR, Kanmani P, Yuvaraj N, Paari KA, Pattukumar V, Arul V. Isolation, characterization and identification of a potential probiont from South Indian fermented foods (kallappam, koozh and mor kuzhambu) and its use as biopreservative. *Probiotics Antimicrob. Proteins* 2010; 2: 145-151.

Kurekci C. Prevalence, antimicrobial resistance, and resistant traits of coagulase negative staphylococci isolated from cheese samples in Turkey. *J. Dairy Sci.* 2015; 99: 2675-2679.

Kusumaningtyas E, Widiastuti R, Kusumaningrum HD, Suhartono MT. Sequence analysis and modeling of antimicrobial peptide from goat milk protein hydrolyzed by bromelain. *Proc. Intsem. LPVT* 2016; 327-335. doi.org/10.14334.

Kwan CK, Ernst JD. HIV and tuberculosis: a deadly human syndemic. *Clin. Microbiol. Rev.* 2011; 24: 351-376.

Laghi L, Zhu C, Campagna G, Rossi G, Bazzano M, Laus F. Probiotic supplementation in trained trotter horses: effect on blood clinical pathology data and urine metabolomic assessed in field. *J. Appl. Physiol.* 2018; 125: 654-660.

Landeta G, Curiel JA, Carrascosa AV, Muñoz R, De las Rivas B. Characterization of coagulase-negative staphylococci isolated from Spanish dry cured meat products. *Meat Sci.* 2013; 93: 387-396.

Laskowski RA, MacArthur MW, Moss DS, Thornton JM. PROCHECK - a program to check the stereochemical quality of protein structures. *J. App. Cryst.* 1993; 26: 283-291.

Lee J, Hwang K, Chung M, Cho D, Park C. Resistance of *Lactobacillus casei* KCTC 3260 to reactive oxygen species (ROS): role for a metal ion chelating effect. *J. Food Sci.* 2005; 70: 388-391.

Lee JW, Shin JG, Kim EH, Kang HE, Yim IB, Kim JY, Joo HG, Woo HJ. Immunomodulatory and antitumor effects *in vivo* by the cytoplasmic fraction of *Lactobacillus casei* and *Bifidobacterium longum*. *J. Vet. Sci.* 2004; 5: 41-48.

Lee NK, Han KJ, Son SH, Eom SJ, Lee SK, Paik HD. Multifunctional effect of probiotic *Lactococcus lactis* KC24 isolated from kimchi. *LWT-Food Sci. Technol.* 2015; 64, 1036-1041.

Lee NK, Kim SY, Han KJ, Eom SJ, Paik HD. Probiotic potential of *Lactobacillus* strains with anti-allergic effects from kimchi for yogurt starters. *LWT-Food Sci. Technol*. 2014; 58: 130-134.

Liang X, Zhang L, Natarajan SK, Becker DF. Proline mechanisms of stress survival. *Antioxid. Redox Sig.* 2013; 19: 998-1011.

Lima MDSF, Souza KMS, Albuquerque WWC, Teixeira JAC, Cavalcanti MTH, Porto ALF. *Saccharomyces cerevisiae* from Brazilian kefir-fermented milk: an *in vitro* evaluation of probiotic properties. *Microb. Pathog.* 2017; 110: 670-677.

London N, Raveh B, Schueler-Furman O. Peptide docking and structure-based characterization of peptide binding: from knowledge to know-how. *Curr. Opin. Struct. Biol.* 2013; 23, 894-902.

Luthy R, Bowie JU, Eisenberg D. Assessment of protein models with three-dimensional profiles. *Nature* 1992; 356: 83-85.

Lv XC, Huang XL, Zhang W, Rao PF, Ni L. Yeast diversity of traditional alcohol fermentation starters for Hong Qug lutinous rice wine brewing, revealed by culture dependent and culture-independent methods. *Food Control* 2013; 34: 183-190.

Ma EL, Choi YJ, Choi J, Pothoulakis C, Rhee SH, Im E. The anticancer effect of probiotic *Bacillus polyfermenticus* on human colon cancer cells is mediated through ErbB2 and ErbB3 inhibition. *Int. J. Cancer* 2010; 127: 780-790.

Macindoe G, Mavridis L, Venkatraman V, Devignes MD, Ritchie DW. HexServer: An FFT-based protein docking server powered by graphics processors. *Nucleic Acids Res.* 2010; 38: W445-W449.

Malothu N, Jaswanth S. Bhandaru, Kulandaivelu U, Jojula M, Adidala RR, Umadevi KR, Dusthackeer AVN, Kaki VR, Akkinepally RR. Synthesis, *in vitro* antimycobacterial evaluation and docking studies of some new 5,6,7,8-tetrahydropyrido[4',3':4,5]thieno[2,3-*d*] pyrimidin-4(3*H*)-one schiff bases. *Bioorg. Med. Chem. Lett.* 2016; 26: 836-840.

Manisseri C, Gudipati M. Prebiotic activity of purified xylobiose obtained from Ragi (*Eleusine coracana*, Indaf-15) Bran. *Indian J. Microbiol.* 2012; 52: 251-257.

Manovina M, Thamaraiselvi B, Gousika T. Isolation and *in vitro* characterization of *Lactobacillus* sp, from traditionally fermented black rice (karupu kavuni arisi) and brown rice (kai kuthal arisi). *Int. J. Innov. Sci. Res. Technol.* 2019; 4: 16-19.

Manzoor A, Ul-Haq I, Baig S, Qazi JI, Seratlic S. Efficacy of locally isolated lactic acid bacteria against antibiotic-resistant uropathogens. *Jundishapur J. Microbiol.* 2016; 9: e18952. doi.org/10.5812/jjm.18952.

Mariam SH. Identification and survival studies of *Mycobacterium tuberculosis* within laboratory-fermented bovine milk. *BMC Res. Notes* 2014; 26: 175. doi.org/10.1186/1756-0500-7-175.

Markus J, Mathiyalagan R, Kim YJ, Abbai R, Singh P, Ahn S, Perez ZEJ, Hurh J, Yang DC. Intracellular synthesis of gold nanoparticles with antioxidant activity by probiotic *Lactobacillus kimchicus* DCY51T isolated from Korean kimchi. *Enzyme Microb. Technol.* 2016; 95: 85-93.

Martín B, Garriga M, Hugas M, Bover-Cid S, Veciana-Noqués MT, Aymerich T. Molecular, technological and safety characterization of gram-positive catalase-positive cocci from slightly fermented sausages. *Int. J. Food Microbiol.* 2006; 107: 148-158.

Marty E, Bodenmann C, Buchs J, Hadorn R, Eugster-Meier E, Lacroix C, Meile L. Prevalence of antibiotic resistance in coagulase-negative staphylococci from spontaneously fermented meat products and safety assessment for new starters. *Int. J. Food Microbiol.* 2012; 159: 74-83.

Matikevičienė V, Grigiškis S, Lubytė E, Dienys G. Partial purification and characterization of bacteriocin-like peptide produced by *Staphylococcus xylosus. Environ. Technol. Resour.* 2017; 3:213-216.

Mauriello G, Casaburi A, Blaiotta G, Villani F. Isolation and technological properties of coagulase negative staphylococci from fermented sausages of Southern Italy. *Meat Sci.* 2004; 67: 149-158.

Meile L, Leisinger T. Purification and properties of the bifunctional ptoline dehydrogenase/1-pyrroline-5-carboxylate dehydrogenase from *Pseudomonas aeruginosa. Eur. J. Biochem.*1982; 129: 67-75.

Menakha M, Sangeetha M, Mani P, Al-Aboody MS, Vijayakumar R. *In silico* prediction of drug molecule from *Ipomoea sepiaria* against Type 2 diabetes. *Prog. Med. Sci.* 2018; 3: 9-14.

Menzel R, Roth J. Purification of the 4. *putA* gene product. *J. Biol. Chem.* 1981; 256: 9755-9761.

Millstone JE, Hurst SJ, Métraux GS, Cutler JI, Mirkin CA. Colloidal gold and silver triangular nanoprisms. *Small* 2009; 5: 646-664.

Miremadi F, Ayyash M, Sherkat F, Stojanovska L. Cholesterol reduction mechanisms and fatty acid composition of cellular membranes of probiotic *Lactobacilli* and *Bifidobacteria*. *J. Funct. Foods* 2014; 9: 295-305.

Mishra V, Prasad D. Application of *in vitro* methods for selection of *Lactobacillus casei* strains as potential probiotics. *Int. J. Food Microbiol.* 2005; 103: 109-115.

Miyazaki Y, Kamiya S, Hanawa T, Fukuda M, Kawakami H, Takahashi H, Yokota H. Effect of probiotic bacterial strains of *Lactobacillus, Bifidobacterium*, and *Enterococcus* on enteroaggregative *Escherichia coli*. *J. Infect. Chemother.* 2010; 16: 10-18.

Monteagudo-Mera A, Rodríguez-Aparicio L, Rúa J, Martínez-Blanco H, Navasa N, García-Armesto MR, Ferrero MA. *In vitro* evaluation of physiological probiotic properties of different lactic acid bacteria strains of dairy and human origin. *J. Funct. Foods* 2012; 4: 531-541.

Montville TJ, Chung HJ, Chikindas ML, Chen Y. Nisin A depletes intracellular ATP and acts in bactericidal manner against *Mycobacterium smegmatis*. *Lett. Appl. Microbiol.* 1999; 28: 189-193.

Moortvedt-Abildgaard CI, Nissen-Meyer J, Jelle B, Grenov B, Skaugen M, Nes IF, Production and pH-dependent bactericidal activity of lactocin S, a lantibiotic from *Lactobacillus sake* L45. *Appl. Environ. Microbiol.* 1995; 61: 175-179.

Mora D, Musacchio F, Fortina MG, Senini L, Manachini PL. Autolytic activity and pediocin induced lysis in *Pediococcus acidilactici* and *Pediococcus pentosaceus* strains. *J. Appl. Microbiol.* 2003; 94: 561-570.

Mosmann T. Rapid colorimetric assay for cellular grow and survival: Application to proliferation and cytotoxicity assays. *J. Immunol. Methods* 1983; 65: 55-63.

Mossallam SF, Amer EI, Dia RG. Potentiated anti-microsporidial activity of *Lactobacillus acidophilus* CH1 bacteriocin using gold nanoparticles. *Exp. Parasitol.* 2014; 144: 14-21.

Mota-Meira M, LaPointe G, Lacroix C, Lavoie MC. MICs of mutacin B-Ny266, nisin A, vancomycin, and oxacillin against bacterial pathogens. *Antimicrob. Agents Chemother.* 2000; 44: 24-29.

Nair B, Pradeep T. Coalescence of nanoclusters and formation of submicron crystallites assisted by *Lactobacillus* strains. *Cryst. Growth Des.* 2002; 2: 293-298.

Nami Y, Abdullah N, Haghshenas B, Radiah D, Rosli R, Khosroushahi AY. Probiotic potential and biotherapeutic effects of newly isolated vaginal *Lactobacillus acidophilus* 36YL strain on cancer cells. *Anaerobe* 2014; 28: 29-36.

Nascimento JS, Fagundes PC, de Paiva Brito MAV, dos Santos KRN, de Freire Bastos MC. Production of bacteriocins by coagulase-negative staphylococci involved in bovine mastitis. *Vet. Microbiol.* 2005; 106: 61-71.

Navartana MA, Sahl HG, Tagg JR. Two component anti- *Staphylococcus aureus* lantibiotic activity produced by *Staphylococcus aureus* C55. *Appl. Environ. Microbiol.* 1998; 64: 4803-4808.

Nazari AG, Mozafari M. Simulation of structural features on mechanochemical synthesis of Al_2O_3-TiB_2 nanocomposite by optimized artificial neural network. *Adv. Polym. Tech.* 2012; 23: 220-227.

Nishito Y, Osana Y, Hachiya T, Popendorf K, Toyoda A, Fujiyama A, Itaya M, Sakakibara Y. Whole genome assembly of a *natto* production strain *Bacillus subtilis natto* from very short read data. *BMC Genomics* 2010; 11: 243-255.

Noriega L, Cuevas I, Margolles A, de los Reyes-Gavilan CG. Deconjugation and bile salts hydrolase activity by *Bifidobacterium* strains with acquired resistance to bile. *Int. Dairy J.* 2006; 16: 850-855.

Ntushelo K, Harrison NA, Elliott ML. Comparison of the ribosomal RNA operon from Texas Phoenix decline and lethal yellowing phytoplasmas. *Eur. J. Plant Pathol.* 2012; 33: 779-782.

Oguntoyinbo FA, Sanni AI, Franz SMAP, Holzapfel WH. *In vitro* fermentation studies for selection and evaluation of *Bacillus* strains as starter cultures for the production of okpehe, a traditional African fermented condiment. *Int. J. Food Microbiol.* 2007; 113: 208-218.

Oh JH, Lee JS. One-pot photochemical synthesis of gold nanoplates using nonionic diblock copolymers and their surface functionalization. *Bull. Korean Chem. Soc.* 2018; 39: 1165-1170.

Orlando A, Messa C, Linsalata M, Cavallini A, Russo F. Effects of *Lactobacillus rhamnosus* GG on proliferation and polyamine metabolism in HGC-27 human gastric and DLD-1 colonic cancer cell lines. *Immunopharmacol. Immunotoxicol.* 2009; 31: 108-116.

Orlando A, Refolo MG, Messa C, Amati L, Lavermicocca P, Guerra V, Russo F. Antiproliferative and proapoptotic effects of viable or heat-killed *Lactobacillus paracasei* IMPC2.1 and *Lactobacillus rhamnosus* GG in HGC-27 gastric and DLD-1 colon cell lines. *Nutr. Cancer* 2012; 64: 1103-1111.

Ørskov ER, McDonald L. The estimation of protein degradability in the rumen from incubation measurements weighted according to the rate of passage. *J. Agr. Sci. Camb.* 1979; 92: 499-503.

Owusu-Kwarteng J, Tano-Debrah K, Akabanda F, Jespersen L. Technological properties and probiotic potential of *Lactobacillus fermentum* strains isolated from West African fermented millet Dough. *BMC Microbiol.* 2015; 15: 261. doi.org/10.1186/s12866-015-0602-6.

Pal I, Brahmkhatri VP, Bera S, Bhattacharyya D, Quirishi Y, Bhunia A, Atreya HS. Enhanced stability and activity of an antimicrobial peptide in conjugation with silver nanoparticle. *J. Colloid Interf. Sci.* 2016; 483: 385-393.

Palaniswamy SK, Govindaswamy V. *In-vitro* probiotic characteristics assessment of feruloyl esterase and glutamate decarboxylase producing *Lactobacillus* spp. isolated from traditional fermented millet porridge (kambu koozh). *LWT-Food Sci. Technol.* 2016; 68: 208-216.

Paradeshi JS, Patil SN, Koli SK, Chaudhari BL. Effect of copper on probiotic properties of *Lactobacillus helveticus* CD6. *Int. J. Dairy Technol.* 2017; 70. doi.org/10.1111/1471-0307.12384.

Parente E, Ricciardi A, Addario G. Influence of pH on growth and bacteriocin production by *Lactococcus lactis* subsp. *lactis* 140NWC during batch fermentation. *Appl. Microbiol. Biotechnol.* 1994; 41: 388-394.

Parkouda C, Nielsen DS, Azokpota P, Ouoba LII, Amoa-Awua WK, Thorsen L, Houhouigan JD, Jensen JS, Tano-Debrah K, Diawara B, Jakobsen M. The microbiology of alkaline-fermentation of indigenous seeds used as food condiments in Africa and Asia. *Crit. Rev. Microbiol.* 2009; 35: 139-156.

Parvez S, Malik KA, Ah Kang S, Kim HY. Probiotics and their fermented food products are beneficial for health. *J. Appl. Microbiol.* 2006; 100: 1171-1185.

Passarini I, Rossiter S, Malkinson J, Zloh M. *In silico* structural evaluation of short cationic antimicrobial peptides. *Pharmaceutics* 2018; 10: 72. doi.org/10.3390/pharmaceutics10030072.

Patel AK, Ahire JJ, Pawar SP, Chaudhari BL, Chincholkar SB. Comparative accounts of probiotic characteristics of *Bacillus* spp. isolated from food wastes. *Food Res. Int.* 2009; 42: 505-510.

Patel K, Kapoor S, Dave DP, Mukherjee T. Synthesis of nanosized silver colloids by microwave dielectric heating. *J. Chem. Sci.* 2015; 117: 53-60.

Patel S, Majumder A, Goyal A. Potentials of exopolysaccharides from lactic acid bacteria. *Indian J. Microbiol.* 2012; 52: 3-12.

Pei J, Li X, Han H, Tao Y. Purification and characterization of plantaricin SLG1, a novel bacteriocin produced by *Lb. plantarum* isolated from yak cheese. *Food Control* 2018; 84: 111-117.

Piraino P, Zotta T, Ricciardi A, McSweeney PLH, Parente E. Acid production, proteolysis, autolytic and inhibitory properties of lactic acid bacteria isolated from pasta filata cheeses: a multivariate screening study. *Int. Dairy J.* 2008; 18: 81-92.

Pisano MB, Viale S, Conti S, Fadda ME, Deplano M, Melis MP, Cosentino S. Preliminary evaluation of probiotic properties of *Lactobacillus* strains isolated from Sardinian dairy products. *Biomed. Res. Int.* 2014; 286390. doi.org/10.1155/2014/286390.

Porel S, Singh S, Radhakrishnan TP. Polygonal gold nanoplates in a polymer matrix. *Chem. Commun.* 2005; 18: 2387-2389.

Potter GD, Arnold FF, Householder DD, Hansen DH, Brown KM. Digestion of starch in the small or large intestine of the equine. *Proc. Europ€aische Konferenz über die Ern€ahrung des Pferdes.* 1992; 107-111.

Prasad K, Jha A, Kulkarni A. *Lactobacillus* assisted synthesis of titanium nanoparticles. *Nanoscale Res. Lett.* 2007; 2: 248-250.

Preetam Raj JP, Purushothaman M, Khusro A, Panicker SG. *In vitro* anticancer and antioxidant activity of gold nanoparticles conjugate with *Tabernaemontana divaricata* flower SMs against MCF -7 Breast cancer cells. *Korean Chem. Eng. Res.* 2016; 54: 75-80.

Ragul K, Kandasamy S, Devi PB, Shetty PH. Safety and stability assessment of potential probiotic strains from fermented mango brine pickle. *Probiotics Antimicrob. Proteins* 2019. doi.org/10.1007/s12602-019-09617-7.

Rajoka MSR, Mehwish HM, Fanga H, Padhiard AA, Zeng X, Khurshid M, He Z, Zhao L. Characterization and anti-tumor activity of exopolysaccharide produced by *Lactobacillus kefiri* isolated from Chinese kefir grains. *J. Funct. Foods* 2019; 63: 103588. doi.org/10.1016/j.jff.2019.103588.

Ramos CL, Thorsen L, Schwan RF, Jespersen L. Strain-specific probiotics properties of *Lactobacillus fermentum, Lactobacillus plantarum* and *Lactobacillus brevis* isolates from Brazilian food products. *Food Microbiol.* 2013; 36: 22-29.

Reith F, Etschmann B, Grosse C. Mechanisms of gold biomineralization in the bacterium *Cupriavidus metallidurans*. *Proc. Natl. Acad. Sci. U. S. A*. 2009; 106: 17757-17762.

Reniero R, Cocconcelli PS, Bottazzi V, Morelli L. High frequency conjugation in *Lactobacillus* mediated by an aggregation promoting factor. *J. Gen. Microbiol.* 1991; 138: 763-768.

Rijnaarts HHM, Norde W, Bouwer EJ, Lyklema J, Zehnder AJB. Bacterial adhesion under static and dynamic conditions. *Appl. Microbiol.* 1993; 59: 3255-3265.

Ritz M., Tholozan JL, Federighi M, Pilet MF. Morphological and physiological characterization of *Listeria monocytogenes* subjected to high hydrostatic pressure. *Appl. Environ. Microbiol.* 2001; 67: 2240-2247.

Rivera J, Vannakambadi G, Höök M, Speziale P. Fibrinogen-binding proteins of gram-positive bacteria. *Thromb. Haemost.* 2007; 98: 503-511.

Roane TM, Pepper IL. Microbial responses to environmentally toxic cadmium. *Microb. Ecol.* 1999; 38: 358-364.

Rodriguez Plaza JG, Rivas-Santiago B, Hernandez-Pando R, Rio GD. Prospective tuberculosis treatment: peptides, immunity and autophagy. *J. Mol. Genet. Med.* 2014; 8: 128. doi.org/10.4172/1747-0862.1000128.

Roessler A, Forssten SD, Glei M, Ouwehand AC, Jahreis G. The effect of probiotics on faecal microbiota and genotoxic activity of faecal water in patients with atopic dermatitis: a randomized, placebo-controlled study. *Clin. Nutr.* 2012; 31: 22-29.

Rosano GL, Ceccarelli EA. Rare codon content affects the solubility of recombinant proteins in a codon bias-adjusted *Escherichia coli* strain. *Microb. Cell Fact.* 2009; 8: 41. doi.org/10.1186/1475-2859-8-41.

Rostamizadeh M, Rizi SMH. Predicting gas flux in silicalite-1 zeolite membrane using artificial neural networks. *J. Membrane Sci*. 2012; 403-404: 146-151.

Rowe JB, Lees MJ, Pethick DW. Prevention of acidosis and laminitis associated with grain feeding in horses. *J. Nutr.* 1994; 124: 2742-2744.

Roy RK. Design of experiments using the Taguchi approach: 16 steps to product and process improvement. John Wiley & Sons, New York, 2001; 560.

Russo F, Orlando A, Linsalata M, Cavallini A, Messa C. Effects of *Lactobacillus rhamnosus* GG on the cell growth and polyamine metabolism in HGC-27 human gastric cancer cells. *Nutr. Cancer* 2007; 59: 106-114.

Saad N, Delattre C, Urdaci M, Schmitter JM, Bressollier P. An overview of the last advances in probiotic and probiotic field. *LWT-Food Sci. Technol.* 2013; 50: 1-16.

Sadrzadeh M, Mohammadi T, Ivakpour J, Kasiri N. Separation of lead ions from wastewater using electrodialysis: Comparing mathematical and neural network modeling. *Chem. Eng. J.* 2008; 144: 431-441.

Saeed S, Ahmad S, Rasool SA. Antimicrobial spectrum, production and mode of action of staphylococcin 188 produced by *Staphylococcus aureus* 188. *Pak. J. Pharm. Sci.* 2004; 17: 1-8.

Samandari-Gikloo T, Mehrabi AA, Jahanbakhsh S, Fazeli A, Tahmasebi Z. Investigation of physiological and biochemical responses and essential oil yield of peppermint under salt stress. *Biosci. Biotechnol. Res. Asia* 2018; 15: 407-418.

Sankari D, Khusro A. Biochemical, molecular characterization and sequence analysis of keratinase producing novel strain of *Bacillus licheniformis* isolated from poultry farm. *Int. J. Pharm. Pharm. Sci.* 2014; 6: 457-461.

Sanni A, Morlon-Guyot J, Guyot J. New efficient amylase-producing strains of *Lactobacillus plantarum* and *L. fermentum* isolated from different Nigerian traditional fermented foods. *Int. J. Food Microbiol.* 2002; 72: 53-62.

Saravanan C, Kavitake D, Kandasamy S, Devi PB, Shetty PH. Production, partial characterization and antioxidant properties of exopolysaccharide a-D-glucan produced by *Leuconostoc lactis* KC117496 isolated from an idli batter. *J. Food Sci. Technol.* 2018; 56: 159-166.

Sarkar P, Lohith Kumar DH, Dhumal C, Panigrahi SS, Choudhary R. Traditional and ayurvedic foods of Indian origin. *J. Ethn. Foods* 2015; 2: 97-109.

SAS. User's guide: statistics. Cary, NC: SAS Institute. 2002; 9.

Sathyabama S, Vijayabharath R, Bruntha Devi P, Ranjith Kumar M, Priyadarisini VB. Screening for probiotic properties of strains isolated from feces of various human groups. *J. Microbiol.* 2012; 50: 603-612.

Sau TK, Rogach AL. Nonspherical noble metal nanoparticles: colloid-chemical synthesis and morphology control. *Adv. Mater.* 2010; 22: 1781-1804.

Sawatari Y, Yokota A. Diversity and mechanisms of alkali tolerance in lactobacilli. *Appl. Environ. Microbiol*. 2007; 73: 3909-3915.

Schmitt EK, Riwanto M, Sambandamurthy V, Roggo S, Miault C, Zwingelstein C, Krastel P, Noble C, Beer D, Rao SPS, Au M, Niyomrattanakit P, Lim V, Zheng J, Jeffery D, Pethe K, Camacho LR. The natural product cyclomarin kills *Mycobacterium tuberculosis* by targeting the ClpC1 subunit of the caseinolytic protease. *Angew. Chem. Int. Ed. Engl.* 2011; 50: 5889-5891.

Sebald W, Friedl P, Schairer HU, Hoppe J. Structure and genetics of the H-conducting F_0 portion of the ATP synthase. *Ann. N. Y. Acad. Sci.* 1982; 402: 28-44.

Servin AL. Antagonist activities of lactobacilli and bifidobacteria against microbial pathogens. *FEMS Microbiol. Rev*. 2004; 28: 405-440.

Shabanzadeh P, Yusof R, Shameli K. Artificial neural network for modeling the size of silver nanoparticles' prepared in montmorillonite/starch bionanocomposites. *J. Ind. Eng. Chem*. 2015; 24: 42-50.

Shah M, Badwaik V, Kherde Y, Waghwani HK, Modi T, Aguilar ZP, Rodgers H, Hamilton W, Marutharaj T, Webb C, Lawrenz MB, Dakshinamurthy R. Gold nanoparticles: Various methods of synthesis and antibacterial applications. *Front. Biosci.* 2014; 19: 1320-1344.

Shahbaz-Mohammadi H, Omidinia E. Screening and characterization of proline dehydrogenase flavoenzyme producing *Pseudomonas entomophila. Iran. J. Microbiol.* 2011; 3: 201-209.

Shahbaz-Mohammadi H, Omidinia E. Isolation, purification and characterization of proline dehydrogenase from a *Pseudomonas putida* POS-F84 isolate. *Iran. J. Biotechnol.* 2012; 10: 111-119.

Shehata AN, Abd El, Aty AA. Optimization of process parameters by statistical experimental designs for the production of Naringinase enzyme by marine fungi. *Int. J. Chem. Eng.* 2014; 273523. doi.org//10.1155/2014/273523.

Shehata MG, El Sohaimy SA, El-Sahn MA, Youssef MM. Screening of isolated potential probiotic lactic acid bacteria for cholesterol lowering property and bile salt hydrolase activity. *Ann. Agric. Sci.* 2016; 61: 65-75.

Shepherd ML, Swecker Jr WS, Jensen RV, Ponder MA. Characterization of the fecal bacteria communities of forage-fed horses by pyrosequencing of 16S rRNA V4 gene amplicons. *FEMS Microbiol. Lett.* 2012; 326: 62-68.

Sieladie DV, Zambou NF, Kaktcham PM, Cresci A, Fonteh F. Probiotic properties of lactobacilli strains isolated from raw cow milk in the western highlands of cameroon. *Innov. Rom. Food Biotechnol.* 2011; 9: 12-28.

Simonova M, Strompfova V, Marcinakova M, Laukova A, Vesterlund S, Moratalla ML, Bover-Cid S, Vidal-Carou C. Characterization of *Staphylococcus xylosus* and *Staphylococcus carnosus* isolated from Slovak meat products. *Meat Sci.* 2006; 73: 559-564.

Singh S, Singh DB, Singh A, Gautam B, Ram G, Dwivedi S, Ramteke PW. An approach for identification of novel drug targets in *Streptococcus pyogenes* sf370 through pathway analysis. *Interdiscipl. Sci. Comput. Life Sci.* 2016; 8: 388-394.

Sivakumar PM, Seenivasan PS, Kumar V, Doble M. Synthesis, antimycobacterial activity evaluation, and QSAR studies of chalcone derivatives. *Bioorgan. Med. Chem. Lett.* 2007; 17: 1695-1700.

Sneath PHA. Gram positive rods. In Bergeys Manual of Systematic Bacteriology, Hensyl, W.M., Ed.; Williams and Wilkins: Philadelphia, PA, USA, 1994; 9: 2106-2111.

Sondergaard AK, Stahnke LH. Growth and aroma production by *Staphylococcus xylosus, S. carnosus* and *S. equorum*-a comparative study in model systems. *Int. J. Food Microbiol.* 2002; 75: 99-109.

Sosunov V, Mischenko V, Eruslanov B, Svetoch E, Shakina Y, Stern N, Majorov K, Sorokoumova G, Selishcheva A, Apt A. Antimicobacterial activity of bacteriocins and their complexes with liposomes. *J. Antimicrob. Chemother.* 2007; 59: 919-925.

Stein K, Borowicki A, Scharlau D, Schettler A, Scheu K, Obst U, Glei M. Effects of synbiotic fermentation products on primary chemoprevention in human colon cells. *J. Nutr. Biochem*. 2012; 23: 777-784.

Stevens HC, Nabors L. Microbial food cultures: A regulatory update. *Food Technol.* 2009; 63: 36-41.

Stutz K, Stephan R, Tasara T. SpA, ClfA, and FnbA genetic variations lead to Staphaurex test-negative phenotypes in bovine mastitis *Staphylococcus aureus* isolates. *J. Clin. Microbiol.* 2011; 49: 638-646.

Subramanian N, Jothimanivannan C, Moorthy K. Antimicrobial activity and preliminary phytochemical screening of *Justicia gendarussa* (Burm. F.) against human pathogens. *Asian J. Pharm. Clin. Res.* 2012; 5: 229-233.

Sung C, Kim BG, Kim S, Joo HS, Kim PI. Probiotic potential of *Staphylococcus hominis* MBBL 2-9 as anti-*Staphylococcus aureus* agent isolated from the vaginal microbiota of a healthy woman. *J. Appl. Microbiol.* 2010; 108: 908-916.

Suryawanshi SK, Chouhan U. Computational approaches for the prediction of antimicrobial potential peptides from *Ocimum tenuiflorum. Asian J. Pharm. Clin. Res.* 2018; 11: 398-401.

Suskovic J, Brkic B, Matosic S, Maric V. *Lactobacillus acidophilus* M92 as potential probiotic strain. *Milchwissenschaft* 1997; 52: 430-435.

Swiecilo A, Zych-Wezyk I. Bacterial stress response as an adaptation to life in a soil environment. *Pol. J. Environ. Stud.* 2013; 22: 1577-1587.

Swyers KL, Burk A, Hartsock T, Ungerfeld E, Shelton J. Effects of direct-fed microbial supplementation on digestibility and fermentation end-products in horses fed low-and high-starch concentrates. *J. Anim. Sci.* 2008; 86: 2596-608.

Tamang JP, Shin DH, Jung SJ, Chae S. Functional properties of microorganisms in fermented foods. *Front. Microbiol.* 2016; 7: 578. doi.org/10.3389/fmicb.2016.00578.

Tamang JP, Watanabe K, Holzapfel WH. Review: Diversity of microorganisms in global fermented foods and beverages. *Front. Microbiol.* 2016; 7: 377. doi.org/10.3389/fmicb.2016.00377.

Tamang JP. Diversity of fermented foods, In: Tamang JP, Kailasapathy K. Eds. Fermented Foods and Beverages of the World, CRC Press, Taylor & Francis Group, New York, 2010; 41-84.

Tamang JP. Naturally fermented ethnic soybean foods of India. *J. Ethn. Foods* 2015; 2: 8-17.

Tamura K, Dudley J, Nei M, Kumar S. MEGA4: Molecular Evolutionary Genetics Analysis (MEGA) software version 4.0. *Mol. Biol. Evol.* 2007; 24: 1596-1599.

Thapa N, Tamang JP. Functionality and therapeutic values of fermented foods. In Health Benefits of Fermented Foods, Ed. J.P. Tamang (New York: CRC Press), 2015: 111-168.

Thapliyal A, Khar RK, Chandra A. Artificial neural network modelling of green synthesised silver nanoparticles in bentonite/starch bio-nanocomposite. *Curr. Nanosci.* 2018; 14: 239-251.

Theodorou MK, Williams BA, Dhanoa MS, McAllan AB, France J. A simple gas production method using a pressure transducer to determine the fermentation kinetics of ruminant feeds. *Anim. Feed Sci. Technol.* 1994; 48: 185-197.

Thirumangaimannan G, Gurumurthy K. A study on the fermentation pattern of common millets in Koozh preparation - A traditional South Indian food. *Indian J. Tradit. Know.* 2013; 12: 512-517.

Todorov SD, Dicks LMT. Screening for bacteriocin-producing lactic acid bacteria from boza, a traditional cereal beverage from Bulgaria comparison of the bacteriocins. *Process Biochem.* 2006; 41: 11-19.

Todorov SD, Franco BD, Wild IJ. *In vitro* study of beneficial properties and safety of lactic acid bacteria isolated from Portuguese fermented meat products. *Benef. Microbes* 2014; 5: 351-366.

Torre LA, Bray F, Siegel RL, Ferlay J, Lortet-Tieulent J, Jemal A. Global cancer statistics 2012. *CA: Cancer J. Clin.* 2015; 65: 87-108.

Um MN, Lee, Ho C. Isolation and identification of *Staphylococcus* sp. from Korean fermented fish products. *J. Microbiol. Biotechnol.* 1996; 6: 340-346

Uma Maheshwari S, Amutha S, Anandham R, Hemalatha G, Senthil N, Kwon SW, Sivakumar N. Characterization of potential probiotic bacteria from 'panchamirtham; A Southern Indian ethinic fermented fruit mix. *LWT-Food Sci. Technol.* 2019; 116: 108540.

Uma Maheshwari S, Amutha S, Hemalatha G, Senthil N, Anandham R, Kumutha K. Characterization of probiotic bacteria from fermented fruit mix. *Int. J. Curr. Microbiol. App. Sci.* 2018; 7: 2236-2242.

Upton M, Cotter P, Tagg J. Antimicrobial peptides as therapeutic agent. *Int. J. Microbiol.* 2012; 326503. doi.org/10.1155/2012/326503.

Vallejo LH, Salem AZM, Kholif AE, Elghangour MMY, Fajardo RC, Rivero N, Bastida AZ, Mariezcurrena MD. Influence of cellulase or xylanase on the *in vitro* rumen gas production and fermentation of corn stover. *Indian J. Anim. Sci.* 2016; 86: 70-74.

Veerapagu M, Jeya KR. Evaluation of probiotic characteristics of bacteria isolated from fermented food. *Pharma. Innov. J.* 2017; 6: 322-325.

Vermorel M, Martin Rosset W. Concepts, scientific bases, structure and validation of the French horse net energy system (UFC). *Livest. Prod. Sci.* 1997; 47: 261-275.

Vicky VM, Rodney S, Ajay S, Hardik R. Introduction to metallic nanoparticles. *J. Pharm. Bioallied Sci.* 2010; 2: 282-289.

Vogel RF, Hammes WP, Habermeyer M, Engel KH, Knorr D, Eisenbrand G. Microbial food cultures-Opinion of the Senate Commission on Food Safety (SKLM) of the German Research Foundation (DFG). *Mol. Nutr. Food Res.* 2011; 55: 654-662.

Wang G. Database-guided discovery of potent peptides to combat HIV-1 or superbugs. *Pharmaceuticals* 2013; 6: 728-758.

Wang J, Zhang H, Chen X, Chen Y, Menghebilige BQ. Selection of potential probiotic lactobacilli for cholesterol-lowering properties and their effect on cholesterol metabolism in rats fed a high-lipid diet. *J. Dairy Sci.* 2012; 95: 1645-1654.

Wang K, Li W, Rui X, Chen X, Jiang M, Dong M. Characterization of a novel exopolysaccharide with antitumor activity from *Lactobacillus plantarum* 70810. *Int. J. Biol. Macromol.* 2013; 63: 133-139.

Wang P, Wang X, Wang L, Hou X, Liu W, Chen C. Interaction of gold nanoparticles with proteins and cells. *Sci. Technol. Adv. Mater.* 2015; 16: 1-15.

Wang Y, Zhao T, Wei D, Strandberg E, Ulrich AS, Ulmschneider JP. How reliable are molecular dynamics simulations of membrane active antimicrobial peptides? *Biochem. Biophys. Acta-Biomembr.* 2014; 1838: 2280-2288.

Weber H. Dry sausages manufacture, the importance of protective cultures and their metabolic products. *Fleischwirtschaft.* 1994; 74: 278-282.

Welin A, Raffetseder J, Eklund D, Stendahl O, Lerm M. Importance of phagosomal functionality for growth restriction of *Mycobacterium tuberculosis* in primary human macrophages. *J. Innate Immun.* 2011; 3: 508-518.

Wen L, Lin Z, Gu P, Zhou J, Yao B, Chen G, Fu J. Extracellular biosynthesis of monodispersed gold nanoparticles by a SAM capping route. *J. Nanopart. Res.* 2009; 11: 279-288.

Widerstrom M, Wistrom J, Sjostedt A, Monsen T. Coagulase-negative staphylococci: update on the molecular epidemiology and clinical presentation, with a focus on *Staphylococcus epidermidis* and *Staphylococcus saprophyticus*. *Eur. J. Clin. Microbiol. Infect. Dis.* 2012; 31: 7-20.

Wilaipun P, Zendo T, Okuda K, Nakayama J, Sonomoto K. Identification of the Nukacin KQU-131, a New Type-A(II) lantibiotic produced by *Staphylococcus hominis* KQU-131 isolated from Thai fermented fish product (Plara). *Biosci. Biotechnol. Biochem.* 2008; 72: 2232-2235.

Williams BA, Verstegen MWA, Tamminga S. Fermentation in the large intestine of single-stomached animals and its relationship to animal health. *Nutr. Res. Rev.* 2001; 14: 207-227.

Wladyka B, Piejko M, Bzowska M, Pieta P, Krzysik M, Mazurek L, Guevara-Lora I, Bukowski M, Sabat AJ, Friedrich AW, Bonar E, Międzobrodzki J, Dubin A, Mak P. A peptide factor secreted by *Staphylococcus pseudintermedius* exhibits properties of both bacteriocins and virulence factors. *Sci. Rep.* 2015; 5: 14569. doi.org/10.1038/srep14569.

World Cancer Report 2014. World Health Organization. 2014. Chapter 5.1. ISBN 92-832-0429-8.

World Health Organization. Global tuberculosis report 2012. Geneva, Switzerland: WHO; 2012.

Wu YC, Kimura B, Fujii T. Comparison of three culture methods for the identification of *Micrococcus* and *Staphylococcus* in fermented squid shiokara. *Fish. Sci.* 2000; 66: 142-146.

Xanthopoulos V, Litopoulou-Tzanetaki E, Tzanetakis N. Characterisation of *Lactobacillus* isolates from infant faeces as dietary adjuncts. *Food Microbiol.* 2000; 17: 205-215.

Xavier AS, Lakshmanan M. Delamanid: A new armor in combating drug-resistant tuberculosis. *J. Pharmacol. Pharmacother.* 2014; 5: 222-224.

Xin H, Ji S, Peng J, Han P, An X, ShanWang, Cao B. Isolation and characterisation of a novel antibacterial peptide from a native swine intestinal tract-derived bacterium. *J. Antimicrob. Agents* 2017; 49: 427-436.

Yadav R, Puniya A, Shukla P. Probiotic properties of *Lactobacillus plantarum* RYPR1 from an indigenous fermented beverage Raabadi. *Front. Microbiol.* 2016; 7: 1683. doi.org/10.3389/fmicb.2016.01683.

Yah N, Marlida Y, Arnim, Yuherman. Antimicrobial activity of lactic acid bacteria thermophilic isolated from hot spring rimbo panti of West Sumatera for food preservatives. *Pakistan J. Nutr.* 2014; 13: 465-472.

Yeh YC, Creran B, Rotello VM. Gold nanoparticles: preparation, properties, and applications in bionanotechnology. *Nanoscale* 2012; 4: 1871-1880.

Yi L, Dang Y, Wu J, Zhang L, Liu X, Liu B, Zhou Y, Lu X. Purification and characterization of a novel bacteriocin produced by *Lactobacillus crustorum* MN047 isolated from koumiss from Xinjiang, China. *J. Dairy Sci.* 2016; 99: 7002-7015.

Zago M, Fornasari ME, Carminati D, Burns P, Suàrez V, Vinderola G, Reinheimer J, Giraffa G. Characterization and probiotic potential of *Lactobacillus plantarum* strains isolated from cheeses. *Food Microbiol.* 2011; 28: 1033-1040.

Zahir I, Houari A, Iraqui M, Ibnsouda S. *Aerococcus* sp. with an antimycobacterial effect. *Afr. J. Biotechnol.* 2011; 10: 19473-19480.

Zheng Y, Lu Y, Wang J, Yang L, Pan C, Huang Y. Probiotic properties of *Lactobacillus* strains isolated from Tibetan Kefir grains. *PLoS One* 2013; 8: e69868. doi.org/10.1371/journal.pone.0069868.

Zhu J, Kan C, Li H, Cao Y, Ding X, Wan J. Synthesis and growth mechanism of gold nanoplates with novel shapes. *J. Cryst. Growth* 2011; 321: 124-130.

Zijlstra P, Chon JWM, Gu M. Five-dimensional optical recording mediated by surface plasmons in gold nanorods. *Nature* 2009; 459: 410-413.

Zinzalla G, Thurston DE. Targeting protein–protein interactions for therapeutic intervention: a challenge for the future. *Future Med. Chem.* 2009; 1: 65-93.

Zuker M, Stiegler P. Optimal computer folding of large RNA sequences using thermodynamics and auxiliary information. *Nucleic Acids Res.* 1981; 9: 133-148.

[A]

Media, Reagents, and Buffer preparation

MRS broth medium (g/L):

Proteose peptone – 10.0

Beef extract – 10.0

Yeast extract – 5.0

Dextrose – 20.0

Polysorbate 80 – 1.0

Ammonium citrate – 2.0

Sodium acetate (CH_3COONa) – 5.0

Magnesium sulphate – 0.1

Manganese sulphate ($MnSO_4$) – 0.05

Dipotassium phosphate – 2.0

Distilled water – 1000 mL

pH – 6.5

*MRS agar medium was prepared by adding 18.0 g of Agar agar into 1 L of distilled water.

Tryptone Soya broth medium (g/L):

Pancreatic digest of casein – 17.0

Papaic digest of soyabean meal – 3.0

Sodium chloride – 5.0

Dextrose – 2.5

Dipotassium phosphate – 2.5

Lowenstein-Jensen medium (g/L):

Potato starch – 30.0

L-Asparagine – 3.5

Monopotassium phosphate (KH_2PO_4) – 2.5

Magnesium citrate ($C_6H_6MgO_7$) – 0.5

Malachite green – 0.5

Magnesium sulphate – 0.25

Glycerol – 12 mL

Egg suspension – 1000 mL

Middlebrook 7H9 broth base (g/L):

Ammonium sulphate – 0.5

Disodium phosphate (Na_2HPO_4) – 2.5

Monopotassium phosphate – 1.0

Sodium citrate ($Na_3C_6H_5O_7$) – 0.1

Magnesium sulphate – 0.05

Calcium chloride – 0.0005

Zinc sulphate – 0.001

Copper sulphate – 0.001

Ferric ammonium citrate ($C_6H_8FeNO_7$) – 0.04

L-Glutamic acid – 0.5

Pyridoxine – 0.001

Biotin – 0.0005

Distilled water – 1000 mL

pH – 6.6±0.2

Ringer solution (g/L):

Calcium chloride – 0.2

Sodium chloride – 6.0

Potassium chloride – 2.0

Sodium bicarbonate – 1.2

Distilled water – 1000 mL

Lugol's iodine:

0.33 % (w/v) iodine was powdered with 0.66 % (w/v) potassium iodide (KI). The mixture was dissolved in certain volume of distilled water.

YT-broth medium (g/L):

Casein enzymic hydrolysate – 16.0

Yeast extract – 10.0

Sodium chloride – 5.0

Distilled water – 1000 mL

pH – 7.0±0.2

DNase agar medium (g/L):

Deoxyribonucleic acid – 2.0

Tryptose – 20.0

Sodium chloride – 5.0

Agar – 18.0

Distilled water – 1000 mL

pH – 7.0±0.2

Nutrient gelatin agar plates (g/L):

Peptone – 5.0

Beef extract – 3.0

Gelatine – 120.0

Sodium chloride – 30.0

Agar – 18.0

Distilled water – 1000 mL

pH – 7.0±0.2

Nutrient broth (g/L):

Peptone – 5.0

Beef extract – 3.0

Yeast extract – 2.0

Sodium chloride – 5.0

Distilled water – 1000 mL

pH – 7.0±0.2

Mueller Hinton broth medium (g/L):

Beef extract – 2.0

Casein acid hydrolysate – 18.0

Starch – 1.5

Distilled water – 1000 mL

pH – 7.2±0.2

Luria Bertani broth (g/L):

Tryptone – 10.0

Yeast extract – 5.0

Sodium chloride – 10.0

Distilled water – 1000 mL

pH – 7.0±0.2

Peptone broth (g/L):

Peptone – 5.0

Distilled water – 1000 mL

pH – 7.0±0.2

Mannitol Salt broth medium (g/L):

Proteose peptone – 10.0

Beef extract – 1.0

Sodium chloride – 75.0

D-Mannitol – 10.0

Phenol red – 0.025

Distilled water – 1000 mL

pH – 7.2±0.2

Brain Heart Infusion broth (g/L):

Calf brain, infusion from – 200.0

Beef heart, infusion from – 250.0

Protease peptone – 10.0

Sodium chloride – 2.0

Disodium phosphate – 5.0

Distilled water – 1000 mL

pH – 7.4 ± 0.2

PBS (g/L):

Sodium chloride – 8.0

Potassium chloride – 0.2

Disodium phosphate – 1.44

Monopotassium phosphate – 0.24

Distilled water – 1000 mL

pH – Adjusted accordingly

Sodium citrate buffer (pH 4.5):

24.1 g of sodium citrate dihydrate was added into 800 mL of distilled water. 3.4 g of citric acid ($C_6H_8O_7$) was added into the solution. The volume was made up to 1 L and pH was adjusted.

TE Buffer:

15.7 g of Tris-Cl (desired pH) was added into the distilled water. 2.92 g of EDTA (pH 8) was added into the solution. The volume was made up to 1 L.

TBE buffer:

Tris – 108.0 g

Boric acid (H_3BO_3) – 55.0 g

Disodium EDTA (0.5M, pH 8.0) – 40 mL

Distilled water – 1000 mL

Tris-HCl buffer (100mM, pH 8.3):

60.5 g of Tris-Base was dissolved in 350 mL of distilled water in a beaker. Slowly, 32.5 mL of 12M HCl was added until the pH reaches 8.3. Volume was made up to 500 mL and filter sterilized before use.

Sodium phosphate buffer (0.1M, pH 7.0):

Solution A: 27.6 g NaH_2PO_4. H_2O was added in 1L of distilled water (0.2 M).

Solution B: 53.65 g Na_2HPO_4. $7H_2O$ was added in 1L of distilled water (0.2 M).

39 mL of Solution A was added into 61 mL of Solution B.

Sodium phosphate buffer (1M, pH 7.0):

Solution A: 138.0 g $NaH_2PO_4.H_2O$ was added in 1L of distilled water.

Solution B: 142.0 g Na_2HPO_4 was added in 1L of distilled water.

423 mL of Solution A was added into 577 mL of Solution B.

Potassium phosphate buffer (0.1M, pH 7.0):

Solution A: 27.2 g KH_2PO_4 was added in 1L of distilled water (0.2 M).

Solution B: 34.8 g K_2HPO_4 was added in 1L of distilled water (0.2 M).

39 mL of Solution A was added into 61 mL of Solution B.

Potassium phosphate buffer (0.1M, pH 6.5):

Solution A: 27.2 g KH_2PO_4 was added in 1L of distilled water (0.2 M).

Solution B: 34.8 g K_2HPO_4 was added in 1L of distilled water (0.2 M).

68.5 mL of Solution A was added into 31.5 mL of Solution B.

[B]

Chemicals and Reagents

2,2-diphenyl-1-picrylhydrazyl: DPPH; $C_{18}H_{12}N_5O_6$

4-(2-hydroxyethyl)-1-piperazineethane sulfonic acid: HEPES; $C_8H_{18}N_2O_4S$

Acetic acid: CH_3COOH

Acetonitrile: C_2H_3N

Acrylamide: C_3H_5NO

Ammonium acetate: $NH_4CH_3CO_2$

Ammonium chloride: NH_4Cl

Ammonium citrate: $C_6H_{11}NO_7$

Ammonium nitrate: NH_4NO_3

Ammonium persulphate: APS; $(NH_4)_2S_2O_8$

Ammonium sulphate: $(NH_4)_2SO_4$

Arabinose: $C_5H_{10}O_5$

Boric acid: H_3BO_3

Calcium chloride: $CaCl_2$

Carbon dioxide: CO_2

Chloramphenicol: $C_{11}H_{12}Cl_2N_2O_5$

Chloroform: $CHCl_3$

Cholesterol: $C_{27}H_{46}O$

Citric acid: $C_6H_8O_7$

Coomassie Brilliant Blue: CBB

Copper sulphate: $CuSO_4$

Dextrose: $C_6H_{12}O_6$

Diethylaminoethyl: DEAE; $C_6H_{15}NO$

Dimethyl sulphoxide: DMSO; C_2H_6OS

Dipotassium phosphate: K_2HPO_4

Disodium phosphate: Na_2HPO_4

Doxorubicin: $C_{27}H_{29}NO_{11}$

Ethanol: C_2H_5OH

Ethyl acetate: $C_4H_8O_2$

Ethylenediaminetetraacetic acid: EDTA; $C_{10}H_{16}N_2O_8$

Ferric ammonium citrate: $C_6H_8FeNO_7$

Ferric chloride: $FeCl_3$

Ferrous sulphate: $FeSO_4$

Fructose: $C_6H_{12}O_6$

Gentamicin: $C_{21}H_{43}N_5O_7$

Glucose: $C_6H_{12}O_6$

Glycerol: $C_3H_8O_3$

Hydrochloric acid: HCl

Hydrogen peroxide: H_2O_2

Kanamycin: $C_{18}H_{38}N_4O_{15}S$

Lactic acid: $C_3H_6O_3$

Lactose: $C_{12}H_{22}O_{11}$

Lead nitrate: $Pb(NO_3)_2$

Magnesium chloride: $MgCl_2$

Magnesium citrate: $C_6H_6MgO_7$

Magnesium sulphate: $MgSO_4$

Maltose: $C_{12}II_{22}O_{11}$

Manganese sulphate: $MnSO_4$

Mannitol: $C_6H_{14}O_6$

Mercaptoethanol: C_2H_6OS

Mercuric chloride: $HgCl_2$

Methanol: CH_3OH

Monopotassium phosphate: KH_2PO_4

Monosodium phosphate: NaH_2PO_4

MTT: $C_{18}H_{17}N_5S$

Nalidixic acid: $C_{12}H_{12}N_2O_3$

Naphthylamine: $C_{10}H_9N$

Ortho-nitrophenyl-β-galactoside: ONPG; $C_{12}H_{15}NO_8$

Orthophosphoric acid: H_3PO_4

Penicillin G: $C_{16}H_{18}N_2O_4S$

Phenol: C_6H_6O

Potassium bromide: KBr

Potassium chloride:	KCl
Potassium iodide:	KI
Potassium nitrate:	KNO_3
Proline:	$C_5H_9NO_2$
Rifampicin:	$C_{43}H_{58}N_4O_{12}$
Silver nitrate:	$AgNO_3$
Sodium acetate:	CH_3COONa
Sodium bicarbonate:	$NaHCO_3$
Sodium carbonate:	Na_2CO_3
Sodium chloride:	$NaCl$
Sodium citrate:	$Na_3C_6H_5O_7$
Sodium dodecyl sulphate:	SDS; $NaC_{12}H_{25}SO_4$
Sodium hydroxide:	$NaOH$
Sodium nitrate:	$NaNO_3$
Sodium pyruvate:	$C_3H_3NaO_3$
Streptomycin:	$C_{21}H_{39}N_7O_{12}$
Sucrose:	$C_{12}H_{22}O_{11}$
Sulphanilic acid:	$C_6H_7NO_3S$
Taurocholic acid:	$C_{26}H_{45}NO_7S$
Tetrachloroauric acid:	$HAuCl_4.3H_2O$
Tetramethylethylenediamine:	TEMED; $C_6H_{16}N_2$
Toluene:	C_7H_8
Trehalose:	$C_{12}H_{22}O_{11}$
Trifluoro acetic acid:	$C_2HF_3O_2$
Tween20:	$C_{58}H_{114}O_{26}$
Tween40:	$C_{44}H_{54}N_7O_8P$
Tween80:	$C_{64}H_{124}O_{26}$
Xylose:	$C_5H_{10}O_5$
Zinc chloride:	$ZnCl_2$
Zinc sulphate:	$ZnSO_4$
α-Cyano-4-hydroxycinnamic acid:	CHCA; $C_{10}H_7NO_3$

[C]

Websites and Software

BLAST - *https://blast.ncbi.nlm.nih.gov/Blast.cgi*

GenBank - *https://www.ncbi.nlm.nih.gov/genbank/submit/*

ORF Finder - *https://www.ncbi.nlm.nih.gov/orffinder/*

Linear regression curve - *https://www.graphpad.com/quickcalcs/linear1/*

MASCOT search program - *http://matrixscience.com*

PEP-FOLD - *http://bioserv.rpbs.univ-paris-diderot.fr/services/PEP-FOLD3/*

iCn3D - *https://www.ncbi.nlm.nih.gov/Structure/icn3d/full.html*

ExPASy-ProtParam tool - *http:// web.expasy.org/protparam*

SOPMA tool - *http://npsa-prabi.ibcp.fr/cgi-bin/npsa_automat.pl?page=npsa_sopma.html*

TMHMM tool - *www.cbs.dtu.dk/services/TMHMM*

Helical Wheel Projections - *http://www.bioinformatics.nl/cgi-bin/emboss/pepwheel*

PubChem - *https://pubchem.ncbi.nlm.nih.gov/*

RCSB PDB - *http://www.rscb.org/pdb*

PROCHECK - *https://servicesn.mbi.ucla.edu/PROCHECK/*

RNAfold web server

Hex 8.0.0 docking software

General Linear Model of Statistical Analysis System (SAS)

Turkey's test

MATLAB R2019a (The Mathworks USA)

MEGA software version 4.0

One way ANOVA

Qualitek-4 (Automatic Design and Analysis of Taguchi Experiment; Nutek Inc. USA)

Design Expert Version 11.0.0 (Stat-Ease Inc., Minneapolis, Minnesota, USA)

Summary

A total of 56 bacteria were isolated from traditionally prepared various fermented foods of Tamil Nadu, India. '*Koozh*' associated 6 CNS strains showed anti-tubercular activities with high RLU reductions (92.4±0.3-97.7±0.4%). Among those isolates, strain MANF2 showed satisfactory probiotic attributes by exhibiting vast array of desirable characteristics. The strain demonstrated good technological characteristics as well as showed negative results towards *in vitro* haemolytic, DNase, and gelatinase tests, thereby revealing non-pathogenicity and safety aspect of this strain for possible development of functional food. As per statistical optimization tools (Taguchi OA design and BBD of RSM), MRS medium of pH 6.5 constituting yeast extract (0.5% w/v), magnesium sulphate (0.1% w/v), and glycerol (1.5% v/v), being further incubated at 30^{0}C showed increased anti-tubercular activity (98.7%) and approximately 4 fold improvement in the biomass yield (8.3 mg/mL) of strain MANF2 with respect to the traditional OFAT method. Anti-tubercular and anticancer protein of molecular mass 7712.3 Da was purified from strain MANF2, which showed sequence homology (95%) with Glyceraldehyde-3-phosphate dehydrogenase of *Staphylococcus* sp., suggesting a new Glyceraldehyde-3-phosphate dehydrogenase-like protein. The molecular mass of the most abundant peptide in the protein was observed as 1922.12 Da, and thus, this peptide was named as NMANF2. *In silico* tools indicated satisfactory stereo-chemical, physiochemical, and functional characteristics of peptide NMANF2. Further, the peptide showed strong affinity with various receptors such as DNA gyrase, ribonucleotide reductase, LysA, alanine racemase, and isocitrate lyase of *M. tuberculosis*. Similarly, among targeted proteins of A540 cell line, peptide NMANF2 revealed potential docking with Bcl-2. On the other hand, the peptide was reported as potential inhibitor of CDK4 among targeted HT-29 cell line receptors. Antimicrobial agents (*M. piperita*, penicillin G, and mercuric chloride) at sub-inhibitory concentration enhancedn total protein content of strain MANF2. The medium containing yeast extract (0.5% w/v) as well as glycerol (1.5% v/v), and supplementation of *M. piperita* (1.5% v/v) at log phase of strain MANF2 revealed maximum protein content of 9.4±0.4 mg/mL using CCD of RSM. Anti-tubercular and anticancer protein (molecular mass - 51293 Da) from strain MANF2 under mild stress of *M. piperita* was purified, which showed 100% homology with ProDH, thereby categorizing it as a new class of ProDH-like protein. The molecular mass of the most abundant peptide in this protein was observed as 2110.87 Da and thus, this peptide was named as SMANF2. *In silico* tools showed satisfactory stereo-chemical, physiochemical, and functional characteristics of peptide SMANF2. Further, the peptide showed the highest affinity with LysA, followed by ribonucleotide reductase, alanine racemase, DNA gyrase, and isocitrate lyase of *M. tuberculosis*. Among targeted proteins of A540 cell lines, peptide SMANF2 showed potential docking ability with Bcl-2. Likewise, the peptide was reported as potential inhibitor of Bcl-xL among targeted HT-29 cell line receptors. Further, some of the functional properties of strain MANF2 growing under mild stress of *M. piperita* varied with respect to the control strain. Statistical optimization tools such as BBD and ANN enhanced the production of microwave irradiation-based AuNPs, which was synthesized using strain MANF2 as reducing agent. The SEM and DLS analyses revealed the synthesis of anisotropic gold nanoplates of 100 nm, particularly pentagonal and square-shaped nanoplates with sharp edges. The protein/gold nanoplates bioconjugate of various concentrations exhibited promising anti-tubercular (against drug sensitive and drug resistant *M. tuberculosis* strains) and anticancer (A540 and HT-29 cancer cell lines) properties. The supplementation of strain MANF2 increased *in vitro* gas production from horse's faeces at different incubation periods. The inclusion of strain MANF2 showed non-significant ($P>0.05$) reductions in the pH values with respect to the control.

In a nutshell, findings of this research work suggested the exemplary biotechnological applications of strain MANF2 not only as auspicious anti-tubercular and anticancer agents for the development of efficacious therapeutic drug in future but also its pivotal role as ideal feed supplement towards improved digestibility and fermentation kinetics of horses.

CPSIA information can be obtained
at www.ICGtesting.com
Printed in the USA
LVHW082357051222
734629LV00016B/1098

9 781805 459842